Register Now for
to Your Book!

MW01505111

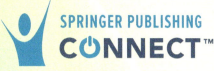

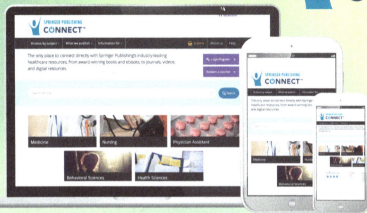

Your print purchase of *Cancer Pharmacology: An Illustrated Manual of Anticancer Drugs, Second Edition,* **includes online access to the contents of your book**—increasing accessibility, portability, and searchability!

Access today at:
http://connect.springerpub.com/content/book/978-0-8261-4933-6
or scan the QR code at the right with your smartphone. Log in or register, then click "Redeem a voucher" and use the code below.

4J0P6GEN

Scan here for quick access.

Having trouble redeeming a voucher code?
Go to https://connect.springerpub.com/redeeming-voucher-code

If you are experiencing problems accessing the digital component of this product, please contact our customer service department at cs@springerpub.com

The online access with your print purchase is available at the publisher's discretion and may be removed at any time without notice.

Publisher's Note: New and used products purchased from third-party sellers are not guaranteed for quality, authenticity, or access to any included digital components. .

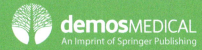

demosMEDICAL
An Imprint of Springer Publishing

SPC®

View all our products at springerpub.com/demosmedical

CANCER PHARMACOLOGY

CANCER PHARMACOLOGY

AN ILLUSTRATED MANUAL OF ANTICANCER DRUGS

Second Edition

Edited by

Ashkan Emadi, MD, PhD

Judith E. Karp, MD

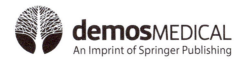

demosMEDICAL
An Imprint of Springer Publishing

Springer Publishing Company, LLC
www.springerpub.com
connect.springerpub.com

Acquisitions Editor: David D'Addona
Compositor: Amnet
Production Editor: Dennis Troutman

ISBN: 978-0-8261-4932-9
ebook ISBN: 978-0-8261-4933-6
DOI: 10.1891/9780826149336

23 24 25 26 27 / 5 4 3 2 1

Medicine is an ever-changing science. Research and clinical experience are continually expanding our knowledge, in particular our understanding of proper treatment and drug therapy. The authors, editors, and publisher have made every effort to ensure that all information in this book is in accordance with the state of knowledge at the time of production of the book. Nevertheless, the authors, editors, and publisher are not responsible for any errors or omissions or for any consequence from application of the information in this book and make no warranty, expressed or implied, with respect to the content of this publication. Every reader should examine carefully the package inserts accompanying each drug and should carefully check whether the dosage schedules therein or the contraindications stated by the manufacturer differ from the statements made in this book. Such examination is particularly important with drugs that are either rarely used or have been newly released on the market. The publisher has no responsibility for the persistence or accuracy of URLs for external or third-party Internet websites referred to in this publication and does not guarantee that any content on such websites is, or will remain, accurate or appropriate.

Library of Congress Cataloging-in-Publication Data

Names: Emadi, Ashkan, editor. | Karp, Judith E., editor.
Title: Cancer pharmacology : an illustrated manual of anticancer drugs / editors, Ashkan Emadi, Judith E. Karp.
Description: Second edition. | New York, NY : Springer Publishing Company, [2024] | Includes bibliographical references and index.
Identifiers: LCCN 2023005637 (print) | LCCN 2023005638 (ebook) | ISBN 9780826149329 (paperback) | ISBN 9780826149336 (ebook)
Subjects: MESH: Antineoplastic Agents—pharmacology | Neoplasms—drug therapy | Molecular Targeted Therapy
Classification: LCC RC271.C5 (print) | LCC RC271.C5 (ebook) | NLM QV 269 | DDC 616.99/4061—dc23/eng/20230429
LC record available at https://lccn.loc.gov/2023005637
LC ebook record available at https://lccn.loc.gov/2023005638

Contact sales@springerpub.com to receive discount rates on bulk purchases.

Publisher's Note: **New and used products purchased from third-party sellers are not guaranteed for quality, authenticity, or access to any included digital components.**

Printed in the United States of America by Hatteras, Inc.

We dedicate this book to the chemists, biologists, pharmacologists, clinicians and clinical investigators, and patients and their families who continue to improve the lives of patients with cancer—and to science and its divinity.

Contents

Contributors

Ciera Bernhardi, PharmD, BCOP
Oncology Clinical Pharmacy Specialist
University of Maryland Greenebaum Comprehensive Cancer Center
Baltimore, Maryland

Alison Duffy, PharmD, BCOP
Associate Professor
University of Maryland School of Pharmacy
Oncology Clinical Pharmacy Specialist
University of Maryland Greenebaum Comprehensive Cancer Center
Baltimore, Maryland

Ashkan Emadi, MD, PhD
Professor of Medicine and Pharmacology
University of Maryland School of Medicine
Associate Director for Clinical Research & Director of Translational Genomics Laboratory
University of Maryland Greenebaum Comprehensive Cancer Center
Baltimore, Maryland

Amy M. Fulton, PhD
Professor Emerita of Pathology
University of Maryland School of Medicine
University of Maryland Greenebaum Comprehensive Cancer Center
Baltimore, Maryland

Gabriel Ghiaur, MD, PhD
Associate Professor of Medicine and Oncology
Department of Oncology
Johns Hopkins University
Baltimore, Maryland

Lukasz P. Gondek, MD, PhD
Assistant Professor
Sidney Kimmel Comprehensive Cancer Center
Johns Hopkins University
Baltimore, Maryland

Molly Graveno, PharmD, BCOP
Oncology Clinical Pharmacy Specialist
Department of Pharmacy
University of Maryland Medical Center
Baltimore, Maryland

Vicky Hsu, PhD
Pharmacologist
U.S. Food and Drug Administration
Division of Clinical Pharmacology I
Office of Clinical Pharmacology
Center for Drug Evaluation and Research
Silver Spring, Maryland

Arif Hussain, MD
Professor of Medicine
University of Maryland Greenebaum Comprehensive Cancer Center
University of Maryland School of Medicine
Veterans Affairs Medical Center
Baltimore, Maryland

S. Percy Ivy, MD
Associate Chief, Investigational Drug Branch/CTEP/DCTD/NCI
Program Director, Experimental Therapeutics Clinical Trials Network
National Cancer Institute
Bethesda, Maryland

Elizabeth Jaffee, MD
The Dana and Albert "Cubby" Broccoli Professor of Oncology
Deputy Director, Sidney Kimmel Comprehensive Cancer Center
Johns Hopkins University School of Medicine
Baltimore, Maryland

Judith E. Karp, MD
Professor Emerita, Oncology and Medicine
Sidney Kimmel Comprehensive Cancer Center
Johns Hopkins University School of Medicine
Baltimore, Maryland

Scott H. Kaufmann, MD, PhD
Professor of Pharmacology and Medicine
Division of Oncology Research
Mayo Clinic
Rochester, Minnesota

Mira A. Kohorst, MD
Assistant Professor of Pediatrics
Department of Pediatrics and Adolescent Medicine
Mayo Clinic
Rochester, Minnesota

Justin Lawson, PharmD, BCOP
Clinical Oncology Speciatlist
University of Maryland Greenebaum Comprehensive Cancer Center
University of Maryland Medical Center
Baltimore, Maryland

Richard F. Little, MD
Senior investigator, Clinical Investigations Branch, CTEP
Division of Cancer Treatment and Diagnosis
National Cancer Institute
National Institutes of Health
Bethesda, Maryland

Yuchen (Jake) Liu, MD
Hematology/Oncology Fellow
University of Maryland
Baltimore, Maryland

Sagar Lonial, MD
Professor and Chair
Department of Hematology and Medical Oncology
Emory University School of Medicine
Atlanta, Georgia

Kathryn Maples, PharmD, BCOP
Clinical Pharmacy Specialist, Winship Cancer Institute
Emory Healthcare
Atlanta, Georgia

Yuya Nagai, MD, PhD
Medical Director of the Department of Hematology
Kobe City Medical Center General Hospital
Kobe, Hyogo, Japan

Vincent C. O. Njar, PhD
Professor of Medicinal Chemistry and Pharmacology
Department of Pharmacology
Center for Biomolecular Therapeutics
University of Maryland Greenebaum Comprehensive Cancer Center
University of Maryland School of Medicine
Baltimore, Maryland

Olanrewaju O. Okusanya, PharmD, MS
Pharmacologist
U.S. Food and Drug Administration
Division of Clinical Pharmacology I
Office of Clinical Pharmacology
Center for Drug Evaluation and Research
Silver Spring, Maryland

Sergiu Pasca, MD
Postdoctoral Fellow
Sidney Kimmel Comprehensive Cancer Center
Johns Hopkins University
Baltimore, Maryland

Donna Przepiorka, MD, PhD
Medical Officer
U.S. Food and Drug Administration
Division of Hematological Malignancies I
Office of Oncologic Diseases
Center for Drug Evaluation and Research
Silver Spring, Maryland

Vedran Radojcic, MD
Medical Director, Syndax Pharmaceuticals, Inc.
Waltham, Massachussetts
Adjunct Assistant Professor
Department of Internal Medicine
University of Utah
Salt Lake City, Utah

Edward A. Sausville, MD, PhD
Retired Clinical Professor of Medicine
University of Maryland Greenebaum Comprehensive Cancer Center
University of Maryland
Baltimore, Maryland

Matthew D. Thompson, PhD, MPH
Pharmacologist
U.S. Food and Drug Administration
Division of Hematology Oncology Toxicology
Office of Oncologic Diseases
Center for Drug Evaluation and Research
Silver Spring, Maryland

Katherine H. R. Tkaczuk, MD
Professor of Medicine
Director, Breast Evaluation and Treatment Program
University of Maryland Greenebaum Comprehensive Cancer Center
University of Maryland School of Medicine
Baltimore, Maryland

Mark Yarchoan, MD
Associate Professor of Oncology
Sidney Kimmel Comprehensive Cancer Center
Johns Hopkins University
Baltimore, Maryland

Joshua F. Zeidner, MD
Associate Professor of Medicine, Department of Medicine
Division of Hematology/Oncology
Lineberger Comprehensive Cancer Center
University of North Carolina
Chapel Hill, North Carolina

Preface

We are living in an exciting time for cancer pharmacology. The fusion of multiple disciplines of basic and clinical science is creating effective, life-prolonging therapies for a growing number of malignancies. The progress is electrifying and the promise for patients is exhilarating!

Historically, the first anticancer agents targeted molecules that are critical to the overall process of cell replications in both normal and malignant cells and, as such, were relatively nondiscriminatory in their cytotoxicity. The revolution in molecular technology that began in the late 1980s is now being brought to bear on the structural design of agents that selectively target tumor-related gene mutations and signaling pathway intermediaries in ways that may augment tumor cell death and spare underlying normal cell populations. In addition to specific tumor cell features, we continue to dissect the complex interactions between the malignant clone and its multifaceted microenvironment and exploit those interactions for therapeutic purposes.

Our first edition of *Cancer Pharmacology* followed the evolution of drug development from the traditional cytotoxic agents that target cell cycle–driving molecules to agents that target genetic, epigenetic, hormonal, and immunobiologic molecules. We created a unique format comprising predominantly illustrations rather than relying on extensive written text. We were fortunate to assemble a stellar group of clinical and molecular scientists to address the challenges and opportunities presented by clinical trials design, development of biomarkers that predict response and survival, and issues related to ultimate drug approval.

The success of our first illustrated edition and the rapid expansion of new targeted agents into the oncology armamentarium led us to develop a second edition with an increased clinical focus and many updates including recent approvals of molecularly targeted agents over the broad spectrum of both solid tumors and hematologic malignancies. Toward this end, we have expanded and extensively updated the existing chapters, incorporated a new chapter on pharmacogenomics, and completely revised our previous chapters on targeted therapies, multiple myeloma as a paradigm for multi-targeted intervention, and transplant-related agents with a focus on graft versus host disease. We have also updated the clinical pearls and multiple-choice questions for each chapter, with increased emphasis on questions relevant to board exams.

In short, cancer pharmacology is the quintessence of bidirectional translational research, moving basic laboratory science into patients and, at the same time, moving clinical observations into the laboratory to achieve an optimal clinical outcome. It is fascinating (and ironic) to realize that this entire field grew out of the field of chemical warfare almost 80 years ago and has evolved over the last 30 years to exploit discrete molecular features of specific cancers and their microenvironmental milieu. We think and hope that the pioneering cancer pharmacologists of the 1940s through 1970s would be thrilled to see how their field has evolved in the 21st century. We hope that we have conveyed to you, our readers, the tremendous knowledge, excitement, and promise that cancer pharmacology encompasses today. We have tried to capture the stunning developments on the basic science level and the soaring translation of those new discoveries into the clinical arena. Looking to the future, we hope to continue revising this book with updates based on structurally new agents targeting newly discovered pathways and new drug approvals. Thank you for sharing this incredible learning journey with us!

Ashkan Emadi
Judith E. Karp

Basic Principles of Cancer Pharmacology and Clinical Drug Development

CHAPTER 1

Drug Development in Oncology

EDWARD A. SAUSVILLE ● ASHKAN EMADI

INTRODUCTION

The notion that cancer might be usefully treated by drugs is a relatively new one, as, in general, surgery historically was the mainstay of therapeutic approaches to cancer, and even when radiation was found to cause useful effects on tumors, its use was as an alternate local treatment (Figure 1.3). However, in the 19th century, the German pathologist Paul Ehrlich posited the possibility of "magic bullet" compounds that would have affinity for neoplastic cells (or infectious organisms), based on his appreciation of the differential capacity of synthetic dyes to stain different cell organelles or cell types. This led to the screening of collections of chemicals, and then extracts of biological sources (plants, bacteria, marine organisms, etc.) for cytotoxic activity against cancer cells and survival of the host organism (usually animals with tumors). A different approach arose from the realization that ablation of certain organs, for example, ovary or testes, could favorably affect tumors such as breast and prostate, respectively. This suggested that understanding the biological mechanisms driving cancer cell growth could lead to useful treatments, prototypic of what is now described as "targeted" treatments for cancer. Cancer treatment has historically been closely tied to an understanding of the pharmacology of the relevant drugs, as in many cases they are used at the highest dose possible to achieve either a cytotoxic effect or fully engage the target of the agent in the tumor cell.

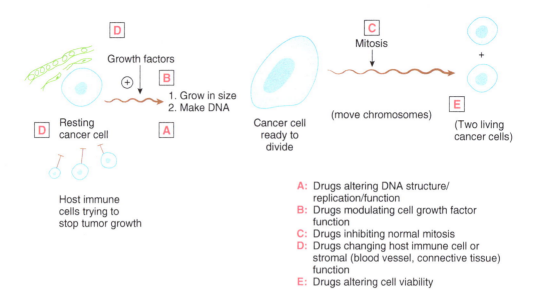

A: Drugs altering DNA structure/replication/function
B: Drugs modulating cell growth factor function
C: Drugs inhibiting normal mitosis
D: Drugs changing host immune cell or stromal (blood vessel, connective tissue) function
E: Drugs altering cell viability

FIGURE 1.1 **Targets for cancer drugs.**

A. Drugs altering DNA structure/replication/function
   1. DNA-directed alkylating agents
   2. Topoisomerase I/II inhibitors
   3. Antimetabolites
      a. Purine/pyrimidine analogs
      b. Antifolates
   4. DNA breaking agents
   5. DNA repair inhibitors
   6. Antitumor antibiotics
B. Growth factor antagonists
   1. Hormone receptor antagonists
      a. Estrogen antagonists
      b. Androgen antagonists
      c. Glucocorticoids
   2. Growth factor receptor antagonists
      a. Tyrosine kinase inhibitors
      b. Multitargeted kinase inhibitors
      c. Antireceptor antibodies
      d. Selective kinase inhibitors
   3. Protein synthesis
      a. Amino acid use
      b. Ribosome translation efficiency
   4. Cell cycle activation
C. Mitosis inhibitors
   1. Microtubule disruptor
   2. Microtubule stabilizer
D. Immune/stromal mediators
   1. Cytokines
   2. T-lymphocyte activator

(continued)

FIGURE 1.1 **Targets for cancer drugs. (*continued*)**

    3. Chimeric antigen receptor acting on T cells
    4. Antitumor antibody
    5. Blood vessel growth inhibitor
        a. Antibodies against vascular endothelial growth factor (VEGF)
        b. VEGF receptor kinase inhibitors
        c. VEGF receptor mimetics
E. Drugs altering cell viability
    1. Differentiating agents
    2. Proteosome inhibitors
    3. Apoptosis modulators

PATHOPHYSIOLOGY OF CANCER, WHERE CANCER DRUGS COME FROM

- Current working model: Clinical cancer is an infection-like process where by the infecting organisms (the cancer cells) are derived from the host (normal cells).
- Cancer cells arise from mutations in normal cell DNA leading to activation of cellular pathways promoting cell growth in a way independent of normal growth regulatory signal.
  - Cancers frequently have distinct subsets of cells with different groups of mutations in each population.
  - "Driver" mutations have a fundamental potency in directly promoting tumor growth; "passenger" mutations have no immediate importance in promoting growth.
- Mutations that characterize a "successful" cancer (i.e., the hallmarks of cancer) can result in:
  - Abnormal proliferative potential
  - Loss of growth suppressor functions including cell differentiation and senescence
  - Indefinite chromosome replication potential
  - Evasion of physiologic cell death signals
  - Ability to make new blood vessels and generate supporting stroma
  - Evasion of immune recognition
  - Responsiveness to tumor-promoting inflammation
  - Tolerance of damage to DNA
  - Change in metabolism to resemble unicellular organisms (e.g., bacteria)
  - An acquired capacity for invasion and metastasis
- Useful cancer drugs affect one or more of these differences between host cells and cancer cells.

HOW DO WE KNOW A CANCER DRUG MIGHT BE USEFUL?

- Phase 1 trials define a tolerable dose and schedule of the drug.
  - Phase 1 trials are open label, nonrandomized, dose escalation, uncontrolled clinical studies.
  - The primary objectives of Phase 1 studies are to evaluate the safety and tolerability of a drug (α) or drugs combination ($\alpha+\beta$) as well as to estimate the maximum

tolerated doses (MTDs) and/or biologically active doses (e.g., recommended Phase 2 doses [RP2Ds]) of α or α+β in patients with newly diagnosed disease X or resistant/refractory/unresponsive to n lines of treatments in one or a few diseases.

- The primary endpoints of Phase 1 studies are usually the incidence of dose/regimen limiting toxicities (DLT/RLT) and incidence of treatment-emergent adverse events (TEAEs).
- One of the most prevalent designs for oncology Phase 1 trials is 3+3 design.
- These clinical studies do not usually have response or survival as a primary endpoint, but they can be noted as secondary endpoints.
- Phase 1 clinical trials in oncology usually have pharmacologic studies as exploratory endpoints.

- Phase 2 trials look for evidence of "treatment" effect (e.g., tumor shrinkage, symptom effect) usually without a control group or, if with a control group with a smaller number of patients, not allowing rigorous statistical conclusions.
  - Phase 2 clinical responses (if accepted as "surrogate endpoints" that reasonably likely can predict meaningful clinical outcomes such as improvement in overall survival) may support "accelerated approval" for sale to public by the U.S. Food and Drug Administration (FDA).
  - Usually in a Phase 2 clinical trial, everyone gets the same dose. But some Phase 2 trials randomly assign subjects to different treatment arms to receive different doses or schedules to provide the best balance of safety and response.
  - Usually (but not always), if enough (definition of enough or adequate must be prespecified) subjects benefit (primary endpoint on response) from the treatment, and the adverse events are acceptable, Phase 3 clinical trials are initiated.
- Phase 3 trials seek to show improvement in a clinically useful endpoint in patients receiving the new drug as compared to patients receiving "standard" or (rarely) no therapy (= control group).
  - Clinically useful endpoints include overall survival (considered the gold standard by many; Figure 1.2), progression-free survival, relief of symptoms.
  - Usually the basis for regulatory agency (e.g., FDA) approval for sale to public
  - Generally multicenter industry/pharma sponsored trials requiring strict protocol compliance with frequent audits and presence of a central monitoring committee
  - Can have noninferiority design
  - Can have run-in design for evaluation of compliance
- Phase 4 clinical studies are postmarketing surveillance, uncontrolled, and observational clinical studies intended to detect long-term, rare adverse events of an FDA-approved agent.
  - Can be mandated by FDA
  - Can be a pharmacoeconomics study
  - Can be for a new indication (i.e., expansion of the label)

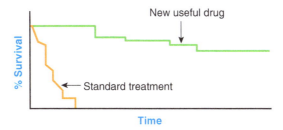

FIGURE 1.2 Kaplan-Meier estimate, a standard format for displaying result of a Phase 3 clinic trial.

Kaplan-Meier estimate is one of the best ways to measure and to depict the fraction of subjects living for a certain time after treatment. In clinical trials, the outcome of an intervention is calculated by measuring the number of subjects who survive after that intervention over a period of time.

The time starting from a defined point (e.g., the day of enrollment or the first day of treatment) to the occurrence of a given event (e.g., death, disease relapse) is called survival time, and the analysis of group data is the survival analysis.

This method can be affected by subjects who discontinued the study for personal reasons or when a fraction of the subjects may not experience the event before the end of the study (although they would have experienced it if observation continued), or when a fraction of subjects are lost to follow-up. These situations are called censored observations. The Kaplan-Meier estimate is the most straightforward and the most prevalent approach for computing the survival over time despite all real world situations associated with subjects on clinical trials.

The two survival curves are compared statistically by testing the null hypothesis that there is no difference regarding survival among two interventions. This null hypothesis is tested by statistical tests called log-rank test and Cox proportional hazards test.

WHY DO CANCER DRUGS WORK AT ALL, STOP WORKING, OR NEVER WORK?

- Classical cytotoxic agents (1940s–1990s): Each exposure to a useful cancer drug treatment kills a constant fraction of "susceptible" cells until all cancer cells are killed OR remaining cells are "dormant" OR are eliminated by the immune system; the available drugs were mainly cytotoxic chemotherapeutic agents (see Chapters 5–9).

- Hormone modulating agents: In 1896, Dr. George Beaston performed surgical oophorectomy for patients with advanced breast cancer and observed significant tumor regression, increased sense of well-being in patients, and reduction in cutaneous metastases (see Chapter 13). In 1941, Dr. Charles Huggins demonstrated that in men with prostate cancer, reducing androgen by performing orchiectomy or administering estrogen can improve symptoms and sense of well-being in patients with widespread metastasis (see Chapter 14).

- Modern view utilizing targeted treatments: Drugs kill cancer cells in preference to normal cells acting processes active in cancer cells as a result of mutations; the drugs are

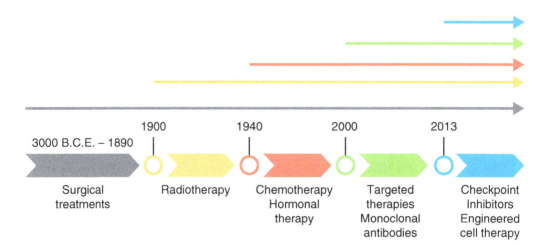

FIGURE 1.3 Timeline of cancer treatment.

preferentially lethal to tumor cells in the context of those mutations by activating cell death programs in tumor cells, similar or identical to physiologic cell death pathways active in normal organism growth or function.

- ○   Successful cancer drugs are therefore "synthetically" lethal with cancer cell mutations and are called targeted therapy (see Chapters 10–12, 15).
- Therefore, cancer cells not possessing synthetic lethal mutations will not be killed by the drug, and will be intrinsically resistant to the drug.
- While the last decade of the 20th century witnessed the advent of monoclonal antibodies (see Chapter 17) and significant improvement in treatment of malignancies such as lymphoma and breast cancer, already in the second decade of the 21st century, we observe revolutionary impact of modern immunotherapy including checkpoint inhibitors and engineered cell therapy such as chimeric antigen receptor (CAR) T-cell therapy (see Chapter 18).

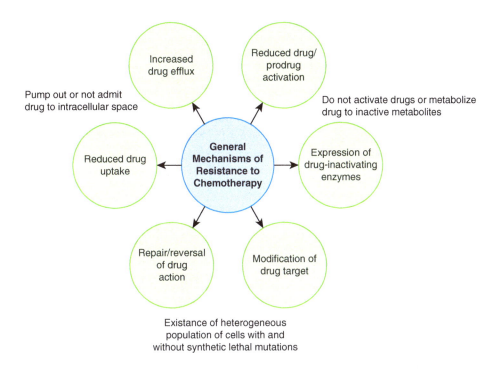

FIGURE 1.4 **Resistance to chemotherapy.**

PHARMACOKINETICS: ACTION OF THE HOST ON AN ADMINISTERED DRUG

The four major components of pharmacokinetics are absorption, distribution, metabolism, and excretion (ADME; Figure 1.5).

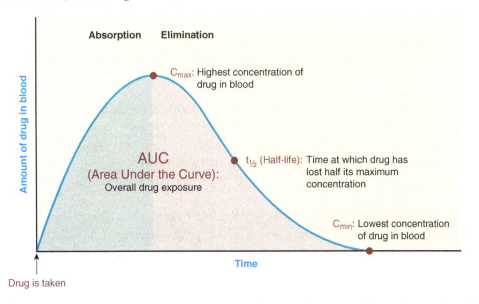

FIGURE 1.5 **Pharmacokinetic endpoints.**

Dosing of cytotoxic antineoplastic agents typically is close to a maximal tolerated dose (MTD) defined as a result of a Phase 1 trial and refined through Phase 2 and 3 trials. Such drugs are usually dosed according to patient size, conventionally estimated by considering the patient's body surface area (BSA).

- There are several formulas for calculation of BSA. The most widely used is the Dubois formula that is equally effective in approximating body fat in obese and nonobese subjects. The Mosteller formula, with a simpler mathematical calculation, is also commonly utilized.

Modification of dosing is typically required for concomitant laboratory abnormalities present in patients with cancer. In addition, dysfunction of organs due to the cancer or to underlying medical conditions affects how the body deals with the administered drug. For example, elevation of bilirubin or transaminases frequently are considered in dosing agents cleared by the liver, and creatinine clearance is estimated to correctly dose patients with altered renal function. Therefore, restating some aspects of clinical pharmacology important in cancer treatment is of import in correctly understanding a basis for optimal drug use.

Drug clearance can occur by **(A)** renal functions (filtration, tubular secretion); **(B)** hepatic actions (cytochrome-mediated oxidation, glucuronidation); or **(C)** tissue or blood metabolism or sequestration (e.g., fat deposition).

Clearance (volume of a sampled compartment from which drug is removed per unit time) is related to the dose and the area under the curve (AUC) as follows:

$$\text{Clearance (volume/time)} = \frac{\text{Dose (mass)}}{\text{AUC (mass/volume)(time)}}$$

- Drugs administered intravenously (IV), orally (PO), or through other routes reach a central compartment (usually blood) from which the drug is distributed to body tissues (including tumor).

The administered drug may be active directly or need further metabolism to an active form. Important examples of drugs requiring metabolism for activation:

- Cyclophosphamide, ifosfamide, irinotecan activated by liver
- Nucleosides (e.g., cytosine arabinoside) phosphorylated by tumor cells

Figure 1.5 illustrates key information that is obtained by measuring drug presence in a body compartment. The highest concentration achieved (peak concentration) is then followed by an elimination phase. The area under the concentration × time curve (AUC) is a more complete estimation of drug exposure than the single peak concentration, and is a key feature in ensuring that the dose and schedule selected can potentially accomplish the needed effect on the drug's target in the tumor cell.

Knowing the drug dose and AUC, the clearance of the drug can be estimated. Clearance from the central compartment reflects all of the ways of removing the drug: renal excretion and bile secretion, metabolism in plasma, uptake by cells of both tumor and host, etc.

- Carboplatin is an example of a drug that is actually dosed according to the achievement of a particular AUC.
- Clearance of a drug can importantly reflect pharmacogenetic aspects (see Chapter 2) of drug-metabolizing enzymes: for example, fatal cytopenias can emerge after "normal" doses of 5-fluorouracil in patients lacking dihydropyrimidine dehydrogenase.
- Clearance can change as dose increases: for example, cytosine arabinoside (ara-C) at low doses (<500 mg/m^2) is predominantly cleared by metabolism by cytidine deaminase; at high doses (e.g., $\geq1,000$ mg/m^2), renal clearance becomes important and therefore the dose of the agent is reduced, particularly in older patients who commonly have decreased creatinine clearance even if creatinine concentration is normal or minimally abnormal.
- The peak effect of a drug can also influence toxicity; for example, it is thought that bolus doses administered over relatively short infusions of anthracyclines correlate with a greater propensity for cardiac damage than lower dose continuous infusions.

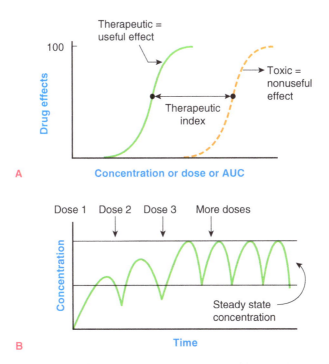

FIGURE 1.6 Pharmacokinetics: Relation to toxicity of achievement of steady state. (A). Therapeutic index is the ratio between drug concentration or dose or AUC (area under the curve) causing toxicity versus therapeutic effect **(B).** Most cancer drugs have a narrow therapeutic index; that is, toxic doses are quite close to therapeutic doses. If drug doses administered before the prior doses are cleared, the drug will ultimately reach a constant concentration (steady state); this is actually desirable, for example, in the use of "targeted agents," which must be present continuously to suppress oncogenic kinase drivers of cell growth.

PHARMACODYNAMICS: ACTION OF AN ADMINISTERED DRUG ON THE HOST

Pharmacodynamic studies include mechanism(s) of action (MOA) studies, exposure-safety relationship, and exposure-efficacy relationship.

- An important example for pharmacodynamic studies is the effect of a drug on cardiac electrophysiology such as QTc intervals.

Drugs can act by the formation of a covalent derivative of its target (e.g., DNA alkylating agent); a noncovalent but tightly bound adduct to alter target function (e.g., microtubule disruptors); or biochemically reversible interaction with a target to alter target function (e.g., various protein kinase inhibitors).

LIMITATIONS TO EFFECTIVE DRUG ACTION

Drug–drug interactions: For example, induction of a cytochrome P450 by drug A may promote the metabolism of drug B (decreasing drug B's effect), or drug A may act to interfere with drug B's metabolism, potentially leading to toxicity from drug B. Consultation with an oncology pharmacy specialist is helpful in adjudicating particular issues.

- An important example of drug–drug interaction is the relative contraindication of venetoclax with strong CYP3A inhibitors at initiation and ramp up of dose due to increased incidence of tumor lysis syndrome. These inhibitors include the antifungal azoles (itraconazole, posaconazole, voriconazole, and ketoconazole).
- Likewise, dose adjustment or avoidance of vincristine in combination with commonly used azole antifungals (itraconazole, posaconazole, voriconazole, and ketoconazole) in patients with hematologic malignancies is necessary to avoid severe vinca–associated neurotoxicity.

Bioavailability (F)

$$F = \frac{\text{Mass of drug reaching effective central compartment}}{\text{Mass of administered drug}}$$

where $0 < F \leq 1$

- Oral bioavailability is typically low (as low as 5%) and variable; it is influenced by food, consumption or antacids.
- Intravenous bioavailability by definition = 1, with circulating blood volume as the central compartment.

Specialized compartments:

- Blood–brain barrier (BBB) is due to extensive tight junctions between endothelial cells of brain microcirculation and drug transporters on endothelial cells.
- BBB is not the sole determinant of distribution of drugs to cerebrospinal fluid (CSF); intrathecal treatment addresses meningeal surface but NOT central nervous system (CNS) parenchymal disease.

ADJUVANT AND NEOADJUVANT THERAPY IN CANCER TREATMENT

The goal of cancer treatment can be definitive (curative) or palliative. For solid tumors, with a few exceptions, surgical resection is the primary and definitive treatment modality. *Adjuvant* therapy is chemotherapy, radiation, hormonal therapy, and/or targeted therapy, which is given in the absence of any objective (surgical or imaging) evidence of remaining cancer, to increase the statistical probabilities of a cure, potentially by eradicating any micrometastases. Some patients might have been cured already by surgical resection alone, and adjuvant therapy would expose them to unnecessary toxicity of chemotherapy. Some patients may have cancer recurrence in spite of the adjuvant therapy, and these patients would not receive any additional benefit from chemotherapy. The decision about whether to offer an adjuvant therapy to any individual patient is based on the risk/benefit analyses results of *randomized clinical trials*.

Neoadjuvant therapy is chemotherapy, radiation, hormonal therapy, and/or targeted therapy that is the first step to shrink a tumor before the main treatment, usually surgery, is given.

CHAPTER SUMMARY

Cancer drugs have emerged from conscientious efforts to optimize the pharmacology of agents that displayed cytotoxic activity, as well as agents designed to interfere with recognized biochemical pathways promoting growth or, more recently, affecting the tumor cell microenvironment including vasculature of the tumor and immune cells. Subsequent chapters will deal with each class of anticancer agents. Cancer treatment when administered as a dose or doses at intervals seeks to maximize the therapeutic ratio between tumor effects and deleterious effects on the host. Understanding the elimination routes and bases for drug interactions is key to the safe and optimal use of the agent. Drugs that are administered on a continuing basis alternatively target a steady state concentration, which is key to assuring that optimal modulation of biochemical pathways governing cell growth is achieved, and also may be affected by drug interactions and metabolism of the agent.

Adjustment of the dosages of cancer chemotherapeutics according to the patient's renal and hepatic functions is a common and day-to-day routine practice in clinical oncology in academic centers, community practice, and clinical trials. Here are dosing guidelines of selected antineoplastic agents for patients with renal and/or hepatic dysfunction.

$$\text{Clearance (volume/time)} = \frac{\text{Dose (mass)}}{\text{AUC (mass/volume)(time)}}$$

$$\text{Bioavailability} = F = \frac{\text{Mass of drug reaching effective central compartment}}{\text{Mass of administered drug}}$$

AGENT	DOSE ADJUSTMENT IN	
	RENAL DYSFUNCTION	HEPATIC DYSFUNCTION
Bendamustine	• Renal impairment: CrCl <40 mL/min, omit	Moderate (transaminase 2.5–10 × ULN and T.Bil 1.5–3 × ULN) or severe (T.Bil >3 × ULN), omit
Bleomycin	• CrCl 40–50 mL/min, 70% of full dose • CrCl 30–40 mL/min, 60% of full dose • CrCl 20–30 mL/min, 55% of full dose • CrCl 10–20 mL/min, 45% of full dose • CrCl 5–10 mL/min, 40% of full dose	No adjustment is required
Capecitabine	• CrCl 30–50 mL/min, 75% of full dose • CrCl <30 mL/min, omit • CrCl <30 mL/min, omit	No adjustment is required
Carboplatin	Dose based on GFR, using Calvert formula: Dose (mg) = target AUC × (GFR + 25). AUC = 5–7 For ESRD patient, • CrCl <30 mL/min, omit	No adjustment is required

(continued)

| AGENT | DOSE ADJUSTMENT IN | |
	RENAL DYSFUNCTION	HEPATIC DYSFUNCTION
Carmustine	• CrCl 45–60 mL/min, 80% of full dose • CrCl 30–45 mL/min, 75% of full dose • CrCl <30 mL/min, 70% of full dose	Dosage adjustment may be necessary; no specific recommendations found
Cisplatin	• CrCl 46–60 mL/min, 50% of full dose • CrCl 31–45 mL/min, 25% of full dose • CrCl ≤30 mL/min, omit	No adjustment is required
Cladribine	• CrCl 10–50 mL/min, 75% of full dose • CrCl <10 mL/min, 50% of full dose	No specific recommendations found
Cyclophosphamide	• CrCl 40–60 mL/min: No adjustment recommended	• T.Bil >3.1–5.0 mg/dL or AST >180 IU/L, 75% of full dose • T.Bil >5.0 mg/dL, omit

Cytarabine	• CrCl 40–60 mL/min:
	  – if dose >2 g/m^2/dose, ↓ to 1 g/m^2/dose
	  – if dose = 0.75–1 g/m^2/dose, ↓ to 0.5 g/m^2/dose
	• CrCl <40 mL/min:
	  – if dose >0.75 g/m^2/dose, give ≤200 mg/m^2/day
		No specific recommendations found. Patient with liver dysfunction receiving cytarabine should be carefully monitored; adjust the dose based on clinical judgment.

Dacarbazine	• CrCl 30–60 mL/min, 75% of full dose • CrCl 10–30 mL/min, 50% of full dose • CrCl <10 mL/min, omit	No specific recommendations found. Patient with liver dysfunction receiving dacarbazine should be carefully monitored; adjust the dose based on clinical judgment.
Daunorubicin	Serum creatinine >3 mg/dL, 50% of full dose	• T.Bil 1.5–3.0 mg/dL or AST 60–180 IU/L, 75% of full dose • T.Bil >3.1–5.0 mg/dL or AST >180 IU/L, 50% of full dose • T.Bil >5.0 mg/dL, omit

(continued)

	DOSE ADJUSTMENT IN	
AGENT	**RENAL DYSFUNCTION**	**HEPATIC DYSFUNCTION**
Docetaxel	No adjustment is required	• Transaminase >1.5 × ULN, **and** ALP >2.5 ULN, the recommended dose is 75 mg/m² • T.Bil > ULN **and/or** trans-aminase >3.5 × ULN associated with ALP >6 × ULN, should not be used unless strictly indicated
Doxorubicin	• CrCl <10 mL/min, 75% of full dose	• T.Bil 1.5–3.0 mg/dL or AST 60–180 IU/L, 50% of full dose • T.Bil >3.1–5.0 mg/dL or AST >180 IU/L, 25% of full dose • T.Bil >5.0 mg/dL, omit
Doxorubicin (liposomal)	No adjustment is required	• T.Bil 1.2–3.0 mg/dL or AST 60–180 IU/L, 50% of full dose • T.Bil >3.0 mg/dL or AST >180 IU/L, 25% of full dose • T.Bil >5.0 mg/dL, omit
Epirubicin	Serum creatinine >5 mg/dL, lower doses should be considered	• T.Bil 1.2–3.0 mg/dL or AST 2–4 × ULN, 50% of full dose • T.Bil >3.0 mg/dL or AST >4 × ULN, 25% of full dose • T.Bil >5.0 mg/dL, omit
Erlotinib	CrCl <10 mL/min, omit	• AST ≥3 × ULN or T.Bil 1–7 mg/dL, 50% of full dose • T.Bil >7.0 mg/dL, omit
Etoposide	• CrCl >15–50 mL/min, 75% of full dose • CrCl <15 mL/min, omit	T.Bil 1.5–3 mg/dL or AST 60–180 IU/L, 50% of of full dose T.Bil ≥3 mg/dL or AST >180 IU/L, omit
Fludarabine	• CrCl 30–70 mL/min, 50% of full dose • CrCl <30 mL/min, omit	No adjustment is required
Fluorouracil	No adjustment is required	• T.Bil >5.0 mg/dL, omit

(continued)

AGENT	DOSE ADJUSTMENT IN	
	RENAL DYSFUNCTION	HEPATIC DYSFUNCTION
Gemcitabine	No specific recommendations found	• Increased AST: no need for dose adjustment • Increased T.Bil: reduce dose by 20% (i.e., from 1,000 to 800 mg/m²) and increase if tolerated
Hydroxyurea/ hydroxycarbamide	• CrCl 10–60 mL/min, 75% of full dose • CrCl <10 mL/min, 50% of full dose	• T.Bil 1.5–5.0 mg/dL or AST 60–180 IU/L, 50% of full dose • T.Bil >5.0 mg/dL or AST >180 IU/L, omit
Idarubicin	• Serum creatinine ≥2.5 mg/dL, dose reduction recommended	• T.Bil 2.5–5.0 mg/dL, 50% of full dose • T.Bil >5.0 mg/dL, omit
Ifosfamide	• CrCl 46–60 mL/min, 80% of full dose • CrCl 31–45 mL/min, 75% of full dose • CrCl 10–30 mL/min, 70% of full dose • CrCl <10 mL/min, omit	No specific recommendations found
Imatinib	• CrCl 40–59 mL/min, doses >600 mg are not recommended • CrCl 20–39 mL/min, 50% of full dose. Dose can be increased up to maximum of 400 mg. • CrCl <20 mL/min, use with caution (In two patients with severe renal impairment, doses of 100 mg/day were tolerated.)	• Initial dose: – severe hepatic impairment, initial dose, 75% of full dose • Hepatic toxicity during treatment – transaminases >5 × ULN or T.Bil >3 × ULN, omit Restart at reduced doses (reduce from 400 mg to 300 mg, from 600 mg to 400 mg, or from 800 mg to 600 mg) when transaminases <2.5 × ULN **and** T.Bil <1.5 × ULN

(continued)

| AGENT | DOSE ADJUSTMENT IN | |
	RENAL DYSFUNCTION	HEPATIC DYSFUNCTION
Irinotecan (weekly, usual dose 125 mg/m² for 4 of 6 weeks)	No adjustment anticipated to be required	• Increased AST: no need for dose adjustment • T.Bil 1.5–3 × ULN **and** ratio of AST to ALT <5 × ULN, 60 mg/m² • T.Bil 3.1–5 × ULN **and** ratio of AST to ALT <5 × ULN, 50 mg/m² • T.Bil <1.5 × ULN **and** ratio of AST to ALT 5.1–20 × ULN, 60 mg/m² • T.Bil 1.5–3 × ULN **and** ratio of AST to ALT 5.1–20 × ULN, 40 mg/m²
Irinotecan **Regimen 1 (weekly):** 125 mg/m² IV infusion over 90 minutes on days 1, 8, 15, 22, then 2 weeks off, then repeat **Regimen 2 (once every 3 weeks):** 350 mg/m² IV infusion over 30-90 minutes every 3 weeks	No adjustment anticipated to be required	• Increased AST: no need for dose adjustment • T.Bil >1.5–3 × ULN, dose = 200 mg/m² • T.Bil >3 × ULN, omit
Ixabepilone (monotherapy)	No specific recommendations found	• T.Bil ≤1.5 × ULN **and** AST <10 ULN **and** ratio AST to ALT <10 × ULN, reduce the dose to 32 mg/m² • T.Bil 1.5–3 × ULN **and** transaminase <10 × ULN, dose 20 mg/m²; may escalate dose up to 30 mg/m² maximum in subsequent cycles, if tolerated
Ixabepilone (in combination with capecitabine)	No specific recommendations found	• T.Bil >ULN or transaminase >25 × ULN, omit

(continued)

	DOSE ADJUSTMENT IN	
AGENT	**RENAL DYSFUNCTION**	**HEPATIC DYSFUNCTION**
Lenalidomide (use for myelodysplastic syndrome [MDS])	• CrCl 30–60 mL/min, 5 mg every 24 h • CrCl <30 mL/min (not requiring dialysis), 5 mg every 48 h • CrCl <30 mL/min (requiring dialysis), 5 mg three times a week after each dialysis	No specific recommendations found
Lenalidomide (use for multiple myeloma [MM])	• CrCl 30–60 mL/min, 10 mg every 24 h • CrCl <30 mL/min (not requiring dialysis), 15 mg every 48 h • CrCl <30 mL/min (requiring dialysis), 5 mg once daily, dose after dialysis on dialysis days	No specific recommendations found
Lomustine	• CrCl 45–60 mL/min, 75% of full dose • CrCl 30–45 mL/min, 70% of full dose • CrCl <30 mL/min, omit	No specific recommendations found
Melphalan	• CrCl 45–60 mL/min, 85% of full dose • CrCl 30–45 mL/min, 75% of full dose • CrCl 10–30 mL/min, 70% of full dose • CrCl <10 mL/min, 50% of full dose	No adjustment is required
Methotrexate	For low dose (<1 g/m^2): • CrCl 30–60 mL/min, 50% of full dose • CrCl <30 mL/min, omit For high dose (>1 g/m^2): consider therapeutic dose monitoring (TDM)	• T.Bil 3.1–5.0 mg/dL or AST >180 IU, 75% of full dose • T.Bil >5.0 mg/dL, omit
Mitomycin C	• CrCl 30–60 mL/min, 75% of full dose • CrCl 10–30 mL/min, 50% of full dose • CrCl <10 mL/min, omit	• T.Bil 1.5–3.0 mg/dL, 50% of full dose • T.Bil >3.0 mg/dL or transaminase >3 × ULN, 25% of full dose

(continued)

	DOSE ADJUSTMENT IN	
AGENT	RENAL DYSFUNCTION	HEPATIC DYSFUNCTION
Mitoxantrone	No adjustment is required	• T.Bil 1.5–3.0 mg/dL, 50% of full dose • T.Bil >3.0 mg/dL, 25% of full dose
Oxaliplatin	CrCl <30 mL/min, omit	No adjustment is required
Paclitaxel (3-h infusion and first course of therapy)	No adjustment is required	• Transaminase <10 × ULN **and** T.Bil 1.26–2 × ULN, dose = 135 mg/m² • Transaminase <10 × ULN **and** T.Bil 2.01–5 × ULN, dose = 90 mg/m² • Transaminase ≥10 × ULN or T.Bil >5 × ULN, omit
Paclitaxel (24-h infusion and first course of therapy)	No adjustment is required	• Transaminase 2–10 × ULN **and** T.Bil <1.5 mg/dL, dose = 100 mg/m² • Transaminase <10 × ULN **and** T.Bil 1.6–7.5 mg/dL, dose = 50 mg/m² • Transaminase ≥10 × ULN or T.Bil >7.5 mg/dL, omit
Pemetrexed	• CrCl <45 mL/min, omit	No specific recommendations found
Pentostatin	• CrCl 45–60 mL/min, 70% of full dose • CrCl 30–45 mL/min, 60% of full dose • CrCl <30 mL/min, consider using alternative drugs if possible	Not applicable
Sorafenib	No adjustment is required	• T.Bil ≤1.5 × ULN, 400 mg twice a day • T.Bil 1.5–3 × ULN, 200 mg twice a day • T.Bil >3 × ULN, omit
Topotecan	• CrCl 30–60 mL/min, 75% of full dose • CrCl 10–30 mL/min, 50% of full dose • CrCl <10 mL/min, omit	No adjustment is required

(continued)

| AGENT | DOSE ADJUSTMENT IN | |
	RENAL DYSFUNCTION	HEPATIC DYSFUNCTION
Vinblastine	No adjustment is required	• T.Bil 1.5–3.0 mg/dL or AST 60–180 IU/L, 50% of full dose • T.Bil >3.1 mg/dL or AST >180 IU/L, omit
Vincristine	No adjustment is required	• T.Bil 1.5–3.0 mg/dL or AST 60–180 IU/L, 50% of full dose • T.Bil >3.1 mg/dL or AST >180 IU/L, omit
Vinorelbine	No adjustment is required	• T.Bil 2.1–3 × ULN, 50% of dose • T.Bil >3 × ULN, 25% of dose

ALT, alanine transaminase; ALP, alkaline phosphatase; AST, aspartate transaminase; AUC, area under the curve; CrCl, creatinine clearance; ESRD, end-stage renal disease; GFR, glomerular filtration rate; T.Bil, total-value bilirubin; ULN, upper limit of normal.

MULTIPLE-CHOICE QUESTIONS

1. Which one of the following statements is correct?

    A. Adjuvant therapy is chemotherapy, radiation therapy, hormone therapy, or immunotherapy given as the first step to shrink a tumor before the main treatment, usually surgery.
    B. Log kill hypothesis describes the action of chemotherapy at a given dose that kills a constant number of cells.
    C. Combination chemotherapy versus monotherapy is used to improve tumor response to therapy, to decrease the probability of drug resistance, and to increase the tolerance for patients.
    D. Decreased drug efflux and augmented drug uptake are two main mechanisms by which resistance to chemotherapy occurs.

2. Assurance of adequate cardiac function is necessary before administration of which one of the following agents?

    A. Irinotecan
    B. Asparaginase
    C. Hydroxyurea
    D. Idarubicin

3. A 42-year-old woman is scheduled to receive docetaxel with cisplatin and fluoroura-cil for untreated, advanced gastric cancer. Which one of the following lab abnormali-ties requires dose modification for receiving docetaxel?

    A. Creatinine greater than 3 mg/dL
    B. Transaminases greater than 2.5 times the upper limit of normal
    C. Elevated IgE level
    D. Serum albumin less than 3.5 g/dL

4. Which one of the following agents has the narrowest therapeutic index?

    A. Bortezomib
    B. Methotrexate
    C. Cytarabine
    D. Hydroxyurea

5. PSC-833 (valspodar) is a nonimmunosuppressive cyclosporine analog that potently inhibits P-glycoprotein (encoded by *MDR1*; P-gp). It has been tested in multiple on-cology clinical trials in combination with other chemotherapeutic agents. What was the rationale for designing these trials?

    A. It catalytically reduces prodrug to drug conversion.
    B. It induces the overexpression of drug-inactivating intracellular enzymes.
    C. It reduces cellular drug uptake.
    D. It decreases cellular drug efflux.

6. Which one of the following agents does have a similar target as bevacizumab?

    A. Ziv-aflibercept
    B. Daratumumab
    C. Ofatumumab
    D. Trastuzumab

7. Which one of the following adverse events can occur after treatment with trastu-zumab and idarubicin and carfilzomib?

    A. Pulmonary fibrosis
    B. Posterior reversible encephalopathy syndrome (PRES)
    C. Torsades de pointes
    D. Cardiomyopathy

8. In which of the following genes do mutations affect cell metabolism in different blood and solid cancers and have clinically available targeted therapies against different of such mutations?

    A. Hexokinase (HK)
    B. Isocitrate dehydrogenase (IDH)
    C. Pyruvate dehydrogenase complex (PDC)
    D. Carnitine palmitoyltransferase I (CPT1)

9. A 69-year-old man, who is a pilot, presents to a clinic for a second opinion on the management of newly diagnosed myelodysplastic syndrome (MDS) confirmed by outside bone marrow aspiration and biopsy examination. The patient reports progressive fatigue and dyspnea on exertion in the last 7 months. The rest of his past medical history, family history, social history, review of systems, and physical examination is unremarkable. The patient only takes an over-the-counter multivitamin. Laboratory tests shows white blood cell count 4,700/μL (with normal differentials), hemoglobin 6.7 g/dL, platelets 212,000/μL. Folate, vitamin B_{12}, copper, zinc, liver enzymes, thyroid function tests are all within normal range. The patient and his wife request discussion about the agents that can improve anemia in MDS. Which of the following agents is not used/designed/approved to increase hemoglobin in patients with MDS?

   A. Luspatercept-aamt
   B. Darbepoetin
   C. Deferasirox
   D. Lenalidomide

10. Before 2013, all-trans retinoic acid (ATRA) with chemotherapy was the standard of care for treatment of acute promyelocytic leukemia (APL), resulting in cure rates greater than 80%. A randomized multicenter Phase 3 clinical trial was conducted to compare the safety and efficacy of the ATRA plus idarubicin regimen with ATRA plus arsenic trioxide regimen for induction and consolidation therapy in patients with APL classified as low-to-intermediate risk. What would be the best design for such clinical trial?

   A. Double-blind design
   B. 2×2 factorial design
   C. Noninferiority design
   D. Cross-over design

ANSWERS TO MULTIPLE-CHOICE QUESTIONS

1. **C.** Oncology chemotherapy regimens generally consist of a few agents. Combining chemotherapeutic agents versus monotherapy is used to improve tumor response to therapy, to decrease the probability of drug resistance, and to increase the tolerance for patients. Chemotherapy, radiation therapy, hormone therapy, targeted therapy, or immunotherapy given as the first step to shrink a tumor before surgery is called neoadjuvant therapy. Log kill hypothesis describes the magnitude of cancer cell kill by antineoplastic agents as a logarithmic function, that is, a given dose of an anticancer drug kills a constant *proportion* of a cell population rather than a constant *number* of cells. Increased drug efflux and decreased drug uptake are two main mechanisms by which resistance to chemotherapy occurs.

2. **D.** Anthracyclines, such as daunorubicin, doxorubicin, idarubicin, and epirubicin, are chemotherapeutic agents used to treat many types of cancers. The main adverse event of anthracyclines is cumulative dose-dependent cardiotoxicity, which may cause heart failure.

3. **B.** Taxanes (e.g., paclitaxel, docetaxel, cabazitaxel, abraxane, or protein-bound paclitaxel) are microtubule polymer stabilizers. They are used for the treatment of many epithelial cancers. Treatment-related mortality increases when taxanes are given in the presence of abnormal liver function. Taxanes should not be given if bilirubin is greater than the upper limit of normal (ULN), or if aspartate transaminase (AST) and/or alanine transaminase (ALT) >1.5 × ULN concomitant with alkaline phosphatase >2.5 × ULN. No dose adjustment in taxanes is necessary in the presence of renal dysfunction.

4. **A.** Bortezomib is a proteasome inhibitor used for the treatment of patients with plasma cell disorders. Bortezomib has a very narrow therapeutic index. The main adverse effect of bortezomib is peripheral neuropathy. Bortezomib can be given intravenously (IV) or subcutaneously (SQ). There is no difference in the response rates between IV and SQ; however, SQ administration is associated with a decreased occurrence of grade 3 or higher adverse effects. An overdose of bortezomib can occur when the usual dose (i.e., 1.3 mg/m^2) is doubled. The overdosed patient usually presents with marked thrombocytopenia and hypotension. Fatal outcomes have been reported from bortezomib overdose.

5. **D.** The energy-dependent multidrug efflux pump P-glycoprotein (P-gp) is widely expressed in human cancers including intrinsically drug-resistant cancers, such as pancreatic, liver, colon, and kidney cancers, and in acquired resistance, such as leukemias, lymphomas, and breast cancer. This multidrug resistance (MDR) significantly decreases the efficacy of anticancer drugs and has been a major challenge in oncology. Based on considerable in vitro success, a combination of P-gp inhibitors with antineoplastic agents was tested in several clinical trials of both solid and hematologic neoplasms. However, there are no agents currently approved to block P-gp–mediated resistance in the clinical arena. The cause might be attributed to serious adverse events, drug–drug interactions, and several pharmacokinetic problems.

6. **A.** Vascular endothelial growth factor (VEGF) is the target of both bevacizumab and ziv-aflibercept. Bevacizumab binds VEGF and interferes with its interaction to its receptors on the surface of endothelial cells leading to the prevention of endothelial cell proliferation and formation of new blood vessel in in vitro models of angiogenesis. Ziv-aflibercept is a VEGF inhibitor. It is a recombinant fusion protein that has a VEGF-binding portion that acts as a soluble receptor that binds to human endogenous ligands VEGF-A and VEGF-B. Ziv-aflibercept can inhibit the binding and activation of VEGF-A and VEGF-B to their cognate receptors culminating in decreased neovascularization and decreased vascular permeability.

7. **D.** Trastuzumab can result in subclinical and clinical cardiomyopathy causing cardiac failure manifesting as congestive heart failure (CHF), and decreased left ventricular ejection fraction (LVEF), with greatest risk when administered concurrently with

anthracyclines (e.g. doxorubicin, daunorubicin, idarubicin, epirubicin). The mechanisms of anthracyclines-induced cardiomyopathy include inhibition of the topoisomerase II (TOP2) enzyme, DNA damage due to formation of reactive oxygen species, induction of apoptosis in cardiomyocytes, and inhibition of cellular protein synthesis. As opposed to boronic acid–based reversible proteasome inhibitors such as bortezomib and ixazomib, carfilzomib structure contains an epoxyketone as the active moiety making it an irreversible proteasome inhibitor through formation of double covalent bonds between the epoxyketone pharmacophore and proteasome. The proposed mechanisms of carfilzomib-associated cardiotoxicity include epoxyketone-generated oxidative stress on cardiac myocytes, endoplasmic reticulum stress, accumulation and crosslinking of ubiquinated proteins, and endothelial dysfunction via irreversible binding. In particular, inhibition of ongoing proteasome-dependent sarcomeric protein turnover appears to be the mechanism of induced apoptosis and cell death. New onset or worsening of preexisting cardiomyopathy (e.g., CHF, pulmonary edema, decreased LVEF) and myocardial ischemia have occurred following administration of carfilzomib.

8. **B.** What are the biological characteristics of mutant isocitrate dehydrogenase (mIDH)? Wild-type IDH1 (in both peroxisomes and cytosol) and IDH2 (in mitochondria) are NADP (nicotinamide adenine dinucleotide phosphate)-dependent enzymes that catalyze the oxidative decarboxylation of isocitrate to α-ketoglutarate (α-KG), with production of NADPH (NADP plus hydrogen). Altered amino acids in mIDH1 and mIDH2 reside in the catalytic pocket and result in a neoenzymatic activity, converting α-KG to 2-hydroxyglutarate (2-HG) with the consumption of NADPH. Heterozygous mutations resulting in a single amino acid change at arginine 132 (R132) of IDH1 and arginine 140 (R140) or arginine 172 (R172) in the active site of the IDH2 enzyme have been reported in glioma, acute myeloid leukemia, intrahepatic cholangiocarcinoma, chondrosarcoma, and angioimmunoblastic T-cell lymphoma. These mutations are always monoallelic, resulting in heterodimer enzymes and causing gain of function, with resultant activity as an oncogene. Mutant IDHs cannot catalyze the normal conversion of isocitrate to α-KG, but instead catalyze an NADPH-dependent reduction of α-KG to an oncometabolite, 2-HG. 2-HG is normally present at very low levels in cells, but IDH mutations lead to the accumulation of 2-HG in cancer cells and potentially in the sera of affected patients. Enasidenib is an IDH2 inhibitor indicated for the treatment of adult patients with relapsed or refractory acute myeloid leukemia with an IDH2 mutation. Ivosidenib is an IDH1 inhibitor indicated for patients with a susceptible IDH1 mutation including (1) newly diagnosed acute myeloid leukemia in combination with azacitidine or as monotherapy for the treatment of adults 75 years or older, or who have comorbidities that preclude use of intensive induction chemotherapy, (2) relapsed or refractory acute myeloid leukemia, and (3) locally advanced or metastatic cholangiocarcinoma.

9. **C.** Luspatercept-aamt is approved for treatment of anemia failing an erythropoiesis stimulating agent (ESA) and requiring 2 or more red blood cell (RBC) units over 8 weeks in adult patients with very low to intermediate-1 risk MDS with ring

sideroblasts (RS) or with myelodysplastic/myeloproliferative neoplasm with ring sideroblasts and thrombocytosis (MDS/MPN-RS-T). Lenalidomide is approved for treatment of transfusion-dependent anemia due to low- or intermediate-1-risk MDS associated with a deletion 5q abnormality with or without additional cytogenetic abnormalities. ESA products are commonly used for treatment of anemia in MDS patients. A Phase 3 randomized placebo-controlled trial of darbepoetin alfa in patients with anemia and low/intermediate-1-risk MDS, hemoglobin ≤10 g/dL, low transfusion burden, and serum erythropoietin (EPO) ≤500 mU/mL showed statistically significant improvement in transfusion incidence from weeks 5 to 24 and erythroid response rates in subjects who received darbepoetin alfa versus placebo. Deferasirox (Jadenu tablet and Exjade for oral suspension) is an iron chelator indicated for the treatment of chronic iron overload due to blood transfusions in patients 2 years of age and older. Iron chelators do not increase hemoglobin levels.

10. **C.** Noninferiority clinical trials examine whether a new treatment is not unacceptably less efficacious than an active control treatment already in use in clinical practice. In contrast to superiority trials, noninferiority design is complex and is based on assumptions that cannot be validated directly. The clinical trial in the question was designed as a noninferiority study to show that the difference between the rates of event-free survival (EFS) at 2 years in the ATRA plus idarubicin and ATRA plus arsenic trioxide was not greater than 5%. Two-year EFS rates were 97% in the ATRA plus arsenic trioxide arm and 86% in the ATRA plus idarubicin arm (95% CI for the difference, 2 to 22 percentage points; $p < .001$ for noninferiority and $p = .02$ for superiority of ATRA plus arsenic trioxide).

SELECTED REFERENCES

Brunton LL, Knollman BC, editors. Goodman & Gilman's: The Pharmacological Basis of Therapeutics. 14th ed. New York: McGraw-Hill Education; 2022.

Budman DR, Calvert AH, Rowinsky EK, editors. Handbook of Anticancer Drug Development. Philadelphia: Lippincott Williams & Wilkins; 2003.

Fathi AT, Wander SA, Faramand R, Emadi A. Biochemical, epigenetic, and metabolic approaches to target IDH mutations in acute myeloid leukemia. Semin Hematol. 2015;52(3):165–71. https://doi.org/10.1053/j.seminhematol.2015.03.002

Hanahan D. Hallmarks of cancer: New dimensions. Cancer Discov. 2022;12(1):31–46. https://doi.org/10.1158/2159-8290.CD-21-1059

Hendrayana T, Wilmer A, Kurth V, et al. Anticancer dose adjustment for patients with renal and hepatic dysfunction: From scientific evidence to clinical application. Sci Pharm. 2017;85(1):8. https://doi.org/10.3390/scipharm85010008

Kaelin WG Jr. Synthetic lethality: A framework for the development of wiser cancer therapeutics. Genome Med. 2009;1(10):99. https://doi.org/10.1186/gm99

Lo-Coco F, Avvisati G, Vignetti M, et al. Retinoic acid and arsenic trioxide for acute promyelocytic leukemia. N Engl J Med. 2013;369(2):111–21. https://doi.org/10.1056/NEJMoa1300874

Marubini E, Valsecchi MG. Analysing Survival Sata From Clinical Trials and Observational Studies. Chichester, UK: John Wiley & Sons; 1995. p. 41–8.

Platzbecker U, Symeonidis A, Oliva EN, et al. A phase 3 randomized placebo-controlled trial of darbepoetin alfa in patients with anemia and lower-risk myelodysplastic syndromes. Leukemia. 2017;31(9):1944–50. https://doi.org/10.1038/leu.2017.192

CHAPTER 2

Pharmacogenomics

MOLLY GRAVENO

INTRODUCTION

Pharmacogenomics (PGx) is the study of the relationship between genetic variations and how the body responds to medications. Along with precision medicine, PGx has expanded over the past 20 years to allow for the tailoring of drug selection and dosing based on a patient's genetic features. Genetic tests can predict response to targeted therapies by identifying targetable mutations, rate of metabolism through different enzymes, and the immune response to medications by testing human leukocyte antigen (HLA) variants. PGx tests can sequence a patient's entire genome or be targeted for a gene specific to a medication or disease state (Tables 2.1 and 2.2). These tests are utilized for many different classes of medications including chemotherapy, antidepressants, antiplatelets, and more. The National Institutes of Health (NIH) funds Pharmacogenomics Knowledgebase (PharmGKB) and the Clinical Pharmacogenetics Implementation Consortium (CPIC) aimed to address the barrier to clinical implementation of PGx testing. PharmGPK also provides annotations of clinical guidelines by CPIC and the Dutch Pharmacogenetics Working Group (DPWG), which provide recommendations for dose adjustments or recommend alternative medications, depending on a person's genetic information. PharmGKB also provides annotations to prescribing information for some drug labels regulated by the U.S. Food and Drug Administration (FDA). This information along with clinical pathways, education resources, and more are located at pharmgkb.org. Currently, 396 drugs have PGx annotations by the FDA with different categories of recommendations including "testing required," "testing recommended," "actionable PGx," and "informative PGx." For example, carbamazepine, clopidogrel, codeine, and antidepressants such as fluoxetine have actionable PGx tests in FDA labeling. Table 2.3 includes a list of other relevant medications with actionable mutations. However, not all medications with PGx variations have clear guidelines for use due to interpersonal variability or lack of evidence. Table 2.4 includes a list of medications with available PGx tests, but a lack of firm data to describe the impact of PGx variability on efficacy or safety.

TYPES OF PHARMACOGENOMIC TESTS

A very important aspect of PGx in cancer patients is the testing for targetable mutations such as an EGFR, HER2, VEGF, or BRAFV600E mutation. Many new targeted therapies are FDA approved along with companion diagnostic tests to identify specific mutations. These somatic mutations are discussed in Chapter 12. This chapter focuses on PGx tests related to the pharmacodynamic or pharmacokinetic properties of drugs related to germline or inherited mutations or polymorphisms.

Pharmacokinetics studies the effect of the body on the drug, including absorption, distribution, metabolism, and elimination. Interindividual variations in metabolic pathways can affect the pharmacokinetics of a medication. PGx can test for both metabolism variations, for example, by assessing the cytochrome P450 (CYP) enzyme activity. Other enzymes used for the activation or breakdown of medications, such as thiopurine methyltransferase for mercaptopurine and analogs, are also clinically relevant. PGx tests for enzymatic activity will report out a genotype and phenotype. The genotype is the individual's variants or alleles, which together determine the diplotype as depicted in Figure 2.1. Each allele or genetic variation is

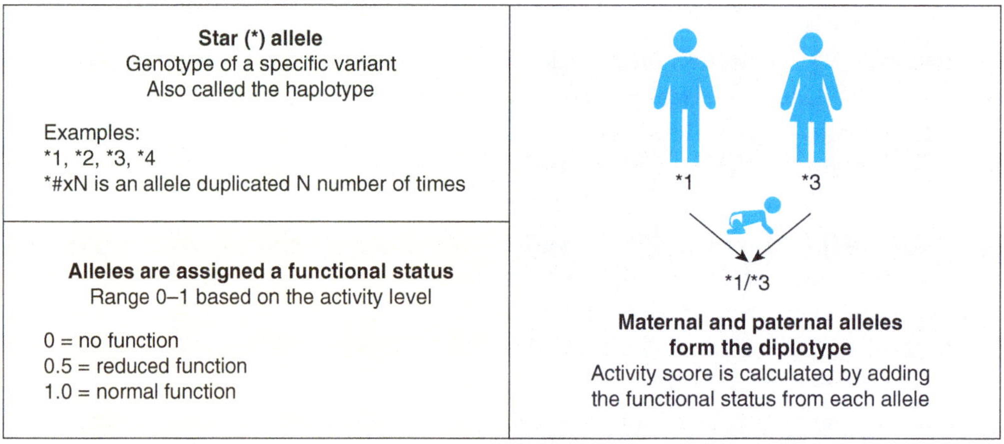

FIGURE 2.1 Nomenclature and activity level for alleles and diplotype.

named using star (*) terminology, and assigned a functional status based on its activity level. The phenotype, or observable trait, is determined by calculating the activity score, which is the sum of the functional status for each allele. Tables 2.1 and 2.2 are examples of an assignment of phenotype based on genotype for an example enzyme.

TABLE 2.1 Example Phenotype, Functional Status, and Activity Score for an Enzyme

*ALLELE	FUNCTIONAL STATUS	ACTIVITY SCORE
*1	Normal function	1.0
*2	Normal function	1.0
*3	Decreased function	0.5
*4	No function	0.0
*2x1	Normal function, additional allele	2.0

TABLE 2.2 Example Phenotype and Genotype for an Enzyme

PHENOTYPE	ACTIVITY SCORE	GENOTYPE	EXAMPLE DIPLOTYPE
Ultrarapid metabolizer	>2.0	Individual with duplicate functional alleles	*1/*1xN, *1/*2xN
Normal metabolizer	1.5–2.0	Two normal function alleles or one normal function and one decreased function allele	*1/*1, *1/*2, *1/*3
Intermediate metabolizer	0.5–1.0	One decreased function and one no function allele, two decreased function alleles, one normal function and one no function allele	*3/*4, *3/*3, *2/*4
Poor metabolizer	0.0	Two no function alleles	*4/*4

PGx can also describe the pharmacodynamic variability between patients, or the impact of the drug on the body. Individuals can have different variant alleles of HLA-B, which can predispose them to serious toxicities depending on the variant and medication. HLA molecules are involved in presenting exogenous and endogenous peptides to T cells for antigen-specific responses. Figure 2.2 demonstrates the interaction between HLA molecules and T cells, leading to an adaptive immune response. HLA-B is normally used to identify exogenous and endogenous peptides; however, different single nucleotide polymorphisms (SNPs) can impact the folding of the HLA active site. As a result, medications fit into the binding pocket and activate the immune system, eliciting adverse reactions. The type of adverse reaction depends on the type of cell involved; for example, keratinocytes are implicated for allopurinol-induced severe cutaneous adverse reactions (SCARs) including Stevens–Johnson syndrome (SJS) and toxic epidermal necrolysis (TEN).

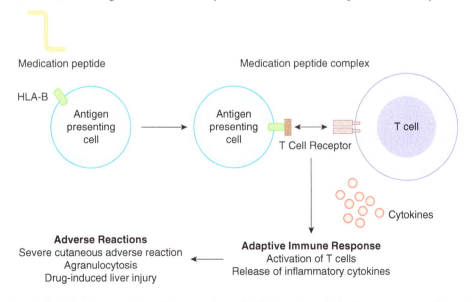

FIGURE 2.2 Activation of adaptive immune response due to medication presentation by human leukocyte antigen (HLA).

TABLE 2.3 Cancer and Supportive Care Medications That Have Data to Support Therapeutic Management Related to PGx Testing

MEDICATION	GENE	DESCRIPTION
Azathioprine	*TPMT* and/or *NUDT15*	Intermediate or poor metabolism results in higher concentrations and an increased risk of adverse reactions. Dose reduction is recommended.
Belinostat	*UGT1A1*	*28/*28 alleles encode for poor metabolism resulting in higher concentrations and an increased risk of adverse reactions. Dose reduction is recommended.
Belzutifan	*CYP2C19* and or *UGT2B17*	Poor metabolism results in higher concentrations an increased risk of adverse reactions. Monitoring is recommended.
Capecitabine	*DPYD*	Intermediate or poor metabolism results in higher concentrations and an increased risk of adverse reactions. Insufficient data for dose reductions in intermediate metabolizers. No dose has been shown to be safe in poor metabolizers. Withhold or discontinue in the presence of early-onset or unusually severe toxicity.
Codeine	*CYP2D6*	Ultrarapid metabolism converts codeine to the active metabolite faster and increases the risk of adverse reactions. Codeine is contraindicated in children under 12 years of age.
Dronabinol	*CYP2C9*	Intermediate or poor metabolism results in higher concentrations and an increased risk of adverse reactions. Monitoring is recommended.
Erdafitinib	*CYP2C9*	*3/*3 alleles encode for poor metabolism resulting in higher concentrations and an increased risk of adverse reactions. Monitoring is recommended.
Fluorouracil	*DPYD*	Intermediate or poor metabolism results in higher concentrations and an increased risk of adverse reactions. Insufficient data are available for dose reduction in intermediate metabolizers. No dosage is safe in poor metabolizers. Withhold or discontinue in the presence of early-onset or unusually severe toxicity.

(*continued*)

TABLE 2.3 Cancer and Supportive Care Medications That Have Data to Support Therapeutic Management Related to PGx Testing (*continued*)

MEDICATION	GENE	DESCRIPTION
Gefitinib	*CYP2D6*	Poor metabolism results in higher concentrations and increased risk of adverse reactions. Monitoring is recommended.
Irinotecan	*UGT1A1*	*28/*28 alleles encode for poor metabolism resulting in higher concentrations and an increased risk of adverse reactions. Reduce the starting dosage by one level and modify based on response.
Metoclopramide	*CYP2D6*	Poor metabolism results in higher concentrations and increased risk of adverse reactions. Monitoring is recommended.
Mercaptopurine	*TPMT* and/or *NUDT15*	Intermediate or poor metabolism results in higher concentrations and an increased risk of adverse reactions. Dosage reduction is recommended.
Pantoprazole	*CYP2C19*	Intermediate or poor metabolism results in higher concentrations and an increased risk of adverse reactions. Monitoring is recommended.
Sacituzumab govitecan-hziy	*UGT1A1*	*28/*28 alleles encode for poor metabolism resulting in higher concentrations and an increased risk of adverse reactions. Monitor for adverse reactions and tolerance to treatment.
Tacrolimus	*CYP3A5*	Intermediate or normal metabolism may result in lower systemic concentrations and lower probability of achieving target concentrations. Monitoring is recommended.
Thioguanine	*TPMT* and/or *NUDT15*	Intermediate or poor metabolism results in higher concentrations and an increased risk of adverse reactions. Dosage reduction is recommended.
Tramadol	*CYP2D6*	Ultrarapid metabolism results in higher systemic concentrations of the active metabolite and an increased risk for toxicity. Contraindicated in children under 12 years old and in adolescents following tonsillectomy/adenoidectomy. Breastfeeding is not recommended during treatment.

TABLE 2.4 Cancer and Supportive Care Medications With Pharmacogenetic Associations for Which the Data Indicate a Potential Impact

PHARMACOGENETIC ASSOCIATIONS FOR WHICH THE DATA INDICATE A POTENTIAL IMPACT ON SAFETY OR RESPONSE		
DRUG NAME	**GENE**	**DESCRIPTION**
Allopurinol	HLA-B	*58:01 allele positive increases risk for severe skin reactions.
Lapatinib	HLA-DRBL1	*07:01 allele positive increases risk of hepatotoxicity. Monitoring LFTs recommended regardless of genotype.
	HLA-DQA1	*02:01 allele positive increases risk of hepatotoxicity.
Nilotinib	UGT1A1	*28/*28 alleles encode for poor metabolism and increased risk of adverse effects including hyperbilirubinemia.
Pazopanib	HLA-B	*57:01 allele increases risk of hepatotoxicity. Monitoring LFTs recommended regardless of genotype.
	UGT1A1	*28/*28 alleles encode for poor metabolism and increased risk of hyperbilirubinemia.
Sulfamethoxazole trimethoprim	Nonspecific NAT	Poor metabolism results in higher concentrations and an increased risk of adverse reactions.
Sulfasalazine	Nonspecific NAT	Poor metabolism results in higher concentrations and an increased risk of adverse reactions.
Voriconazole	CYP2C19	Intermediate or poor metabolism results in higher concentrations and an increased risk of adverse reactions.
PHARMACOGENETIC ASSOCIATIONS FOR WHICH THE DATA DEMONSTRATE A POTENTIAL IMPACT ON PHARMACOKINETIC PROPERTIES ONLY		
Tamoxifen	CYP2D6	Intermediate or poor metabolism results in lower systemic concentrations of active metabolite. The impact of CYP2D6 intermediate or poor metabolism on efficacy is not well established.

LFTs, liver function tests.

UGT1A1—IRINOTECAN AND SACITUZUMAB GOVITECAN

Irinotecan is a campthotecan analog derived from *Camptotheca acuminata*, and exhibits its anticancer activity by binding to and inhibiting topoisomerase I. Further details regarding the mechanism of irinotecan can be found in Chapter 9. Irinotecan is a prodrug that requires activation through carboxylesterases (CES) to the active metabolite, SN-38. Irinotecan and SN-38 rely on cellular transport through ATP (adenosine triphosphate)-binding cassette (ABC) transporters and glucuronidation or detoxification though uridine diphosphate (UDP) glucuronosyltransferase (UGT) enzymes, such as UGT1A1, to SN-38 glucuronide as described in Figure 2.3. Irinotecan can also be metabolized in hepatic cells to SN-38 via CYP3A4 and CYP3A5.

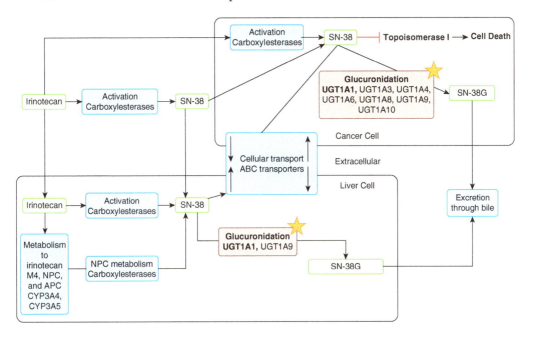

FIGURE 2.3 Activation, transportation, and metabolism of irinotecan.

UGT, uridine diphosphate glucuronosyltransferase.

Interpersonal variability in the activity of carboxylesterases, CYP3A4/5, and ABC transporters can lead to variations in concentrations of active and inactive metabolites of irinotecan. However, UGT1A1 activity variation is the most studied polymorphism linked to toxicity associated with irinotecan. The most common variant allele associated with decreased function is *UGT1A1*28*. This allele leads to reduced glucuronidation, buildup of SN-38, and increased toxicities such as myelosuppression and diarrhea as depicted in Figure 2.4.

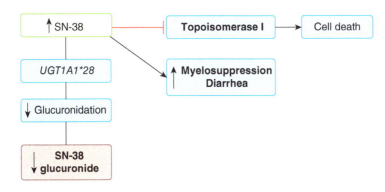

FIGURE 2.4 Impact of decreased glucuronidation on SN-38 concentration and toxicity.

*UGT1A1*6* allele is also associated with decreased function. Homozygous and heterozygous *6 and *28 alleles can affect the metabolic rate of UGT1A1. Given the severity of toxicities seen with decreased function alleles of UGT1A1, PGx testing and dose adjustments can be considered. Current FDA labeling for irinotecan (Camptosar) suggests dose reductions for patients with known homozygous *UGT1A1*28* alleles, but does not require testing prior to treatment. Labeling for liposomal irinotecan (Onivyde) recommends reducing the dose from 70 mg/m^2 to 50 mg/m^2 every 2 weeks for patients who are homozygous for the *UGT1A1*28* allele, with the option to increase the dose as tolerated for subsequent cycles. This is described in Table 2.5.

Sacituzumab govitecan-hziy is a trophoblast cell surface antigen-2 (Trop-2)-directed antibody drug conjugate. It has activity against epithelial cancers and is FDA approved for locally advanced or metastatic, relapsed, or refractory breast cancer and locally advanced or metastatic urothelial cancer, which is also discussed in Chapter 17. The Trop-2 monoclonal antibody is attached to a cleavable linker that once hydrolyzed, releases SN-38 which exhibits its anticancer effect as a topoisomerase I inhibitor. SN-38, is glucuronidated by UGT1A1 to SN-38 glucuronide to be eliminated in the bile. Similar to what is observed with irinotecan, patients with reduced activity of UGT1A1 receiving sacituzumab govitecan are at risk for SN-38–related myelosuppression and diarrhea. The same PGx tests utilized for irinotecan are therefore applicable to those receiving sacituzumab govitecan. FDA labeling for sacituzumab govitecan is summarized in Table 2.5.

TABLE 2.5 U.S. Food and Drug Administration (FDA) Labeling for Sacituzumab Govitecan Pharmocogenomics (PGx) Testing

FDA Labeling for Sacituzumab Govitecan (Trodelvy):
Actionable PGx
Genetic variants of the *UGT1A1* gene such as the *UGT1A1*28* allele lead to reduced UGT1A1 enzyme activity. Individuals who are homozygous for the *UGT1A1*28* allele are at increased risk for neutropenia [from sacituzumab govitecan] *(see Warnings and Precautions [5.5])*. Approximately 20% of the Black or African American population, 10% of the White population, and 2% of the East Asian population are homozygous for the *UGT1A1*28* allele. Decreased function alleles other than *UGT1A1*28* may be present in certain populations.

TABLE 2.6 U.S. Food and Drug Administration (FDA) Labeling for Irinotecan Pharmacogenomics (PGx) Testing

FDA Labeling for Irinotecan (Camptosar): Actionable PGx When administered in combination with other agents or as a single-agent, a reduction in the starting dose by at least one level of [irinotecan] should be considered for patients known to be homozygous for the *UGT1A1*28* allele. However, the precise dose reduction in this patient population is not known and subsequent dose modifications should be considered based on individual patient tolerance to treatment. (Pfizer, 2014, p. 11)
FDA Labeling for Liposomal Irinotecan (Onivyde): Actionable PGx The recommended dose of liposomal irinotecan is 70 mg/m^2 administered by intravenous infusion over 90 minutes every 2 weeks. The recommended starting dose of liposomal irinotecan in patients known to be homozygous for the *UGT1A1*28* allele is 50 mg/m^2 administered by intravenous infusion over 90 minutes. Increase the dose of [liposomal irinotecan] to 70 mg/m^2 as tolerated in subsequent cycles.

DIHYDROPYRIMIDINE DEHYDROGENASE AND FLUOROPYRIMIDINE DOSING

The drug fluorouracil and its prodrugs capecitabine and tegafur are discussed more thoroughly in Chapter 6. However, these agents also have important PGx testing considerations and "actionable PGx" per the FDA labeling. The enzyme dihydropyrimidine dehydrogenase (DPD) is encoded for by the dihydropyrimidine dehydrogenase gene (*DPYD*). DPD is the rate-limiting enzyme in fluorouracil catabolism and polymorphisms in *DPYD* lead to interindividual variations in activity levels. DPD function can be classified as normal, intermediate, or poor, with poor and intermediate function responsible for decreased elimination of the active metabolite and therefore an increased risk for toxicities including myelosuppression and mucositis. **Figure 2.5** shows the metabolic pathway for the catabolism of fluorouracil through DPD.

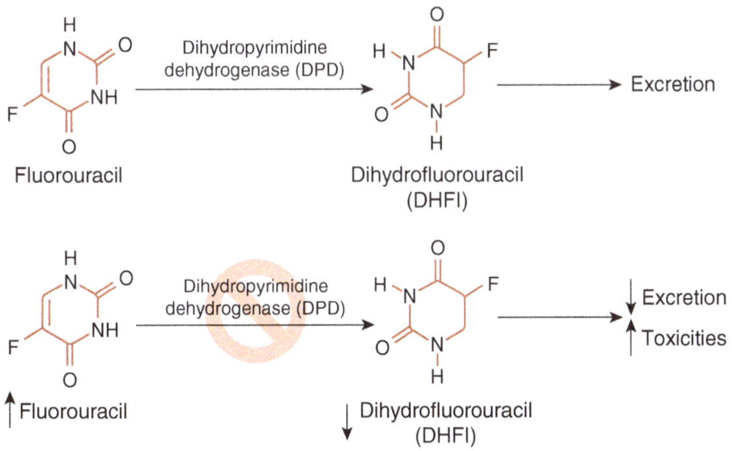

FIGURE 2.5 DPD-dependent catabolism of fluorouracil.

Many variations of *DPYD* have been identified that vary from no impact on function to nonfunctional DPD. The most common and well-established decrease function variants are c.190511G>A, c.1679T>G, c.2846A>T, c.1129–5923C>G. Some variations have not yet established a relationship between the variant and functional status. This limits the utility of star (*) allele nomenclature; thus, only some known variants have been assigned a star (*) allele. Due to the variability in evidence, an allele functionality table also includes a comment on the quality of evidence to support the activity score. Ultimately, the PGx test will report out the likely phenotype based on the best evidence available as detailed in Tables 2.7 and 2.8.

TABLE 2.7 2017 CPIC Recommendations for Fluoropyrimidine Dosing by DPD Phenotype (Abbreviated)

PHENOTYPE	DOSING RECOMMENDATION	CLASSIFICATION OF RECOMMENDATION
DPYD **normal** metabolizer	No dose adjustment recommended	Strong
DPYD **intermediate** metabolizer DPD activity 30%–70%	Reduce based on activity score followed by titration based on tolerability Activity score 1: reduce by 50% Activity score 1.5: reduce dose by 25%–50%	Activity score 1: strong Activity score 1.5: moderate
DPYD **poor** metabolizer Complete DPD deficiency	Activity score 0.5: avoid use; if unavoidable, 5-fluorouracil should be administered at a strongly reduced dose with early therapeutic drug monitoring Activity score 0: avoid use	Strong

CPIC, Clinical Pharmacogenetics Implementation Consortium; DPD, dihydropyrimidine dehydrogenase.

TABLE 2.8 Labeling for Fluoropyrimidines Pharmacogenomics (PGx) Testing

FDA Labeling for Fluorouracil:
Increased Risk of Serious or Fatal Adverse Reactions in Patients With Low or Absent Dihydropyrimidine Dehydrogenase (DPD) Activity: Based on postmarketing reports, patients with certain homozygous or certain compound heterozygous mutations in the DPD gene that result in complete or near complete absence of DPD activity are at increased risk for acute early-onset of toxicity and severe, life-threatening, or fatal adverse reactions caused by fluorouracil (e.g., mucositis, diarrhea, neutropenia, and neurotoxicity). Patients with partial DPD activity may also have increased risk of severe, life-threatening, or fatal adverse reactions caused by fluorouracil.

FDA Labeling for Capecitabine (Xeloda):
Increased Risk of Severe or Fatal Adverse Reactions in Patients With Low or Absent Dihydropyrimidine Dehydrogenase (DPD) Activity: Withhold or permanently discontinue capecitabine in patients with evidence of acute early-onset or unusually severe toxicity, which may indicate near complete or total absence of DPD activity. No capecitabine dose has been proved safe in patients with absent DPD activity.

(continued)

TABLE 2.8 Labeling for Fluoropyrimidines Pharmacogenomics (PGx) Testing (*continued*)

EMA Labeling for Tegafur/Gimeracil/Oteracil (Teysuno):*
Patients with complete DPD deficiency are at high risk of life-threatening or fatal toxicity
  and must not be treated with tegafur. Patients with partial DPD deficiency are at increased
  risk of severe and potentially life-threatening toxicity. A reduced starting dose should be
  considered to limit this toxicity.

*Teysuno is not FDA approved.
EMA, European Medicines Agency; FDA, U.S. Food and Drug Administration.

THIOPURINE METHYLTRANSFERASE, NUDIX-TYPE MOTIF 15, AND THIOPURINES

Thiopurines including mercaptopurine, azathioprine, a prodrug for mercaptopurine, and thioguanine are used for a variety of leukemia, lymphoma, and rheumatologic or immunologic conditions. These agents are discussed more completely in Chapter 6. However, their metabolism and relevant PGx are discussed in this chapter.

Thiopurines are catabolized by thiopurine methyltransferase (TPMT) and nudix-type motif 15 (NUDT15); therefore, patients with genetic variations leading to reduced activity are at a higher risk for toxicities and may require dose adjustments. TPMT functions by adding a methyl group to the thiopurine base, as demonstrated in Figure 2.6. TPMT metabolizes mercaptopurine to an inactive methylmercaptopurine base, which decreases the amount of mercaptopurine that can be metabolized to thioguanine nucleotides, an active metabolite. TPMT metabolizes thioguanine to an inactive methylthioguanine base. Thioguanine has less affinity for TPMT as compared to mercaptopurine or azathioprine, but it is still susceptible to alterations in function since it does not have a second active metabolite.

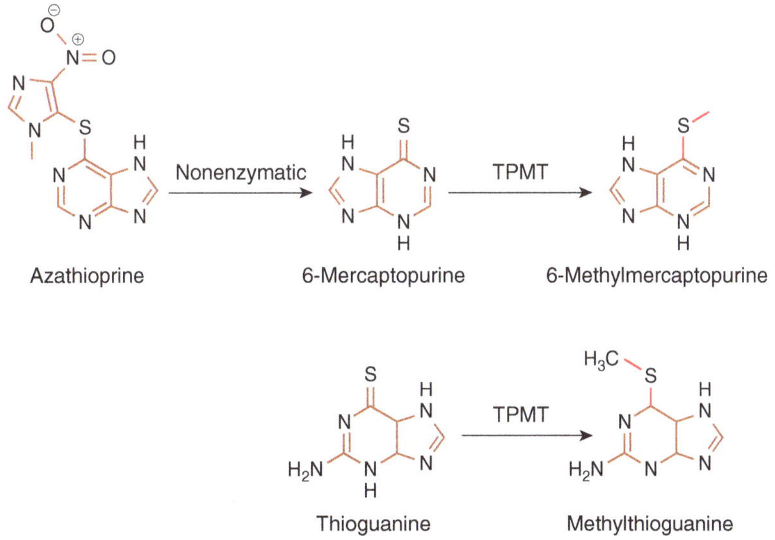

FIGURE 2.6 Activity of thiopurine methyltransferase (TPMT) of thiopurines.

TPMT activity is dependent on SNPs that are inherited by means of autosomal codominance. Homozygous TPMT deficiency has a high predictive value for thiopurine-related toxicity, but is very rare. They are found in approximately 5% of Caucasians, 3% of Asian populations, and 6% of Black populations. TPMT heterozygotes have more variability in response and tolerability at least in part due to variations in metabolism through other enzymes involved in the metabolism and catabolism of thiopurines.

The other enzyme heavily involved in the metabolism of thiopurines is NUDT15, which converts the active metabolites thioguanine triphosphate (TGTP) to thioguanine monophosphate (TGMP). TGMP cannot be incorporated into RNA. NUDT15 also converts thio-deoxyguanosine triphosphate (TdGTP) to thio-deoxyguanosine monophosphate (TdGMP), which cannot be incorporated into DNA (**Figure 2.7**).

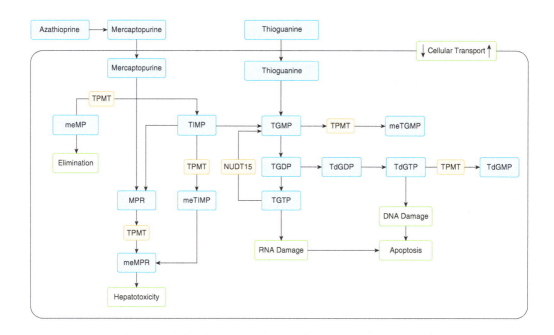

FIGURE 2.7 **Metabolic pathway for azathioprine, mercaptopurine, and thioguanine.**

meMP, methylmercaptopurine; meMPR, meMP ribonucleotides; meTGMP, methylthioguanosine monophosphate; meTIMP, methylthioinosine monophosphate; MPR, mercaptopurine ribonucleotides; TdGDP, 6-thio-deoxy-guanosine diphosphate; TdGMP, 6-thio-deoxy-guanosine monophosphate; TdGTP, 6-thio-deoxy-guanosine triphosphate; TGDP, thioguanosine diphosphate; TGMP, thioguanosine monophosphate; TGTP, thioguanosine triphosphate; TIMP, thioinosine monophosphate; TPMT, thiopurine methyltransferase.

Both TPMT and NUDT15 deficiencies block the continued metabolism of mercaptopurine and thioguanine leading to higher concentrations of active metabolites and an increase in toxicities. Studies have demonstrated a decrease in adverse effects without a compromise in efficacy when medications are empirically dose adjusted based on TPMT and NUDT15 phenotype. Table 2.9 reports examples of starting doses for mercaptopurine and thioguanine based on TPMT and NUDT15 phenotype per CPIC Guidelines. Patients with concomitant intermediate metabolizer phenotypes for both NUDT15 and TPMT have been reported to

TABLE 2.9 2018 CPIC Guidelines for Adjustments for Azathioprine, Mercaptopurine, and Thioguanine Based on TPMT and NUDT15 Phenotype (Abbreviated)

PHENOTYPE	AZATHIOPRINE	MERCAPTOPURINE	THIOGUANINE
TPMT **normal** metabolizer or NUDT15 **normal** metabolizer	Start with normal recommended dose		
TPMT **intermediate** or possible intermediate metabolizer	Start with 30%–80% of recommended starting dose	Strong doses (≥75 mg/ m^2/day): start at 30%–80% of normal starting dose If starting dose <75 mg/m^2: no empiric dose reduction recommended	Start with 50%–80% of recommended starting dose
TPMT **poor** metabolizer	Consider alternative Reduce dose by 10-fold, dose three times weekly rather than daily	Consider alternative Reduce dose by 10-fold, dose three times weekly rather than daily	Reduce dose by 10-fold, dose three times weekly rather than daily
NUDT15 **intermediate** or possible intermediate metabolizer	Start with 30%–80% of recommended starting dose	Strong doses (≥75 mg/ m^2/day): start at 30%–80% of normal starting dose If starting dose <75 mg/m^2: no empiric dose reduction recommended	Start with 50%–80% of recommended starting dose
NUDT15 **poor** metabolizer	Consider alternative Reduce daily dose by 10-fold	Consider alternative Start at 10 mg/m^2	Consider alternative Start with 25% of recommended starting dose

CPIC, Clinical Pharmacogenetics Implementation Consortium; NUDT15, nudix-type motif 15; TPMT, thiopurine methyltransferase.

have decreased tolerance as compared to patients with a single intermediate metabolizer phenotype and may require additional dose adjustments. For conditions other than malignancies that require thiopurines, such as Crohn's disease or rheumatoid arthritis, it is recommended to select alternative agents when a patient has a known deficiency. Table 2.10 describes the labeling related to the PGx tests for azathioprine, mercaptopurine, and thioguanine.

TABLE 2.10 FDA Labeling for Thiopurine Pharmacogenomics Testing

FDA Labeling for Azathioprine (Imuran):

Testing Recommended

Consider alternative therapy in patients with homozygous TPMT or NUDT15 deficiency and reduced dosages in patients with heterozygous deficiency.

Because of the risk of increased toxicity, dosage reduction is recommended in patients known to have heterozygous deficiency of TPMT or NUDT15. Patients who are heterozygous for both TPMT and NUDT15 deficiency may require more substantial dosage reductions.

FDA Labeling for Mercaptopurine (Purixan):

Testing Recommended

Homozygous deficiency in either TPMT or NUDT15: Patients with homozygous deficiency of either enzyme typically require 10% or less of the standard mercaptopurine dosage. Reduce initial dosage in patients who are known to have homozygous TPMT or NUDT15 deficiency.

Heterozygous deficiency in TPMT and/or NUDT15: Reduce the mercaptopurine dosage based on tolerability. Most patients with heterozygous TPMT or NUDT15 deficiency tolerate recommended mercaptopurine doses, but some require dose reduction based on toxicities. Patients who are heterozygous for both TPMT and NUDT15 may require more substantial dosage reductions.

FDA Labeling for Thioguanine (Tabloid):

Testing Recommended

Patients with homozygous deficiency of either TPMT or NUDT15 enzyme typically require 10% or less of the standard thioguanine dosage. Reduce initial dosage in patients who are known to have homozygous TPMT or NUDT15 deficiency. Most patients with heterozygous TPMT or NUDT15 deficiency tolerate recommended thioguanine doses, but some require dose reduction based on toxicities. Patients who are heterozygous for both TPMT and NUDT15 may require more substantial dosage reductions. Reduce the dosage based on tolerability.

FDA, U.S. Food and Drug Administration; NUDT15, nudix-type motif 15; TPMT, thiopurine methyltransferase.

TAMOXIFEN AND CYP2D6

Tamoxifen is a selective estrogen modulator used for the treatment of hormone sensitive breast cancer and is discussed more completely in Chapter 13. Tamoxifen displays interpersonal variability because it relies on enzymatic activation to 4-hydroxytamoxifen and 4-hydroxy-*N*-desmethyltamoxifen (endoxifen) which are 100-fold more potent than tamoxifen. Tamoxifen can be activated by *N*-demethylation by CYP3A4 to *N*-desmethyltamoxifen followed by 4-hydroxylation by CYP2D6 to endoxifen as seen in Figure 2.8. This pathway is highly susceptible to variations in CYP2D6 activity and CYP2D6 inhibitors. Unlike with previous agents discussed in this chapter, poor metabolizers are at risk for subtherapeutic concentrations and treatment failure rather than supratherapeutic levels and increased risk of toxicities.

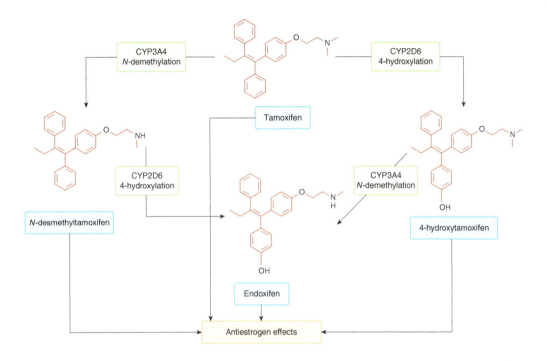

FIGURE 2.8 Activation of tamoxifen through CYP3A4 and CYP2D6.

As depicted in Figure 2.8, metabolism requires both CYP3A4 and CYP2D6. *N*-Demethylation through CYP3A4 can also occur through CYP3A5 and CYP2C19, and therefore, activation of tamoxifen is not reliant on CYP3A4 activity alone. On the other hand, 4-hydroxylation of *N*-desmethyltamoxifen to endoxifen solely goes through CYP2D6; therefore, variable activity of CYP2D6 significantly impacts concentrations of endoxifen, the more potent form of tamoxifen.

Many variations of CYP2D6 have been evaluated and grouped into normal function (*1 and *2), decreased function (*9, *10, *17, and *41), and no function (*3, *4, *5, and *6). Normal function alleles are assigned an activity score of 1.0, decreased function alleles are assigned 0.5, and no function alleles are assigned 0. CYP2D6 is also subject to gene deletions, duplications, and multiplications denoted as *xN*. Table 2.11 depicts the phenotypes with example diplotypes for CYP2D6 along with dosage recommendations for tamoxifen (see Table 2.12).

TABLE 2.11 Assignment of CYP2D6 Phenotype Based on Genotype

PHENOTYPE	EXAMPLE DIPLOTYPE	THERAPEUTIC RECOMMENDATION	STRENGTH OF EVIDENCE
Ultrarapid metabolizer Activity score >2.0	*1/*1xN, *1/*2xN	Start at recommended dose, 20 mg/day	Strong
Normal metabolizer Activity score 1.5–2.0	*1/*1, *2/*2, *1/*9	Start at recommended dose, 20 mg/day	Strong

(continued)

TABLE 2.11 Assignment of CYP2D6 Phenotype Based on Genotype (*continued*)

PHENOTYPE	EXAMPLE DIPLOTYPE	THERAPEUTIC RECOMMENDATION	STRENGTH OF EVIDENCE
Normal-intermediate metabolizer Activity score 1.0	*1/*4, *1/*5, *9/*9	Consider alternative Consider starting at higher dose, 40 mg/day	Optional
Intermediate metabolizer Activity score 0.5	*4/*9, *5/*10	Consider alternative Consider starting at higher dose, 40 mg/day	Moderate
Poor metabolizer Activity score 0	*3/*4, *5/*5	Recommend alternative Recommend starting at higher dose, 40 mg/day	Strong

TABLE 2.12 U.S. Food and Drug Administration (FDA) Labeling for Tamoxifen Pharmacogenomics (PGx) Testing

FDA Labeling for Tamoxifen (Soltamox):
Actionable PGx The impact of CYP2D6 polymorphisms on the efficacy of tamoxifen is not well established, but CYP2D6 poor metabolizers who have lower endoxifen concentrations are compared to intermediate, normal, or ultrarapid metabolizers.

CHAPTER SUMMARY

PGx testing can help anticipate or explain interpersonal variations in pharmacodynamic and pharmacokinetic responses to medications. Tests can describe the rate of metabolism, detect the presence of targetable somatic mutations, and predict immune responses to medications through HLA-B alleles. PGx tests can sequence a patient's entire genome or be specific to a single gene for a prespecified medication. Many FDA-approved medications now have PGx testing annotations in the medication labeling including chemotherapy and relevant supportive care medications. These annotations include recommendations for dose modifications or monitoring. Chemotherapy including irinotecan, sacituzumab govitecan, fluoropyrimidines, thiopurines, and tamoxifen have PGx labeling annotations in FDA labeling. Patients who are poor metabolizers of SN-38 are more likely to have dose-limiting myelosuppression and diarrhea from irinotecan and sacituzumab govitecan. Similarly, slow metabolizers of TPMT or NUDT15 and DPD are more likely to experience side effects to thiopurines and fluoropyrimidines, respectively. Alternatively, medications that require activation through an enzyme are at risk for decreased efficacy if a patient has a slow metabolizer phenotype, as seen with tamoxifen and CYP2D6. Pharmacokinetic and pharmacodynamic pathways and annotations are available through the PharmGKB at PharmGKB.org. CPIC Guidelines provides dosing recommendations for several commonly used medications in patients with cancer. CPIC is not designed to provide recommendations on when PGx testing should be done, but rather focuses on evidence-based guidelines for how to modify treatment based on PGx test results.

CLINICAL PEARLS

- PGx testing can be done to predict a response to a medication based on germline mutations that impact the metabolism or elimination of a medication, as well as the possible immune response, as seen with allopurinol-induced severe skin reactions in patients with HLA-B*58:01.
- SN-38 is the active metabolite of irinotecan, which is detoxified through UGT1A1. Poor metabolizers of UGT1A1, including those with homozygous or heterozygous *UGT1A1*28*, are subject to higher systemic concentrations of SN-38 and increased risk for severe myelosuppression and diarrhea.
- DPD is the rate-limiting enzyme involved in the breakdown of fluoropyrimidines including fluorouracil, capecitabine, and tegafur. Patients with *DPYD* deficiency will have a buildup of fluorouracil, which leads to increased risk for toxicities such as myelosuppression, mucositis, diarrhea, and more.
- Thiopurines including mercaptopurine, azathioprine, and thioguanine require TPMT and NUDT15 for catabolism. Deficiency in either TPMT or NUDT15 predisposes patients to increased myelosuppression and other adverse effects.
- Tamoxifen requires activation to the more potent metabolite, endoxifen, through CYP2D6. PGx testing of CYP2D6 can identify poor metabolizers who would be at risk for decreased concentration of endoxifen and decreased efficacy.

MULTIPLE-CHOICE QUESTIONS

1. Patient KS is a 39-year-old, premenopausal female who is diagnosed with Stage IIB hormone receptor positive, human epidermal growth factor receptor 2 negative (HER2⁻) breast cancer. She underwent lumpectomy and radiation and presented to her medical oncologist's office to discuss hormonal therapy. Her oncologist recommends she receive adjuvant treatment with tamoxifen for at least 5 years. KS was previously taking duloxetine for depression and anxiety, which she was counseled to stop due to an interaction with tamoxifen. KS goes home and researches this interaction and finds information about the variability in CYP2D6 impacting tamoxifen response. She discusses this with her oncologist, who orders a PGx test for CYP2D6 activity. The test reveals she is a poor metabolizer for CYP2D6; which of the following is most likely to happen if she were to start standard dose tamoxifen?

    A. Increased risk of toxicity including flushing, peripheral edema, and hot flashes
    B. Increased efficacy and decreased risk of breast cancer recurrence
    C. Decreased absorption of tamoxifen and increased risk of diarrhea
    D. Decreased efficacy and increased risk of breast cancer recurrence

2. Unfortunately, KS has breast cancer recurrence 3 years later detected on routine imaging. Her biopsy results demonstrate she is now hormone receptor negative and she is still HER2⁻. She undergoes treatment with doxorubicin with stable disease, and her oncologist switches her to paclitaxel to which she develops a grade 3 hypersensitivity reaction. Her oncologist recommends KS now start therapy with sacituzumab govitecan. KS is cautious of new therapies given her reaction to paclitaxel. Which of the

following PGx tests could you recommend to ensure that KS is not at an increased risk of toxicities from sacituzumab govitecan?

A. UGT1A1
B. DPD
C. TPMT
D. CYP3A4

3. KS is found to be an appropriate candidate for treatment with sacituzumab govitecan and has an excellent response. She continues on treatment days 1 and 8 every 21 days and wants to use her experience to help the rest of the breast cancer community. She is talking with some other women on a social media page and shares her experience with PGx testing. KS wants to reply to another woman's post asking for resources for women who want to learn more about precision medicine and PGx testing. Which of the following resources would be appropriate for KS to include in her response?

A. CPIC
B. PharmGKB
C. Centers for Disease Control and Prevention (CDC)
D. Answers A and B

4. CF is a fit, 61-year-old male with no past medical history diagnosed with borderline resectable pancreatic cancer. He elected to complete neoadjuvant chemotherapy to increase the probability of a complete resection. He discussed with his oncologist and started treatment with FOLFIRINOX (fluorouracil, irinotecan, and oxaliplatin). He received the first cycle of treatment in the infusion center without incident but presented to the ED 2 days later with 10 bowel movements per day, fever, and general malaise. He is found to have a white blood cell count of 900/μL and an acute kidney injury. The team discusses potential causes and sends PGx tests for DPD and UGT1A1 activity. The results show he is *DPYD* normal metabolizer and he is homozygous for *UGT1A1*28.* Which of his medications likely led to this presentation?

A. Fluorouracil
B. Irinotecan
C. Oxaliplatin
D. Premedications including ondansetron and dexamethasone

5. CF completes his neoadjuvant treatment without irinotecan (FOLFOX) without complication and undergoes successful resection of his pancreatic mass. After recovery from surgery, his oncologist starts to discuss adjuvant treatment with gemcitabine and capecitabine given his intolerance to irinotecan. He becomes concerned when he hears that diarrhea is a side effect of capecitabine and asks if he is at an increased risk like he was with irinotecan. Which of the following is an appropriate response?

A. Yes, since you are homozygous for *UGT1A1*28,* you are at an increased risk for diarrhea but we will dose reduce capecitabine.
B. Yes, capecitabine causes excessive diarrhea in all patients regardless of PGx variations.
C. No, your risk is not increased based on your PGx data since you are a DPD normal metabolizer.

DPYD

6. AP is a 23-year-old female who presented to the ED with diffuse rash and gum bleeding. Her lab test results revealed pancytopenia for which she underwent a bone marrow biopsy consistent with Philadelphia chromosome negative, B-cell acute lymphoblastic leukemia (Ph⁻ B-ALL). She plans to start treatment with a pediatric inspired regimen and completes pretreatment testing including an echocardiogram, hepatitis B serologic tests, and TPMT and NUDT15 activity tests. Her tests results show her as a TPMT intermediate metabolizer and NUDT15 normal metabolizer. After completion of induction therapy, she is set to start consolidation treatment with mercaptopurine 80 mg/m² daily in combination with other chemotherapy. Knowing her TPMT and NUDT15 status, what should be done to her mercaptopurine dose?

A. Continue with mercaptopurine 80 mg/m², which is a low dose and intermediate metabolizers do not need dose reductions.
B. Decrease mercaptopurine dose by 50% to 40 mg/m² daily.
C. Switch mercaptopurine to thioguanine to prevent any interaction with TPMT metabolism.
D. Omit mercaptopurine completely; adherence to chemotherapy schedules for ALL treatment does not impact clinical outcomes.

7. AP tolerates initial treatment with mercaptopurine and is preparing for her next phase of treatment. She is discussing the oral chemotherapy with the clinical pharmacist who reviews the administration and side effects for thioguanine. AP realizes it sounds similar to how she took the mercaptopurine and asked if the tests she did before starting treatment regarding her genetics relate to thioguanine as well. What would be an appropriate response?

A. No, thioguanine is similar to mercaptopurine but is only processed through NUDT15 instead of NUDT15 and TPMT.
B. Yes, thioguanine is also metabolized through TPMT and we should empirically reduce the dose.
C. Yes, thioguanine is activated through TPMT so we should empirically increase the dose.
D. No, thioguanine is not related to mercaptopurine.

8. LP is a 59-year-old male who is diagnosed with hyperleukocytosis with a final diagnosis pending laboratory tests. He was started on hydroxyurea for cytoreduction and allopurinol for tumor lysis prophylaxis. He continues on his home amlodipine, sertraline, and simvastatin. The following day, his white blood cell count trended down, but he develops a severe maculopapular rash with erosions covering 75% to 90% of his body surface area. Dermatology is consulted and diagnoses him with Stevens-Johnson syndrome (SJS). Which of his medications could have a PGx link to his presentation of SJS?

A. Allopurinol
B. Hydroxyurea
C. Sertraline
D. Simvastatin

9. LP is transferred to the medical ICU for supportive care for SJS. He is ultimately diagnosed with acute myeloid leukemia and has some residual skin lesions that the team wants to confirm are not leukemia cutis. A skin biopsy is done that is inconclusive. Is there a blood test that could help determine if allopurinol is involved in the development of the rash?

   A. No, no tests are available for allopurinol-induced adverse effects.
   B. Yes, a blood test can identify if LP is a poor metabolizer of CYP2C19.
   C. No, a skin biopsy test would be required to look for *HLA-B*58:01*.
   D. Yes, a blood test could be used to identify *HLA-B*58:01*.

MULTIPLE-CHOICE QUESTION ANSWERS

1. **D.** Tamoxifen requires activation through CYP2D6 to the more potent metabolite, endoxifen. Poor metabolizers will have lower levels of endoxifen and therefore a decreased estrogen inhibition. Tamoxifen has been proved to reduce the risk of breast cancer recurrence in premenopausal women; therefore, without adequate activity of tamoxifen, KS will be at a higher risk of recurrence. Answer choices A and B are incorrect as this would be the case if tamoxifen required CYP2D6 for elimination. Answer choice C is incorrect because CYP2D6-mediated metabolism does not impact absorption of the medication.

2. **A.** Sacituzumab govitecan is an antibody–drug conjugate that releases SN-38. SN-38 is eliminated through UGT1A1; therefore, PGx tests examining the activity of UGT1A1 can predict if patients are at increased risk for toxicities. B, C, and D are incorrect as these enzymes are not involved in the processing of sacituzumab govitecan.

3. **D.** Both CPIC and PharmGKB are resources for healthcare providers to learn more about PGx testing. CPIC guidelines provide recommendations for therapy modifications based on available PGx tests. PharmGKB has detailed pharmacokinetic and pharmacodynamic pathways. While most of these resources are geared toward healthcare providers, they have patient-specific resources as well. Answer choice C is incorrect as the CDC does not provide resources for PGx testing.

4. **B.** Irinotecan is activated to SN-38, which is broken down by UGT1A1. *UGT1A1*28* allele is known to have decreased function and leads to increased concentrations of SN-38, responsible for this patient's presentation of diarrhea and myelosuppression. Answer choice A is incorrect, as fluorouracil is broken down by DPD, found to have normal activity in this patient. Answer choices C and D are incorrect because these medications do not have relevant PGx testing and are not impacted by UGT1A1.

5. **C.** Since CF was previously found to have *DPYD* normal metabolism and tolerated fluorouracil, he is not at any increased risk of capecitabine-induced diarrhea due to his PGx variants. Answer choice A is incorrect since capecitabine is not metabolized through UGT1A1. B is incorrect because capecitabine is subject to PGx variations through DPD with poor or intermediate metabolizers at an increased risk for toxicities due to accumulation of active moieties.

6. **B.** Intermediate metabolizers of TMPT or NUDT15 are recommended to reduce the starting dose by 30% to 80% due to the increased risk of myelosuppression and hepatotoxicity with the standard dose of thiopurine. This recommendation is specific to strong doses, defined as >75 mg/m^2. Answer choice C is incorrect as thioguanine is also metabolized by TPMT and would have the same dose adjustment recommendations. Answer choice D is incorrect since studies have shown that adherence to chemotherapy regimens in adolescents and young adults significantly improve outcomes.

7. **B.** Thioguanine, mercaptopurine, and azathioprine are all dependent on TMPT and NUDT15 for metabolism. Intermediate and poor metabolizers will be at an increased risk for toxicities; intermediate metabolizers of TPMT are recommended to start at 50% to 80% of the recommended starting thioguanine dose. Answer choice A is incorrect since thioguanine is metabolized through both enzymes. Answer choice C is incorrect since poor metabolizers will have higher systemic concentrations and increased risk of toxicity.

8. **A.** Some medications are able to elicit an immune response through activation of HLA. For example, allopurinol can trigger severe cutaneous skin reactions (SCARs) through HLA-B leading to release of cytokines from T cells and through an immune cascade and can lead to either SJS or toxic epidermal necrolysis (TEN). Patients with *HLA-B*58:01* allele are a significantly higher risk of developing SCARs.

9. **D.** As above, if LP is found to have *HLA-B*58:01*, then it would increase the probability that the presentation is related to allopurinol use. Answer C is incorrect as most PGx tests are blood tests, so a skin biopsy is not required. Answer B is incorrect since allopurinol is not metabolized through CYP2C19.

SELECTED REFERENCES

Amstutz U, Henricks LM, Offer SM, et al. Clinical Pharmacogenetics Implementation Consortium (CPIC) guideline for dihydropyrimidine dehydrogenase genotype and fluoropyrimidine dosing: 2017 update. Clin Pharmacol Ther. 2018;103(2):210–6. https://doi.org/10.1002/cpt.911

Aspen Global Inc. Thioguanine (Tabloid) [package insert]. May 2018. U.S. Food and Drug Administration website. Available from: https://www.accessdata.fda.gov/drugsatfda_docs/label/2018/012429s028lbl.pdf

Bardia A, Messersmith WA, Kio EA, et al. Sacituzumab govitecan, a Trop-2-directed antibody-drug conjugate, for patients with epithelial cancer: Final safety and efficacy results from the phase I/II IMMU-132-01 basket trial. Ann Oncol. 2021;32(6):746–56. https://doi.org/10.1016/j.annonc.2021.03.005

Dean L, Kane M. Allopurinol therapy and HLA-B* 58:01 genotype. In: Pratt VM, Scott SA, Pirmohamed M, et al., editors. Medical Genetics Summaries. Bethesda: National Center for Biotechnology Information; 2013.

Genentech USA, Inc. Capecitabine (Xeloda) [package insert]. U.S. Food and Drug Administration website. Available from: https://www.accessdata.fda.gov/drugsatfda_docs/label/2021/020896s043lbl.pdf

Goetz MP, Sangkuhl K, Guchelaar HJ, et al. Clinical Pharmacogenetics Implementation Consortium (CPIC) guideline for CYP2D6 and tamoxifen therapy. Clin Pharmacol Ther. 2018;103(5):770–7. https://doi.org/10.1002/cpt.1007

Guo C, Xie X, Li J, et al. Pharmacogenomics guidelines: Current status and future development. Clin Exp Pharmacol Physiol. 2019;46(8):689–93. https://doi.org/10.1111/1440-1681.13097

Immunomedics, Inc. Sacituzumab govitecan-hziy (Trodelvy) [package insert]. April 2021. U.S. Food and Drug Administration website. Available from: https://www.accessdata.fda.gov/drugsatfda_docs /label/2021/761115s009lbl.pdf

Kalman LV, Agúndez J, Appell ML, et al. Pharmacogenetic allele nomenclature: International workgroup recommendations for test result reporting. Clin Pharmacol Ther. 2016;99(2):172–85. https://doi.org/10.1002/cpt.280

Klein DJ, Thorn CF, Desta Z, et al. PharmGKB summary: Tamoxifen pathway, pharmacokinetics. Pharmacogenet Genomics. 2013;23(11):643–7. https://doi.org/10.1097/FPC.0b013e3283656bc1

Marsh S, Hoskins JM. Irinotecan pharmacogenomics. Pharmacogenomics. 2010;11(7):1003–10. https://doi.org/10.2217/pgs.10.95

Nelson RS, Seligson ND, Bottiglieri S, et al. UGT1A1 guided cancer therapy: Review of the evidence and considerations for clinical implementation. Cancers (Basel). 2021;13(7):1566. https://doi.org /10.3390/cancers13071566

Nordic Pharma BV. Tegafur, gimeracil, oteracil (Teysuno) [package insert]. European Medicines Agency website. Available from: https://www.ema.europa.eu/en/documents/product-information /teysuno-epar-product-information_en.pdf

Nova Laboratories. Mercaptopurine (Purixan) [package insert]. April 2020. U.S. Food and Drug Administration website. Available from: https://www.accessdata.fda.gov/drugsatfda_docs/ label/2020/205919s004lbl.pdf

Pfizer. Injectables. Irinotecan (Camptosar) [package insert]. Revised December 2014. U.S. Food and Drug Administration website. Available from: https://www.accessdata.fda.gov/drugsatfda_docs/ label/2022/020571Orig1s053lbl.pdf

Relling MV, Klein TE. CPIC: Clinical Pharmacogenetics Implementation Consortium of the Pharmacogenomics Research Network. Clin Pharmacol Ther. 2011;89(3):464–7. https://doi.org /10.1038/clpt.2010.279

Relling MV, Schwab M, Whirl-Carrillo M, et al. Clinical Pharmacogenetics Implementation Consortium guideline for thiopurine dosing based on TPMT and NUDT15 genotypes: 2018 update. Clin Pharmacol Ther. 2019;105(5):1095–105. https://doi.org/10.1002/cpt.1304

Rosemont Pharmaceuticals Ltd. Tamoxifen (Soltamox) [package insert]. April 2019. U.S. Food and Drug Administration website. Available from: https://www.accessdata.fda.gov/drugsatfda_docs/label /2019/021807s006lbl.pdf

Saito Y, Stamp LK, Caudle KE, et al. Clinical Pharmacogenetics Implementation Consortium (CPIC) guidelines for human leukocyte antigen B (HLA-B) genotype and allopurinol dosing: 2015 update. Clin Pharmacol Ther. 2016;99(1):36–7. https://doi.org/10.1002/cpt.161

Sebela Pharmaceuticals. Azathioprine (Imuran) [package insert]. 2018. U.S. Food and Drug Administration website. Available from: https://www.accessdata.fda.gov/drugsatfda_docs/label/2018/016324s039lbl .pdf

Spectrum Pharmaceuticals, Inc. Fluorouracil [package insert]. July 2016. U.S. Food and Drug Administration website. Available from: https://www.accessdata.fda.gov/drugsatfda_docs/label/ 2016/012209s040lbl.pdf

Thorn CF, Marsh S, Carrillo MW, et al. PharmGKB summary: Fluoropyrimidine pathways. Pharmacogenet Genomics. 2011;21(4):237–42. https://doi.org/10.1097/FPC.0b013e32833c6107

Whirl-Carrillo M, Huddart R, Gong L, et al. An evidence-based framework for evaluating pharmacogenomics knowledge for personalized medicine. Clin Pharmacol Ther. 2021;110(3):563– 72. https://doi.org/10.1002/cpt.2350

Zaza G, Cheok M, Krynetskaia N, et al. Thiopurine pathway. Pharmacogenet Genomics. 2010;20(9):573– 4. https://doi.org/10.1097/FPC.0b013e328334338f

Critical Components of Clinical Trials Development: From Bench to Bedside and Back

S. PERCY IVY • RICHARD F. LITTLE • JOSHUA F. ZEIDNER

INTRODUCTION

Converting a molecular entity from bench to a usable drug at bedside is an onerous process that poses many challenges. Academic institutions and pharmaceutical companies expend tremendous time and energy conducting a multistep process to ensure that each agent/future drug meets the safety and efficacy standards of the regulatory agencies (Figure 3.1). After identification/synthesis of a molecule that can reliably target a valid target, in vitro and in vivo studies including pharmacokinetics and pharmacodynamics in different animal species can lead a molecular entity to clinical arena. Phase 1 trials test the safety of a drug in specific patient populations. Phase 2 trials ensure drug safety and efficacy in patients. Phase 3 trials demonstrate efficacy in a larger group of patients and compare the drug in question to standard of care or placebo. Prognostic and predictive biomarkers that correlate with disease outcome and predict a patient's response to specific therapies are integral parts of drug development and clinical trial design (Figure 3.2). In the first portion of this chapter, we will discuss the phases of the clinical trial including preclinical model studies, their challenges, how results are interpreted, and study endpoints germane to oncology (Figures 3.1–3.10 and Tables 3.1–3.4). Thereafter, we will address the processes by which clinical biomarkers are identified, characterized, and validated with regard to their clinical application (Figures 3.11–3.16 and Table 3.4).

PATHWAYS TO DRUG DEVELOPMENT: MOLECULAR DETERMINANTS

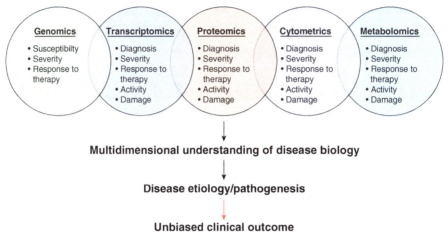

FIGURE 3.1 **The landscape of drug development and discovery has changed dramatically in the last decade.**
Advances in "-omics" have identified new tools for target characterization and analysis. The molecular characterization of tumors has enhanced the basic understanding of disease-specific cancer biology, etiology, and pathogenesis. The in-depth understanding of biology allows for a more comprehensive evaluation of tumor resistance and sensitivity. The tools allow assessment analysis of direct and indirect functional effects of novel drugs on tumors. The emergence of well-characterized resistant tumor clones may provide a path forward for future phases of therapy. Selection of the correct "-omics" tool for biomarker identification depends on the drug effect and the cancer biology–drug relationship. The "-omics" biomarker can be used for diagnosis, patient selection, and evaluation of mechanistic response to therapy.

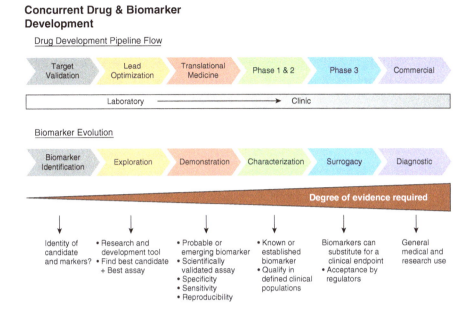

FIGURE 3.2 Concurrent measurements of biomarkers in clinical trials include identification of the specific biomarker and its targets as well as technical and clinical validation of the assays employed for patient selection and monitoring on study. In this instance surrogacy refers to predictive or prognostic biomarkers.

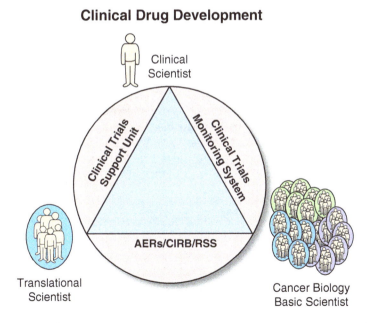

FIGURE 3.3 Clinical drug development triad.

AER, adverse event reporting; CIRB, Central Institutional Review Board; RSS, regulatory support system.

The clinical drug development triad rests on the understanding of basic cancer biology that informs selection of potential molecular features of the tumor to be translated into potential druggable targets and pathways for therapy **Figure 3.3**. Based on the findings of basic and translational scientists, the clinical scientist prioritizes the best scientific opportunities and develops statistically robust clinical trials to advance therapeutics (**Figure 3.4**).

Clinical Translational Research and Cancer Biology: Bedside to Bench and Back

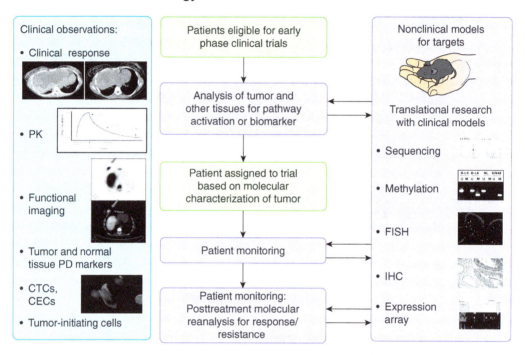

FIGURE 3.4 **Basic and translation approach to clinical trials.**

Using basic and translation underpinnings, the clinical research scientist develops a study represented by the flow diagram in the center of the figure to identify patients selected for treatment and to interrogate the specimens collected during the conduct of early-phase clinical trials of targeted novel therapeutics. Studies such as these add to the understanding of the clinical trial outcomes.

CEC, circulating endothelial cell; CTC, circulating tumor cell; FISH, fluorescent in situ hybridization; IHC immunohistochemistry; PD, pharmacodynamics; PK, pharmacokinetics.

PHASES OF CLINICAL TRIALS

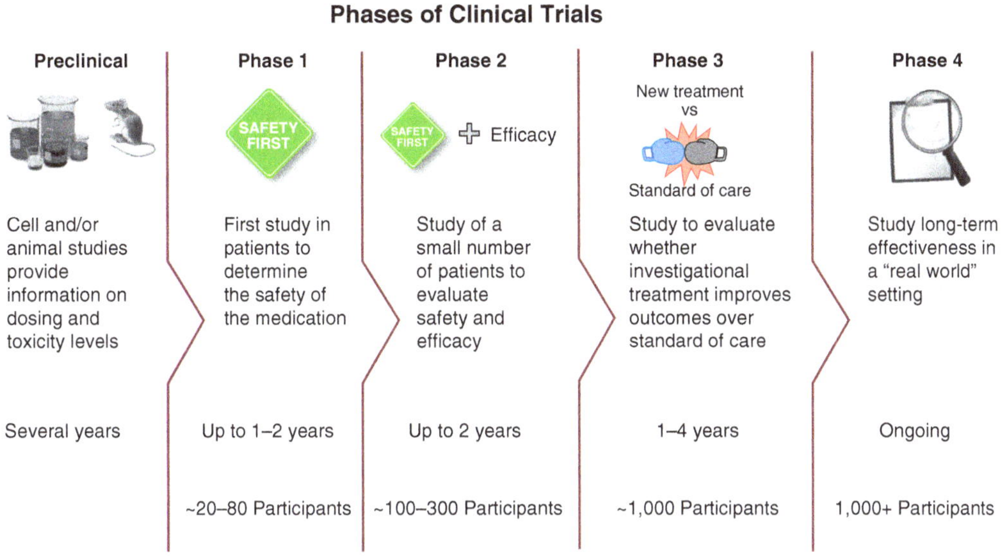
Phases of Clinical Trials
Preclinical
Phase 1
Phase 2
Phase 3
Phase 4
SAFETY FIRST
SAFETY FIRST
Efficacy
New treatment
VS
Standard of care
Cell and/or animal studies provide information on dosing and toxicity levels
First study in patients to determine the safety of the medication
Study of a small number of patients to evaluate safety and efficacy
Study to evaluate whether investigational treatment improves outcomes over standard of care
Study long-term effectiveness in a "real world" setting
Several years
Up to 1–2 years
Up to 2 years
1–4 years
Ongoing
~20–80 Participants
~100–300 Participants
~1,000 Participants
1,000+ Participants

***FIGURE 3.5* Cell and animal studies serve as preliminary data to test a potential investigational agent.**

Once there are enough supporting scientific and safety data, a Phase 1 clinical trial will assess the safety of the agent with the primary goal of determining the maximal tolerated dose (MTD) and/or recommended Phase 2 dosing (RP2D) in humans. A Phase 2 clinical trial can then be implemented if there are enough safety data and preliminary evidence for clinical activity in order to determine whether there is enough efficacy to move on to a larger phase clinical trial. The intent of a Phase 3 trial is to evaluate the efficacy of an agent or combination of agents with a larger cohort in comparison with placebo or standard of care. Phase 3 studies are typically conducted as randomized controlled trials. Phase 4 studies are conducted after a study drug has received approval from the U.S. Food and Drug Administration (FDA). The goal of a Phase 4 study is to determine the long-term effects of the drug.

Source: Stein EM, DiNardo CD, Pollyea DA, et al., Blood, 2017.

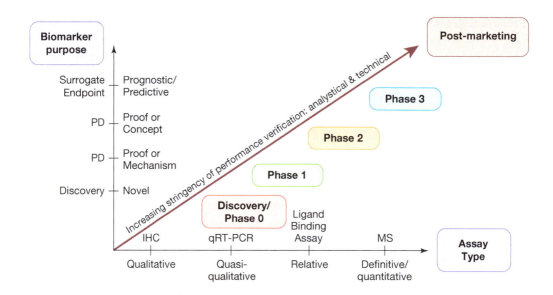

FIGURE 3.6 Development of biomarkers based on their intended use. The development of the biomarker purpose and assay type progresses from discovery throughout clinical development.

Biomarkers rely on appropriately designed clinical trials for establishing their intended use.

IHC, immunohistochemistry; MS, mass spectrometry; PCR, polymerase chain reaction; PD, pharmacodynamics; qRT, quantitative reverse transcription.

Source: Cummings J, Raynaud F, Jones L, et al., Br J Cancer, 2010.

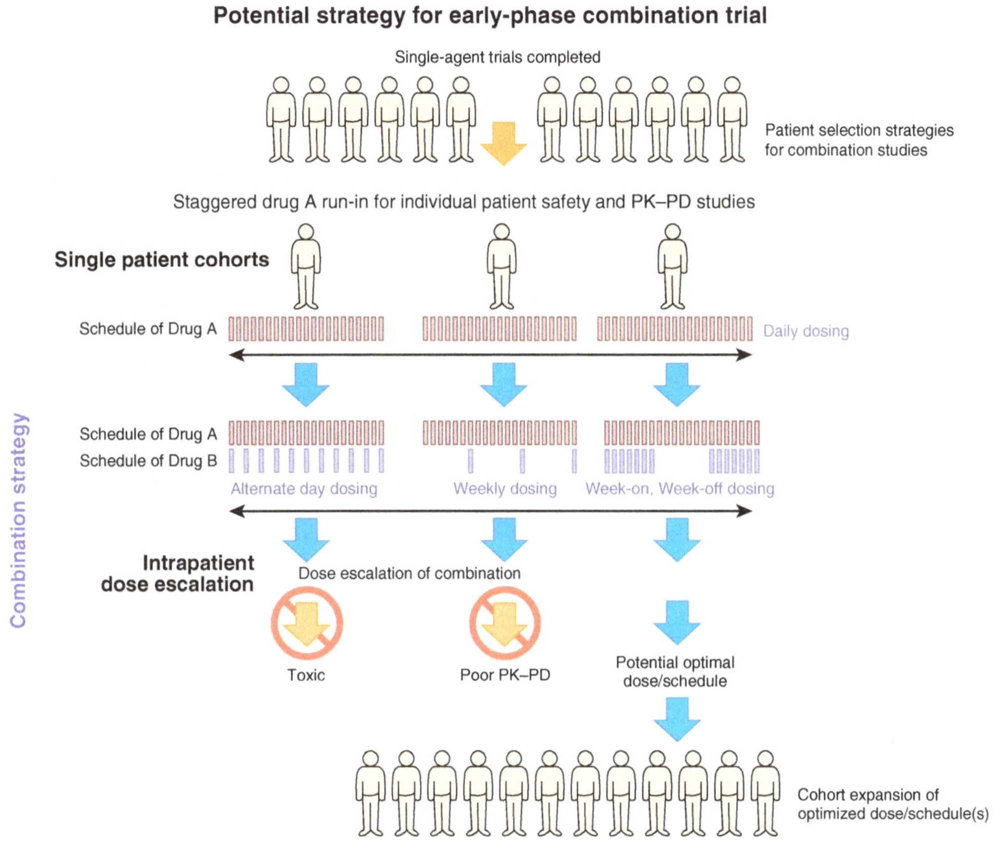

Potential strategy for early-phase combination trial

FIGURE 3.7 **Design of early-phase clinical trials.**
The use of efficient adaptive statistical designs to perform early-phase clinical trials integrating PK and PD studies to minimize the number of patients needed to determine the optimal dose and schedule of two novel agents. Patients are used as their own controls during the dose escalation. In the expansion cohort, the patients are further analyzed for the safety and tolerability of the dose and schedule selected. The PD studies may be used to interrogate the proposed mechanism of action and to identify biomarkers that may be useful for patient selection in later-phase trials. This is one example; more comprehensive reviews of early-phase trial design can be found in the literature.

PD, pharmacodynamics; PK, pharmacokinetics.

Source: Banerji U, Workman P., Semin Oncol, 2016; Rossanese O, Eccles S, Springer C, et al., Drug Discov Today Dis Models, 2016; Yap TA, Sandhu SK, Workman P, de Bono JS., Nat Rev Cancer, 2010.

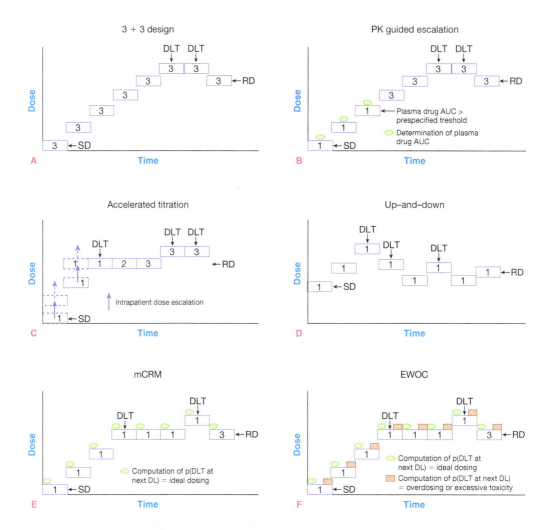

FIGURE 3.8 **Early-phase clinical trials using adaptive designs.**
Panels (A–F) describe several early-phase trial designs that may be used to determine dose and schedule. The design chosen for the trial determining dose and schedule should be based on the known preclinical pharmacology and toxicology. Panel (**A**) presents a "standard" three-patient cohort dose escalation schema. Panel (**B**) uses the PK of a drug to target a specific dose level and effect. Panel (**C**) uses an accelerated titration design to minimize the number of patients treated at nontherapeutic levels of a novel agent. Panel (**D**) provides a statistical design for a drug that has a known dosing range and the recommended phase dose is tightly determined. Panel (**E**) uses another adaptive design using a continual reassessment statistical model. Panel (**F**) uses a statistical design in which the therapeutic index of a drug is very narrow and overdosing the patient is a concern.

AUC, area under the curve; DL, dose level; DLT, dose-limiting toxicity; EWOC, escalation with overdose control; mCRM, modified continual reassessment method; PK, pharmacokinetics; p(DLT at next DL), probability of dose-limiting toxicity at the next dose level; RD, recommended dose; SD, starting dose.

Source: Le Tourneau C, Lee JJ, Siu LL., J Natl Cancer Inst, 2009.

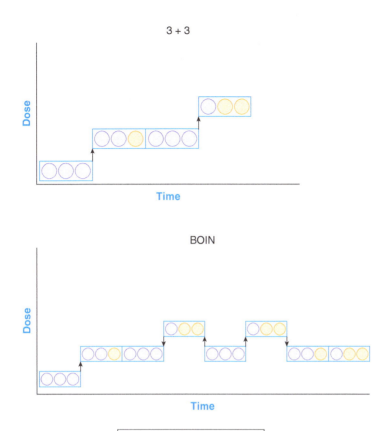

FIGURE 3.9 Bayesian optimal interval (BOIN) design versus 3 + 3 statistical design.

DLT, dose-limiting toxicity.

Source: Hess KR, Fellman BM., Phase I Oncology Drug Development, 2020.

TABLE 3.1 Clinical Trials Definitions

TERMS	DEFINITION
Patient population	Based on inclusion/exclusion criteria. Ensures that patients are similar to reduce variability of results
Control	Treatment against placebo or new active compound Historical control—outcome compared to a previous series of similar subjects Placebo control—used as a control treatment to resemble the treatment being investigated

(continued)

TABLE 3.1 Clinical Trials Definitions (*continued*)

TERMS	DEFINITION
Objectives	Evaluate and establish the effect of a specific intervention. For Phase 1, establish the maximal tolerated dose (MTD) and the recommended Phase 2 dose (RP2D). For Phase 2, define clinical activity with respect to efficacy, safety, and feasibility. For Phase 3, establish clinical activity in comparison with placebo or standard regimens.
Endpoints: Patient population	Primary: the endpoint for which patients are randomized and for which the study is powered. Primary endpoints measure the main clinical effects of a drug or regimen. For Phase 1 trials, primary endpoints are safety and toxicity; for Phase 2 and 3 trials, primary endpoints are efficacy and survival. Secondary: used to evaluate additional therapeutic effects not addressed with the primary endpoint. For Phase 1 trials, secondary endpoints are measurements of survival; for Phase 2 and 3 trials, secondary endpoints are safety and toxicity. Exploratory: These measurements are not planned prospectively; they may be used for unplanned subgroup analysis and hypothesis generation for subsequent studies.
Survival endpoints: Measures of efficacy	Overall survival (OS): time from treatment initiation or randomization to death Disease-free survival (DFS): time from documentation of first response to time of relapse or death Event-free survival: (EFS): time from treatment initiation to treatment failure (i.e., no response), relapse, or death Progression-free survival (PFS): time between treatment initiation and tumor/disease progression or death from any cause Time to treatment failure (TTF): time from treatment initiation to discontinuation (progression, patient choice, death) Health-related quality of life (QOL): QOL with respect to health status over time (complements OS)
Response endpoints	Objective response rate (ORR): proportion of patients achieving complete or partial response) to therapy Complete response (CR): no evidence of tumor based on clinical, histopathologic, and radiographic criteria Disease control rate: percentage of patients with CR, partial response, or stable disease as a result of therapy Duration of response: time from randomization to progression or death for patients achieving measurable response See also Table 3.3 for less-than-complete response definitions (partial response, stable disease).
Bias elimination	Achieved with randomization, stratification, and blinding Single-blind study—patient does not know the identity of the treatment Double-blind study—patient and investigator do not know the identity of the treatment Open-label study—both the researchers and participants know the identity of the treatment
Population size	Powered to show a significant difference between the historical drug and new drug

PATIENT SELECTION AND STUDY DESIGN

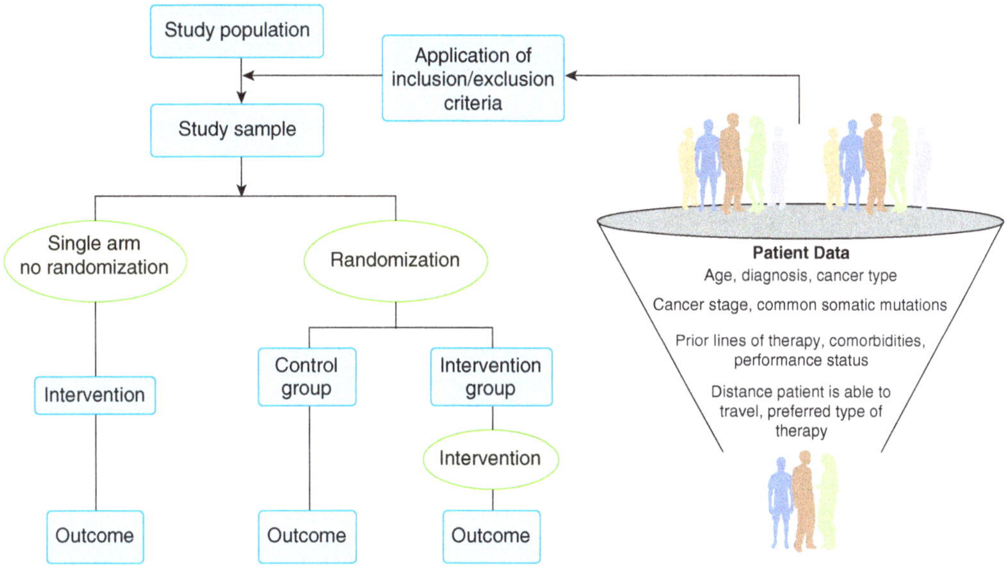

FIGURE 3.10 **Patients with a specified disease type constitute a study population.** Inclusion/exclusion criteria typically include diverse patient characteristics, including age, cancer type and stage, prior therapies, and organ function. These criteria are used to create a study sample that is similar enough to allow the drug in question to serve as the variable. Based on the study design, study sample cohorts can be part of Phase 1 and/or 2 single-arm study where the intervention will be analyzed for safety and outcome. Patient cohorts can also be randomized in Phase 2 and/or 3 studies to a test group or a control group. The control group will receive the standard of care or placebo if acceptable for a given condition, while the test group will receive the experimental medication or treatment to be evaluated. These groups can be "double-blinded," where neither the treating doctors nor the patients know if the patient is receiving the standard treatment versus the experimental treatment. Double-blinding allows the treating healthcare team and patient to make unbiased observations about the progress and effectiveness of the treatment being evaluated. Randomized, double-blind, placebo, or standard-of-care controlled studies are the gold standard for Phase 3 clinical trials.

TABLE 3.2 **Adverse Event Reporting: Common Terminology Criteria for Adverse Events Version 5.0**

GRADES	ADVERSE EVENTS
Grade 1	Mild; asymptomatic or mild symptoms; clinical or diagnostic observation only; intervention not indicated
Grade 2	Moderate; minimal, local, or noninvasive intervention indicated; limiting age-appropriate instrumental ADLs*

(continued)

TABLE 3.2 Adverse Event Reporting: Common Terminology Criteria for Adverse Events Version 5.0 (*continued*)

Grade 3	Severe or medically significant but not immediately life-threatening; hospitalization or prolongation of hospitalization indicated; disabling; limiting self-care ADLs[†]
Grade 4	Life-threatening consequences or urgent intervention indicated
Grade 5	Death related to an adverse event

*Instrumental activites of daily living (ADLs) refer to preparing meals, shopping for groceries or clothes, using the telephone, managing money, etc.
[†]Self-care ADLs refer to bathing, dressing and undressing oneself, using the toilet, taking medication, and not being bedridden.

Note: The Common Terminology Criteria for Adverse Events (CTCAE) is a widely accepted standard classification and severity scale for adverse events in cancer therapy clinical trials. An adverse event is defined as any unfavorable and unintended sign (including an abnormal laboratory finding), symptom, or disease temporally associated with the use of a medical treatment or procedure that may or may *not* be considered related to the medical treatment or procedure. Adverse events are graded based on severity. Grading is provided for each organ system. These criteria are used for the management of chemotherapy dosing and to provide standardization among clinical trial toxicity-related events.

TABLE 3.3 Assessment of Response in Solid Tumor Trials: Comparison of RECIST 1.1, WHO, and Immune-Related Response Criteria (IRRC)

RESPONSE	RECIST	WHO	IRRC
New, measurable lesions (i.e., ≥5 × 5 mm)	Always represent PD	Always represent PD	Incorporated into tumor burden
New, nonmeasurable lesions (i.e., >5 × 5 mm)	Always represent PD	Always represent PD	Do not define progression (but preclude irRC)
Nonindex lesions	Changes contribute to defining BOR of CR, PR, SD, and PD	Changes contribute to defining BOR of CR, PR, SD, and PD	Contribute to defining irRC (complete disappearance required)
Complete response (CR)	Disappearance of all lesions in one observation in randomized studies. Confirmation is needed for nonrandomized studies, according to study protocol.	Disappearance of all lesions in two consecutive observations not less than 4 weeks apart	Disappearance of all lesions in two consecutive observations not less than 4 weeks apart

(continued)

TABLE 3.3 Assessment of Response in Solid Tumor Trials: Comparison of RECIST 1.1, WHO, and Immune-Related Response Criteria (IRRC) (*continued*)

RESPONSE	RECIST	WHO	IRRC
Partial response (PR)	At least a 30% decrease in the sum of diameters of target lesions, taking as reference the baseline sum diameters, in the absence of new lesions or unequivocal progression of nonindex lesions	A ≥50% decrease in SPD of all index lesions compared with baseline in two observations at least 4 weeks apart, in the absence of new lesions or unequivocal progression of nonindex lesions	A ≥50% decrease in tumor burden compared with baseline in two observations at least 4 weeks apart
Stable disease (SD)	Neither sufficient shrinkage to qualify for PR nor sufficient increase to qualify for PD, taking as reference the smallest sum of diameters, in the absence of new lesions or unequivocal progression of nonindex lesions	A 50% decrease in SPD compared with baseline cannot be established nor 25% increase compared with nadir, in the absence of new lesions or unequivocal progression of nonindex lesions	A 50% decrease in tumor burden compared with baseline cannot be established nor 25% increase compared with nadir
Progressive disease (PD)	At least a 20% decrease in the sum of diameters of target lesions, taking as reference the smallest sum on study. The sum must also demonstrate an absolute increase of at least 5 mm. The appearance of one or more new lesions is also considered progression.	At least 25% increase in SPD compared with nadir and/or unequivocal progression of nonindex lesions and/or appearance of new lesions (at any single time point)	At least 25% increase in tumor burden compared with nadir (at any single time point) in two consecutive observations at least 4 weeks apart

Note: In the 1960s, there were early attempts to standardize tumor response to treatment agents. In 1979, the World Health Organization (WHO) published standardized criteria for disease assessment. In 2000, new criteria were presented at the American Society of Clinical Oncology meeting and called response evaluation criteria in solid tumors (RECIST). RECIST provides guidelines that allow physicians to determine if patient is responding to therapy. Immuno-oncology agents have a vastly different mechanism of action than conventional cytotoxic chemotherapy agents for oncology indications. Thus, a modified response assessment is required, known as immune-related response criteria (irRC). The main difference is in categorizing the total tumor burden versus the measurable lesions in WHO and RECIST. The irRC now serves as the gold standard for evaluating immunologic agents.

BOR, best overall response; SPD, sum of the product of the greatest diameters.

Source: Ades F, Yamaguchi N., Ecancermedicalscience, 2015.

BIOMARKER IDENTIFICATION, VALIDATION, AND APPLICATION

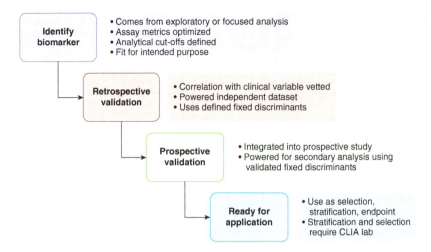

FIGURE 3.11 **When planning to use a biomarker in a clinical trial, it is important to consider how the biomarker was identified and how the assay to detect the biomarker was developed.**
This step is the technical validation and testing of a biomarker for use in a clinical trial. The next step for biomarker development is retrospective clinical validation. Once complete, the biomarker moves to prospective validation in a clinical trial where it is integrated in the study to characterize and analyze the biomarker's relationship to positive outcome events. If there is a clear correlation between response and/or outcome event such as progression-free survival (PFS), overall survival (OS), or both, the biomarker can be used for patient selection. This integral biomarker can now be used for patient selection, stratification, or as an endpoint. Analysis of an integral biomarker must occur in a CLIA environment.

CLIA, Clinical Laboratory Improvement Amendments.

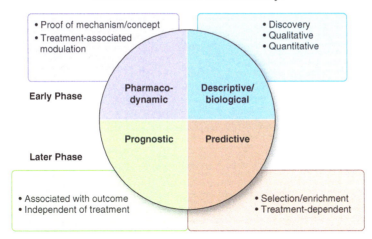

FIGURE 3.12 **Pharmacodynamic and descriptive/biological biomarkers can be important or critical components of early-phase clinical trials when they are rationally employed.**
In later-phase trials, biomarkers related to prognosis or prediction of treatment-related outcomes are used as integral or integrated biomarkers for statistical designs, including patient selection or stratification.

CHARACTERIZATION AND SELECTION OF BIOMARKERS

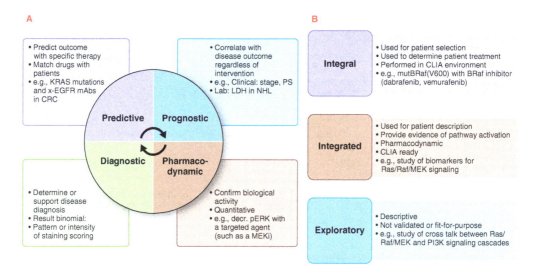

FIGURE 3.13 **Biomarker informed trials require an understanding of the types of biomarkers and appropriate biomarker selection depending on the study goals.** Panel **(A):** definitions and descriptions of functional biomarkers. In early-phase trials, the distinction between predictive and prognostic status of given biomarkers may not be known. Later-phase trials are often required to make this determination. Panel **(B)** shows the trajectory of the types of studies needed to make the determination of a biomarker's ultimate utility. Exploratory biomarker studies may suggest hypotheses that can then be tested in a subsequent clinical trial that helps to determine the biomarker's clinical utility. Ultimately, a biomarker with validated clinical utility can be used in a clinical trial as an integral biomarker.

CLIA, Clinical Laboratory Improvement Amendments; CRC, colorectal cancer; EGFR, epidermal growth factor receptor; LDH, lactate dehydrogenase; mAbs, monoclonal antibodies; MEK, mitogen-activated extracellular signal-regulated kinase; MEKi, MEK inhibitor; NHL, non-Hodgkin lymphoma; PI3K, phosphoinositide 3-kinase; PS, performance status.

PROGNOSTIC BIOMARKER

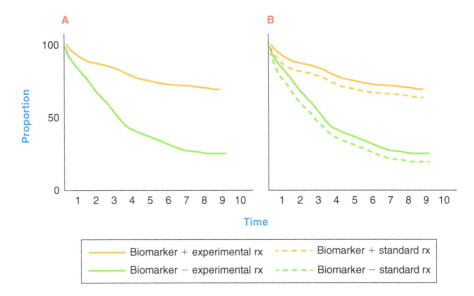

FIGURE 3.14 Example of a biomarker that is prognostic but not predictive.
The randomization of patients to an experimental versus a standard therapy
(rx) can be used to determine whether a biomarker is predictive of a treatment
effect or whether it is merely prognostic of outcome. Panel **(A)** shows that
for patients receiving the experimental therapy, those who are biomarker-
positive (solid orange curve) survive longer than those who are negative for the
biomarker (solid green curve). Looking at these data alone would not allow the
ability to determine if the biomarker is prognostic, predictive, or both. Panel **(B)**
shows how the randomization allows this determination. The biomarker-positive
patients have the same survival regardless of therapy; the biomarker-negative
patients have the same survival regardless of therapy. Therefore, the biomarker
is prognostic. The biomarker is not predictive for benefit of the experimental
therapy (solid curves) relative to the standard therapy (dashed curves) because
within each biomarker subgroup the survival distribution is the same regardless
of the treatment received.

Source: Ballman KV., J Clin Oncol, 2015.

PREDICTIVE BIOMARKER

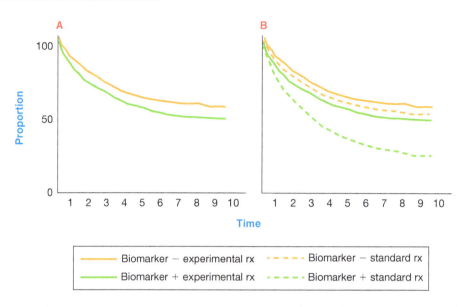

FIGURE 3.15 Example of a biomarker that is both negatively prognostic and predictive.

Panel **(A)** shows the survival curves for patients receiving the experimental therapy (rx). The survival curves are very similar regardless of biomarker status. Panel **(B)** shows that for patients receiving the standard therapy, those who are positive for the biomarker have shorter survival (orange dashed curve) compared to those who are negative for the biomarker (green dashed curve); therefore, the biomarker is negatively prognostic. The biomarker is also predictive for benefit of the experimental therapy (solid curves) relative to the standard therapy (dashed curves) because survival for patients who are positive for the biomarker is substantially longer for those receiving the experimental therapy (orange solid curve) compared to standard therapy (orange dashed curve), whereas for patients who are negative for the biomarker (green curve), the survival distribution is the same regardless of the treatment received.

Source: Ballman KV., J Clin Oncol, 2015.

TABLE 3.4 **Biomarker Challenges and Opportunities**

CHALLENGES	OPPORTUNITIES
Selecting which biomarker(s) and assay(s) to move from exploratory observation to testable entity	Optimize selection and stratification to identify best use for prognostic or predictive purposes
Validating assay metrics and quality control to yield locked-in discriminant	Allow development of database relative to actionable subsets
Defining appropriate application to patients and trials: not all events can be described by a single analysis	Allows for precision and personalization of care planning
Proving that a specific biomarker works on a per-patient basis	A predictive biomarker per se may serve as a novel therapeutic target

The use of biomarkers in both early and late phase clinical trials can pose diverse challenges. For instance, selecting the appropriate testable analytes requires technical and clinical validation. The assay must be "locked-in," reliable, and reproducible. The tissue in which the biomarker will be used must be tested and the assay further validated. The preanalytics should be known and standardized. Nonetheless, the opportunities for the use of highly selective biomarkers in clinical investigation and treatment planning are extensive and include patient selection and stratification, prediction of response to therapy, precision and personalization of cancer care, and providing a novel target for drug development.

THE PHARMACOLOGIC AUDIT TRIAL

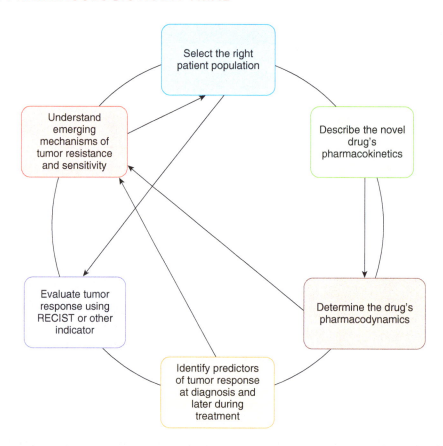

FIGURE 3.16 PhAT outlines key questions that deal with the use of biomarkers. Rigorous implementation of the PhAT ensures discovery and clinical development of high-quality drug candidates and helps optimize clinical trials using biomarkers by guiding informed clinical decisions: **(1)** Select the appropriate patient population, **(2)** describe the drug's **pharmacokinetics**, what the body does to the drug, **(3)** determine the drug's **pharmacodynamics**, what the drug does to the body, **(4)** predict tumor response at an intermediate time point to evaluate the effect, **(5)** assess tumor response at end of treatment using standard morphometric measure and/or mechanistic effects, and **(6)** understand **tumor resistance** and sensitivity paradigms.

PhAT, pharmacological audit trail; RECIST, response evaluation criteria in solid tumors.

Source: Banerji U, Workman P., Semin Oncol, 2016; Rossanese O, Eccles S, Springer C, et al., Drug Discov Today Dis Models, 2016.

CHAPTER SUMMARY

The rapid pace of scientific advances is enabling a greater understanding of disease processes and bringing forth new drug discovery. From start to finish, clinical trials require the concerted effort of a multidisciplinary team of physicians, researchers, and patients to ensure each step proceeds according to plan. In the initial part of this chapter, we discuss basic drug development from predevelopment to the final phases of drug approval. We address the various barriers to clinical trials, including cost, patient misconceptions, and patient participation. Finally, we delve into clinical trial study design with randomized clinical trials, adverse event reporting, response assessment, and study endpoints with Kaplan–Meier curves. In the second part of the chapter, we discuss the use and role of biomarkers in clinical trials and what they mean from the perspective of the patient, the individual clinical trial and clinical trials using the same drug, and biomarker, referred to as aggregated analysis. Biomarkers require an increasing level of stringent performance that requires technical and analytical validation as they are used in later-phase trials. The goal is to develop biomarkers that are fit-for-purpose, that can help select patients for trials, and are predictive of treatment outcome. Prognostic and predictive biomarkers are defined and described based on their clinical utility. The use of a systems-based approach to a patient's tumor evaluation allows for the multidimensional evaluation of disease biology, pathogenesis, and unbiased clinical outcome.

CLINICAL PEARLS

Any clinical protocol at any phase of development should be designed to address the following questions:

- What hypotheses are being tested? (Objectives)
- Why are these hypotheses worth testing? (Background and Rationale)
- In whom will these hypotheses be tested? (Patient Eligibility)
- How will the testing be conducted? (Treatment Schema and Details, Correlates)
- How will the resultant data be analyzed and interpreted? (Statistics)

Objectives and endpoints are not identical. Objectives define the specific aims of the protocol with respect to the questions being asked and the hypotheses being tested. Endpoints, on the other hand, are the ways in which the outcomes will be measured.

Biomarkers that correlate with diverse facets of the underlying disease (prognostic) or treatment intervention (predictive) are critical components of early- and late-phase clinical trial designs.

Exploratory studies are descriptive in nature and are intended to generate hypotheses that can be tested in subsequent trials. The biomarker assay itself may be investigational and the relationship to disease prognosis and/or response prediction may be unknown. Exploratory studies commonly accompany Phase 1 and small Phase 2 clinical trials and serve to identify potentially useful biomarkers.

Integrated studies test a specific hypothesis and are aimed at validating the clinical utility of a specific assay or biomarker for use in later-phase (e.g., large randomized Phase 2 and Phase 3) clinical trials aimed at defining the efficacy of specific treatment regimens. Biomarker validation through the integrated studies can serve as secondary objectives.

Integral studies require that the assays be Clinical Laboratory Improvement Amendments (CLIA)-approved and validated with respect to clinical utility and must be performed on all clinical trial participants in real time on fresh tissue. Integral biomarkers accompany randomized Phase 2 and Phase 3 trials and are used to establish patient eligibility and for randomization and stratification prior to assignment to specific treatment arm. In addition, integral biomarkers may serve as acceptable surrogate measures for clinical endpoints.

MULTIPLE-CHOICE QUESTIONS

1. Which of the following is TRUE about Phase 1 trials?

    A. Drugs are tested in the lab or with mice to determine toxicities.
    B. They are designed to investigate the safety/tolerability of an investigational drug on humans.
    C. They use a single, standard predetermined drug dose.
    D. Participants who enroll have alternative highly effective standard of care treatment options.

2. Which of the following is TRUE about Phase 2 trials?

    A. The primary endpoint usually involves assessing the activity of an investigational agent or combination.
    B. All Phase 2 trials are randomized clinical trials.
    C. They typically involve dose escalation of an investigational agent with the goal to determine a maximal tolerated dose.
    D. It must always proceed to a Phase 3 trial for FDA approval.

3. Which of the following is TRUE about Phase 3 trials?

    A. It is a small trial that tests a drug in a specific cancer type.
    B. It tests long-term effects after the study drug has been FDA approved.
    C. A study designed to assess the effectiveness of an investigational agent or combination is compared against the current standard of care.
    D. It is the first human clinical experience with the new agent in a disease type.

4. 4. All of the following are examples of an adverse event *except*.

    A. Irreversible damage to the liver
    B. Drop in white blood cell count or platelets
    C. Patient lost to follow-up
    D. Death

5. What is overall survival?

    A. The time between treatment initiation and tumor progression or death from any cause
    B. The length of time from date of diagnosis or start of treatment of disease to death

C. The percentage of patients whose cancer shrinks or disappears after treatment

D. The length of time between treatment and relapse

6. Which of the following is not used to measure disease response?

A. RECIST criteria

B. WHO criteria

C. irRC

D. CTCAE

7. Development of a predictive biomarker requires all of the following except:

A. Identification of candidate molecules/pathways

B. Characterization in selected patient populations

C. Assay validation and reproducibility

D. Tumor specificity

8. A clinically useful prognostic biomarker is defined by its ability to:

A. Generate new hypotheses related to drug resistance

B. Determine patient selection for specific treatments

C. Relate to disease outcome independent of treatment

D. Confirm biologic activity of a targeted agent

ANSWERS TO MULTIPLE-CHOICE QUESTIONS

1. **B.** Phase 1 trials represent the initial phase of human clinical testing and are designed as dose-escalation trials to define the dose-limiting toxicity (DLT) profile, the maximum tolerated dose (MTD), and the recommended Phase 2 dose (RP2D) for an investigational agent alone or in combination with other drugs. A Phase 1 trial can be conducted in a broad spectrum of diseases (e.g., advanced solid tumors, usually as a single agent) or in specific disease entities (relapsed/refractory leukemias, in combination with other agents).

2. **A.** The primary objective of a Phase 2 trial is to define the clinical efficacy of the investigational agent alone or in combination with other agents for a specific disease or a set of related disease entities. The Phase 2 trial can consist of a single arm, where all patients receive the drug or combinatorial regimen in the same dose and schedule, or can be randomized to compare a standard regimen or drug by itself with the regimen or drug combined with the investigational agent.

3. **C.** Phase 3 trials are large-scale, comparative, randomized trials that are conducted by multiple institutions or cooperative groups. Phase 3 trials compare the clinical efficacy of the investigational agent or combination with the efficacy of the current standard of care in a specific disease or disease subset, and often serve as the basis for FDA approval if the investigational agent or combination proves to be superior to the standard regimen.

4. **C.** Adverse events are unfavorable consequences that occur during treatment with the investigational agent alone or in combination with other drugs, whether such events are directly due to treatment or to the underlying disease. The occurrence of severe adverse events that are deemed probably or definitely related to the investigational agent or combination form the basis for defining DLT.

5. **B.** While overall survival begins with the date of diagnosis or start of treatment and ends with the patient's death, event-free survival (EFS) measures the time from treatment initiation to tumor progression/disease relapse or death from any cause, and disease-free survival (DFS) measures the duration of response from the time that remission is achieved until relapse or death.

6. **D.** CTCAE represents the Common Terminology Criteria for Adverse Events and serves as a standardized classification system used across all clinical trials to grade severity and attribution of organ-specific adverse events occurring during treatment.

7. **D.** Predictive biomarkers relate to some aspect of response to treatment and can be completely independent of disease-specific features.

8. **C.** Prognostic biomarkers correlate with overall outcome on the basis of disease-related features rather than treatment-related features.

SELECTED REFERENCES

Ades F, Yamaguchi N. WHO, RECIST, and immune-related response criteria: Is it time to revisit pembrolizumab results? Ecancermedicalscience. 2015;9:604. https://doi.org/10.3332/ecancer.2015.604

Amur S. Biomarker Terminology: Speaking the Same Language. U.S. Food and Drug Administration. Available from: https://fda.report/media/102547/BIOMARKER-TERMINOLOGY-SPEAKING-THE-SAME-LANGUAGE.pdf

Babiarz JC, Pisano DJ. Overview of FDA and drug development. In: Pisano DJ, Mantus DS, editors. FDA Regulatory Affairs. A Guide for Prescription Drugs, Medical Devices, and Biologics, 2nd ed. New York: CRC Press; 2008.

Bai JPF, Melas IN, Hur J, Guo E. Advances in omics for informed pharmaceutical research and development in the era of systems medicine. Expert Opin Drug Discov. 2018;13(1):1–4. https://doi.org/10.1080/17460441.2018.1394839

Ballman KV. Biomarker: Predictive or prognostic? J Clin Oncol. 2015;33(33):3968–71. https://doi.org/10.1200/JCO.2015.63.3651

Banerji U, Workman P. Critical parameters in targeted drug development: The pharmacological audit trail. Semin Oncol. 2016;43(4):436–45. https://doi.org/10.1053/j.seminoncol.2016.06.001

Cancer Research UK. What Are Targeted Cancer Drugs? Available from: https://www.cancerresearchuk.org/about-cancer/cancer-in-general/treatment/targeted-cancer-drugs/what-are-targeted-cancer-drugs

Center for Drug Evaluation and Research. Guidance for Industry Codevelopment of Two or More Unmarketed Investigational Drugs for Use in Combination. U.S. Food and Drug Administration; 2010. Available from: https://www.c-path.org/pdf/FDADraftGuidanceCoDevelopment.pdf

Cowan KJ. Implementing fit-for-purpose biomarker assay approaches: A bioanalytical perspective. Bioanalysis. 2016;8(12):1221–3. https://doi.org/10.4155/bio-2016-0070

Cummings J, Raynaud F, Jones L, et al. Fit-for-purpose biomarker method validation for application in clinical trials of anticancer drugs. Br J Cancer. 2010;103(9):1313–7. https://doi.org/10.1038/sj.bjc.6605910

Daidone MG, Foekens JA, Harbeck N, et al. Identification, validation and clinical implementation of cancer biomarkers: Translational strategies of the EORTC PathoBiology Group. Eur J Cancer Suppl. 2012;10(1):120–7. https://doi.org/10.1016/S1359-6349(12)70021-6

Dancey JE, Chen HX. Strategies for optimizing combinations of molecularly targeted anticancer agents. Nat Rev Drug Discov. 2006;5(8):649–59. https://doi.org/10.1038/nrd2089

Delgado A, Guddati AK. Clinical endpoints in oncology—A primer. Am J Cancer Res. 2021;11(4):1121–31.

FDA-NIH Biomarker Working Group. BEST (Biomarkers, EndpointS, and other Tools) Resource. Bethesda, MD: National Center for Biotechnology Information; 2016. https://www.ncbi.nlm.nih.gov/books/NBK326791

Freidlin B, McShane LM, Korn EL. Randomized clinical trials with biomarkers: Design issues. J Natl Cancer Inst. 2010;102(3):152–60. https://doi.org/10.1093/jnci/djp477

Henry NL, Hayes DF. Cancer biomarkers. Mol Oncol. 2012;6(2):140–6. https://doi.org/10.1016/j.molonc.2012.01.010

Hess KR, Fellman BM. Examining performance of Phase I designs: 3+3 versus Bayesian optimal interval (BOIN). In: Yap TA, Rodon J, David S, editors. Phase I Oncology Drug Development. Switzerland: Springer Nature; 2020. https://doi.org/10.1007/978-3-030-47682-3

Hopkins AL, Groom CR. The druggable genome. Nat Rev Drug Discov. 2002;1(9):727–30. https://doi.org/10.1038/nrd892

Ilyin SE, Belkowski SM, Plata-Salamán CR. Biomarker discovery and validation: Technologies and integrative approaches. Trends Biotechnol. 2004;22(8):411–6. https://doi.org/10.1016/j.tibtech.2004.06.005

International Conference on Harmonization. General Considerations for Clinical Trials E8; 2021. Available from: http://www.ich.org/fileadmin/Public_Web_Site/ICH_Products/Guidelines/Efficacy/E8/Step4/E8_Guideline.pdf

International Conference on Harmonization. Quality Guidelines; 2012. Available from: http://www.ich.org/products/guidelines/quality/article/quality-guidelines.html

IQVIA Institute. Global Oncology Trends 2017: Advances, Complexity and Cost; 2017. Available from: https://www.iqvia.com/insights/the-iqvia-institute/reports/global-oncology-trends-2017-advances-complexity-and-cost

Kulasingam V, Diamandis EP. Strategies for discovering novel cancer biomarkers through utilization of emerging technologies. Nat Clin Pract Oncol. 2008;5(10):588–99. https://doi.org/10.1038/ncponc1187

Kummar S, Chen HX, Wright J, et al. Utilizing targeted cancer therapeutic agents in combination: Novel approaches and urgent requirements. Nat Rev Drug Discov. 2010;9(11):843–56. https://doi.org/10.1038/nrd3216

Le Tourneau C, Lee JJ, Siu LL. Dose escalation methods in phase I cancer clinical trials. J Natl Cancer Inst. 2009;101(10):708–20. https://doi.org/10.1093/jnci/djp079

LoRusso PM, Canetta RM, Wagner JA, et al. Accelerating cancer therapy development: The importance of combination strategies and collaboration. Summary of an Institute of Medicine workshop. Clin Cancer Res. 2012;18(22):6101–9. https://doi.org/10.1158/1078-0432.CCR-12-2455

Matthews H, Hanison J, Nirmalan N. "Omics"-informed drug and biomarker discovery: Opportunities, challenges and future perspectives. Proteomes. 2016;4(3):28. https://doi.org/10.3390/proteomes4030028

McShane LM. In pursuit of greater reproducibility and credibility of early clinical biomarker research. Clin Transl Sci. 2017;10(2):58–60. https://doi.org/10.1111/cts.12449

McShane LM, Cavenagh MM, Lively TG, et al. Criteria for the use of omics-based predictors in clinical trials. Nature. 2013;502(7471):317–20. https://doi.org/10.1038/nature12564

National Cancer Institute. Dictionary of Cancer Terms. Available from: https://www.cancer.gov/publications/dictionaries/cancerterms/def/biomarker

National Cancer Institute. Targeted Cancer Therapies. Available from: https://www.cancer.gov/about-cancer/treatment/types/targeted-therapies/targeted-therapies-fact-sheet

National Cancer Institute. Tumor Markers. Available from: https://www.cancer.gov/about-cancer /diagnosis-staging/diagnosis/tumor-markers-fact-sheet

NCI Common Terminology Criteria for Adverse Events. 2018. Available from: https://evs.nci.nih .gov/ftp1/CTCAE/About.html

Neely RJ. Evolution of fit-for-purpose biomarker validations: An LBA perspective. Bioanalysis. 2018;10(12):905–7. https://doi.org/10.4155/bio-2017-0267

Paller CJ, Bradbury PA, Ivy SP, et al. Design of phase I combination trials: Recommendations of the clinical trial design task force of the NCI Investigational Drug Steering Committee. Clin Cancer Res. 2014;20(16):4210–7. https://doi.org/10.1158/1078-0432.CCR-14-0521

Rossanese O, Eccles S, Springer C, et al. The pharmacological audit trail (PhAT): Use of tumor models to address critical issues in the preclinical development of targeted anticancer drugs. Drug Discov Today Dis Models. 2016;21:23–32. https://doi.org/10.1016/j.ddmod.2017.07.002

Sawyers C. Targeted cancer therapy. Nature. 2004;432(7015):294–7. https://doi.org/10.1038 /nature03095

Stein EM, DiNardo CD, Pollyea DA, et al. Enasidenib in mutant IDH2 relapsed or refractory acute myeloid leukemia. Blood. 2017;130(6):722–31. https://doi.org/10.1182/blood-2017-04-779405

Strimbu K, Tavel JA. What are biomarkers? Curr Opin HIV AIDS. 2010;5(6):463–6. https://doi .org/10.1097/COH.0b013e32833ed177

United States Code. Title 21, Part 312, Investigational Drug Application. Available from: http://www .accessdata.fda.gov/scripts/cdrh/cfdocs/cfcfr/CFRSearch.cfm?CFRPart=312

U.S. Food and Drug Administration. The Drug Development Process [Internet]; April 2018. Available from: https://www.fda.gov/forpatients/approvals/drugs/

Workman P, Al-Lazikani B. Drugging cancer genomes. Nat Rev Drug Discov. 2013;12(12):889–90. https://doi.org/10.1038/nrd4184

Yap TA, Sandhu SK, Workman P, de Bono JS. Envisioning the future of early anticancer drug development. Nat Rev Cancer. 2010;10(7):514–23. https://doi.org/10.1038/nrc2870

Yuan Y, Hess KR, Hilsenbeck SG, Gilbert MR. Bayesian optimal interval design: A simple and well-performing design for Phase I oncology trials. Clin Cancer Res. 2016;22(17):4291–301. https://doi .org/10.1158/1078-0432.CCR-16-0592

Zhou Y, Li R, Yan F, et al. A comparative study of Bayesian optimal interval (BOIN) design with interval 3 + 3 (i3+3) design for phase 1 oncology dose-finding trials. Stat Biopharm Res. 2021;13(2):147–55. https://doi.org/10.1080/19466315.2020.1811147

CHAPTER 4

Drug Development and Regulatory Considerations

VICKY HSU • MATTHEW D. THOMPSON • DONNA PRZEPIORKA •
OLANREWAJU O. OKUSANYA

INTRODUCTION

Patients with cancer come from all age groups and include individuals with disease- or age-related organ dysfunction as well as those requiring concurrent use of medications for diseases or disorders unrelated to their cancer. Such heterogeneity in factors that affect drug dosing is especially challenging for cancer drugs for which toxicity is frequent and the therapeutic index is narrow. A robust drug development program is critical to ensure the safety of the study subjects and to establish the dosage that provides the desired therapeutic effect while minimizing toxicity for the entire population.

Clinical and nonclinical pharmacology information is used throughout the drug development program. Figure 4.1 describes the nonclinical studies needed to support submission of an investigational new drug (IND) application to the U.S. Food and Drug Administration (FDA) for a first-in-human (FIH) study of a cancer drug. Figure 4.2 highlights elements that are critical to the safe conduct of dose-escalation trials in humans and factors that are important in the selection of the dose for further clinical development. Figure 4.3 provides an overview of the additional studies that contribute to dose modifications, and Figure 4.4 outlines the additional information relevant to the pharmacology of the drug that is expected prior to start of the clinical trial intended to support licensure and/or at the time of submission of a marketing application.

IND-ENABLING NONCLINICAL STUDIES

Depending on the type of application, the nonclinical pharmacology and toxicology studies described in Figure 4.1 are typically submitted to the FDA as part of a nonclinical package. The pivotal repeat-dose toxicology studies in rodents and nonrodents should follow good laboratory practice (GLP; 21 C.F.R. 58). The FDA will provide feedback during the review of IND applications and marketing applications (new drug applications [NDAs] and biologics license applications [BLAs]) using a flexible, science-based approach. Guidance documents cited in this chapter describe the FDA's current thinking on a topic and are generally viewed as recommendations.

Pharmacology
- ❏ Mechanism(s) of action
- ❏ Proof of principle
- ❏ Secondary pharmacodynamics
- ❏ Antitumor activity
- ❏ Selection of test species
- ❏ Start dose selection
- ❏ Justification for drug combinations

Safety Pharmacology
- ❏ Electrocardiographic measurements in nonrodents (as part of 1-month GLP repeat-dose study)
  - – assessing effects on the cardiovascular, respiratory, and central nervous systems

General Toxicology
- ❏ 1-month general toxicology study in a rodent species (GLP repeat-dose)
  - • Histopathology
  - • Toxicokinetics
  - • Hematology
  - • Clinical chemistry
- ❏ 1-month general toxicology study in a nonrodent species (GLP repeat-dose)
  - • Histopathology
  - • Toxicokinetics
  - • Electrocardiographic measurements
  - • Hematology
  - • Clinical chemistry

Useful Guidance Documents
- *ICH S9 Nonclinical Evaluation for Anticancer Pharmaceuticals*
- *ICH S6(R1) Preclinical Safety Evaluation of Biotechnology-Derived Pharmaceuticals*
- *Preclinical Assessment of Investigational Cellular and Gene Therapy Products*
- *Estimating the Maximum Safe Starting Dose in Initial Clinical Trials for Therapeutics in Adult Healthy Volunteers*

FIGURE 4.1 **IND-enabling nonclinical studies for cancer drugs.**

GLP, good laboratory practice; IND, investigational new drug.

The primary guidance document used for nonclinical evaluations in oncology is *S9 Nonclinical Evaluation for Anticancer Pharmaceuticals*. *S9* provides recommendations for nonclinical studies to support the development of anticancer pharmaceuticals for the treatment of patients with advanced disease. Based on this patient population, the type and timing of nonclinical studies often differ from other therapeutic areas. For additional information on conducting trials for nononcology therapeutics, consult *M3(R2) Nonclinical Safety Studies for the Conduct of Human Clinical Trials and Marketing Authorization for Pharmaceuticals* or the guidance *Severely Debilitating or Life-Threatening Hematologic Disorders: Nonclinical Development of Pharmaceuticals*. When following *S9*, nonclinical studies support initial clinical trials by helping to characterize pharmacologic properties of the new drug, setting the starting dose for the first human exposure, and establishing the toxicologic profile. Additional nonclinical studies (e.g., developmental and reproductive toxicology studies) inform patient safety and labeling. Nonclinical development for biologics often differs from small molecule drugs. As an example, genotoxicity studies for biotechnology-derived pharmaceuticals are not needed. For additional guidance on biologics, consult *S6(R1) Preclinical Safety Evaluation of Biotechnology-Derived Pharmaceuticals*.

Dose Finding

The primary objective of the Phase 1 or initial dose-escalation trial (i.e., an FIH trial) is to determine the recommended Phase 2 dose (RP2D) or range of doses to be taken forward in subsequent clinical trials (**Figure 4.2**). The nonclinical studies provide the key information for designing the early-phase clinical dose-escalation trials in a way that protects the study subjects. For example, certain patients may need to be excluded in the initial trial due

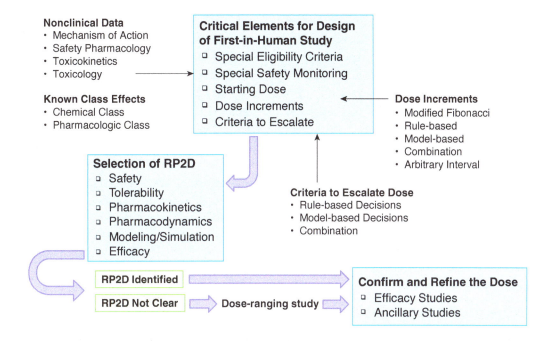

FIGURE 4.2 Getting to the recommended Phase 2 dose (RP2D).

to a potential high risk for toxicity when in vitro or in silico studies of the new drug predict an effect on cardiac repolarization (QTc) or the potential for serious drug–drug interactions. Special safety monitoring may be required when the toxicology studies suggest unusual risks, such as retinal toxicity, or when the mechanism of action (or known effects of drugs in the same class based on mechanism of action) suggests specific off-target or off-tumor toxicities.

Although the nonclinical toxicology studies are essential for establishing the safe starting dose for the FIH trial, the dose–response data in the nonclinical studies as described in Figure 4.1 are also useful for planning the increment in dosing among cohorts during the escalation in the clinical trial (Figure 4.2). Drugs with a steep dose–toxicity curve, such as cytotoxic drugs, warrant use of a scheme with rapidly reducing increments between cohorts (e.g., modified Fibonacci sequence), while drugs with little or no expected toxicity may be tested using dose increments on a log scale. Many targeted therapies fall between these two extremes, and real-time examination of the clinical data in addition to nonclinical information may be used to choose the dose increments, but in such cases, whether based on mathematical modeling or following rules triggered by observed toxicity (e.g., reduce increment to no more than 25% when the first grade 2 adverse reaction occurs), the prespecified details of how the increment in dose would be determined are expected to show that the study subjects are protected from undue risk.

In the historical experience of cancer drug development, the observed steepness of the dose–efficacy relationship for cytotoxic agents led to the expectation that adverse reactions would limit dose escalation prior to the plateau of the dose–efficacy curve. Hence, in order to ensure maximal efficacy, escalation to the maximum tolerated dose (MTD) in the first cycle of treatment was accepted practice. For outpatient therapies, MTD was defined as the highest dose with no more than one of six patients developing a dose-escalation limiting toxicity

(DLT; serious, life-threatening or fatal adverse reactions or grades 3–5 by the National Cancer Institute criteria) in the first cycle, and escalation decisions were guided by the "3+3 rule."

With the introduction of targeted agents and nontoxic monoclonal antibodies where the dose–efficacy curve may plateau before the dose–toxicity curve, escalation to the MTD is not appropriate, because the maximal efficacy of the drug may be (or will likely be) achieved at doses with lower levels of toxicity, compared to cytotoxic drugs. Instead, escalation decisions are guided in real time by a set of rules or a mathematical model based on the combinations of pharmacokinetics (e.g., achievement of a selected therapeutic drug concentration, change in exposure), pharmacodynamics (e.g., receptor occupancy, measures of target inhibition), and clinical activity (e.g., tumor shrinkage). Clinical toxicity is always included in the escalation decision so as not to overshoot the accepted level of toxicity for the intended population and therapeutic setting. Sponsors may request advice from the FDA in a pre-IND meeting to discuss their proposed dose-escalation trial design.

Dose Optimization

It is prudent to have objective minimal criteria for an acceptable RP2D outlined at the start of a dose-escalation trial, especially when using a complex mathematical model to guide selection of dose increments and escalation decisions during the DLT observation period. However, the calculus for selecting the RP2D at the end of the trial should also include tolerability; that is, most patients can continue treatment at the selected dose for multiple cycles (beyond the DLT observation period) without treatment interruptions or dose reductions.

It should also be noted that when there are only few patients in each dose cohort and there is a high degree of variability in the outcomes of the selection parameters for the RP2D, important differences between doses are often not detectable. In such a circumstance, a dose-ranging study, such as a randomization between two or more candidate doses, may be useful prior to embarking on later phase trials. Such trials need not be powered to assess for differences between arms in clinical efficacy outcomes but rather to generate sufficient clinical and pharmacokinetic data to support the selected RP2D. Sponsors may request feedback from the FDA in an end-of-Phase 1 meeting to discuss the RP2D they have selected for further development.

Clinical pharmacology is leveraged in all phases of drug development to ensure that the drug is administered to the right patient with the right dose at the right time. Clinical pharmacology characterizes sources of interindividual variability in drug response, which may affect efficacy and safety in different patient populations.

A core aspect of drug development is underpinned by the relationship between drug exposure and the observed effects (exposure–response). When one considers a randomized dose-finding study, a key objective is to determine if "exposure" to a drug resulted in an efficacious response and to what extent "exposure" results in a safety concern. Exposure can be quantified as dose or as a pharmacokinetic parameter such as maximum concentration (Cmax) or area under the time-concentration curve (AUC). As shown in Figure 4.3, the expectation is that with an increase in exposure, there is an improvement in the degree of response. The improvement in the degree of response can be rapid or steep, with a small change in dose resulting in near-maximum effect. On the other hand, the response can be shallow, with only a slight increase in efficacy with increases in exposures. While we typically have

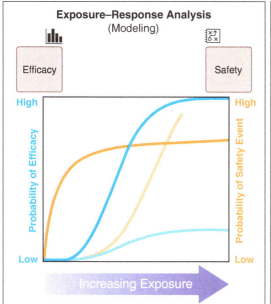
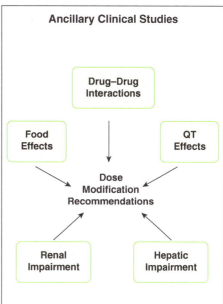

FIGURE 4.3 Studies use models to determine optimal dose selection (left) and consider several factors in dose modifications for specific populations (right).

a few independent measures that are associated with efficacy, there are many independent measures that are associated with safety, and these safety measures are related to exposure as well. Similar to what is observed with efficacy, yet noting that many safety events can be independent, these relationships for safety can be steep and shallow. However, frequently, the exposure–response relationships for safety and efficacy for a drug are quite dissimilar in steepness. The differences in these relationships create the opportunity to define a therapeutic window.

A randomized trial using only one dose level considers exposure–response by evaluating the probability of efficacy and different independent safety events at one exposure value. As such, information on whether a higher or lower dose will provide an adequate risk–benefit assessment is obscured without adequate data at different exposures characterizing the exposure–response curve for efficacy and safety. Thus, it is important to design trials to understand the exposure–response curve for efficacy as well as for safety in order to better understand where the optimal risk–benefit ratio lies and how to mitigate unacceptable toxicity while preserving efficacy.

Clinical pharmacology studies, including pharmacokinetics characterization in FIH, food effect, renal/hepatic impairment, drug–drug interaction, relative bioavailability, and QT studies, should be conducted, as applicable, early in drug development to guide dose selection prior to initiating the trial(s) intended to demonstrate safety and efficacy in support of a marketing application (**Figure 4.3**). These studies provide information on how these intrinsic and extrinsic factors affect the exposure of the study drug and inform us on the increase in safety risk or potential decrease in efficacy.

Food effect: Drugs can be affected by food in many ways. Taking a drug with food can increase or decrease the amount of drug that gets into systemic circulation and, as such, result in efficacy or safety concerns. In addition, taking a drug with food can also reduce gastrointestinal-related adverse reactions that may improve the tolerability of the drug. It is therefore important to understand the effect of food on drugs given orally before the study drug is marketed.

Drug–drug interaction: Many drugs affect the activity, metabolism, or the transport across cell membranes of other drugs. These interactions can be caused by the study drug, or the study drug can be affected by other concomitant medications. Many interactions result in changes in exposures that have an impact on the safety and efficacy of the study drug. For example, a concomitant drug that inhibits metabolic enzymes responsible for the metabolism of the affected drug may result in increased toxicity in the affected drug, thus warranting a dose reduction in the affected drug. It is important to evaluate the impact of other drugs on concomitant administration of the study drug and the impact of the study drug on other drugs administered concurrently.

QT prolongation: Many drugs can cause prolongation of the QT/QTc interval, increasing the risk for sudden death. It is important to understand the concentration–QT relationship of a study drug to enable assessment of risk of QT prolongation with increased exposure.

Renal impairment: If renal excretion is a primary elimination pathway for the study drug, renal impairment may lead to increased exposure and toxicity. It is important to understand the effect of renal impairment on the study drug to determine appropriate dose adjustments for patients with renal impairment.

Hepatic impairment: Many drugs are metabolized in the liver. Hepatic impairment may lead to changes in the metabolism of the study drug and the binding of the drug to various proteins produced by the liver. As such, hepatic impairment may lead to increased exposure and toxicity. It is important to understand the effect of hepatic impairment on the study drug to determine appropriate dose adjustments for patients with hepatic impairment.

Following selection of RP2D based on the totality of clinical pharmacokinetic, pharmacodynamic, activity, safety, and nonclinical pharmacology data at midstage clinical development, sparse pharmacokinetic samples and biomarker data (when available) should be collected from all patients enrolled in trials intended to demonstrate safety and efficacy at late-stage clinical development. These data would provide an opportunity for population pharmacokinetics analyses to understand the contribution of covariates (e.g., age, sex, body weight/size, disease, organ impairment, genetics, concomitant medications, antidrug antibodies for biologics) to interindividual variability in drug exposure and exposure–response analyses to correlate drug exposure with clinical outcomes and safety.

A major goal of the pivotal clinical trial of a new cancer drug is to demonstrate safety and efficacy of the dose and schedule to be described in the prescribing information. Longer-term repeat-dose toxicology studies are conducted to determine if additional safety monitoring is needed for the pivotal trial, and all relevant dose refinement studies should be completed to justify the dose to be studied. For example, if the intended population is expected to have a high proportion of patients with renal impairment, the renal impairment study should be completed first in order to inform dose modifications to be tested in the pivotal trial.

Marketing Applications

By the time of submission of the marketing application, the pharmacologic class should be established, and studies of genotoxicity as well as nonclinical embryofetal and reproductive toxicology should be completed. For more information on reproductive toxicology, consult the draft guidance *S5(R3) Detection of Toxicity to Reproduction.* Also consult the draft guidance *Oncology Pharmaceuticals: Reproductive Toxicity Testing and Labeling Recommendations.* Additionally, the pharmacokinetics of the drug should be well-characterized, and there should be adequate data to justify the recommended dose. Figure 4.4 lists several guidances

Nonclinical Pharmacology
- Established pharmacologic class

Nonclinical Toxicology
- 3-month general toxicology studies
  (GLP repeat-dose study, prior to Phase 3)
- Genotoxicity
- Embryofetal developmental toxicity
  - Typically, two species for small molecule
    drug; one pharmacologically relevant
    species for biopharmaceuticals

Clinical Pharmacology
- Analytical assay validation
- ADME
- Recommended dose justification
  - Exposure–response analyses
  - Effects of intrinsic factors
    - Renal impairment, hepatic
      impairment, age, sex, weight
  - Effects of extrinsic factors
    - Food effects, drug interactions
- Effects on cardiac repolarization (QT)
- Effects of antidrug antibodies on PK

Useful Guidance Documents
- *Oncology Pharmaceuticals: Reproductive Toxicity Testing and Labeling Recommendations*
- *S5(R3) Detection of Toxicity to Reproduction*
- *M10 Bioanalytical Method Validation and Study Sample Analysis*
- *Exposure–Response Relationships – Study Design, Data Analysis, and Regulatory Applications*
- *Population Pharmacokinetics*
- *In Vitro Drug Interaction Studies – Cytochrome P450 Enzyme and Transporter-Mediated Drug Interactions*
- *Clinical Drug Interaction Studies – Cytochrome P450 Enzyme and Transporter-Mediated Drug Interactions*
- *Pharmacokinetics in Patients with Impaired Renal Function: Study Design, Data Analysis, and Impact on Dosing and Labeling*
- *Pharmacokinetics in Patients with Impaired Hepatic Function: Study Design, Data Analysis, and Impact on Dosing and Labeling*
- *E14 Clinical Evaluation of QT/QTc Interval Prolongation and Proarrhythmic Potential for Non-Antiarrhythmic Drugs*
- *Food-Effect Bioavailability and Fed Bioequivalence Studies*
- *Bioavailability and Bioequivalence Studies Submitted in NDAs or INDs – General Consideraion*
- *Assessing the Effects of Food on Drugs in INDs and NDAs – Clinical Pharmacology Considerations*
- *Immunogenicity Assessment for Therapeutic Protein Products*
- *Immunogenicity Testing of Therapeutic Protein Products – Developing and Validating Assays for Anti-Drug Antibody Detection*

FIGURE 4.4 Additional pharmacology considerations for cancer drug marketing applications.

ADME, absorption, distribution, metabolism, and excretion; GLP, good laboratory practice; INDs, investigational new drugs; NDAs, new drug applications; PK, pharmacokinetics.

that provide advice on how the required studies can be designed and conducted, but sponsors may request feedback from the FDA in a pre-NDA meeting to discuss the proposed pharmacology information to be submitted in the marketing application.

CHAPTER SUMMARY

This chapter describes the nonclinical studies needed to support submission of an investigational new drug application with a first-in-human study of a cancer drug. It highlights elements critical to safe conduct of the dose-escalation trial in humans and factors important in the selection of the dose for further clinical development. The chapter outlines the additional information relevant to pharmacology that are expected prior to the start of the clinical trial to support licensure. Clinical and nonclinical pharmacology studies are essential for optimal drug development. The available regulatory guidances help identify the pharmacology information needed for design of safe first-in-human trials, how to optimize dosing for all patients in the intended population using clinical pharmacology data as it emerges from early-phase trials, how to confirm safety and effectiveness of the recommended dose, and how manufacturers or sponsor-investigators can obtain advice from FDA throughout the drug development process.

MULTIPLE-CHOICE QUESTIONS

1. The U.S. Food and Drug Administration (FDA) approval of an investigational agent considers all of the following except:

   A. Nonclinical pharmacology and toxicology studies
   B. Studies leading to the definition of recommended Phase 2 dose (RP2D)
   C. Drug pricing
   D. Dose modifications in the presence of renal and/or hepatic dysfunction

2. Exposure–response analysis is a critical component of clinical pharmacology because:

   A. It describes the mechanism of action of the investigational agent.
   B. It supports the selection of a safe starting dose for Phase 1 testing of a new investigational agent.
   C. It relies exclusively on the presence of drug–drug interactions.
   D. It provides information regarding the relationship between efficacy and safety (i.e., the risk–benefit ratio) over the dosing spectrum.

3. Which of the following is true for the nonclinical pharmacology and toxicology studies of a new drug?

   A. The mechanism of action may identify safety issues based on the pharmacologic class.
   B. The toxicities observed in the animal studies may suggest the need for special safety monitoring tests in the clinical trials.
   C. The steepness of the dose–toxicity curve in animals informs the dose-escalation plan in the first-in-human study.
   D. All of the above

4. Which of the following is true?

    A. How well an oral drug is absorbed may depend on whether it is taken with or without food.
    B. The clinical efficacy of a drug is never affected by concomitant medications.
    C. Impairment of renal or hepatic function usually decreases drug exposure.
    D. All of the above

5. The maximum tolerated dose (MTD) in the Phase 1 trial is always the dose recommended for study in further clinical trials for a new anticancer drug.

    A. True
    B. False

6. For a Phase 1 dose-escalation trial of a new anticancer drug, the doses in consecutive cohorts should always increase by 100%.

    A. True
    B. False

7. For a Phase 1 dose-escalation trial of a new anticancer drug, the decision to escalate to the next higher dose level should always be based solely whether a dose-limiting toxicity (DLT) occurred.

    A. True
    B. False

8. Population pharmacokinetics analyses help to understand what patient-related factors, such as age or sex, might contribute to the interindividual variability in drug exposure.

    A. True
    B. False

9. Patients with any renal or liver function abnormalities are never eligible for trials of anticancer drugs.

    A. True
    B. False

10. A major goal of the pivotal clinical trial of a new anticancer drug is to demonstrate safety and efficacy of the dose and schedule to be described in the prescribing information.

    A. True
    B. False

ANSWERS TO MULTIPLE-CHOICE QUESTIONS

1. C. The FDA assesses all aspects of preclinical and clinical testing when evaluating an investigational agent for new drug application (NDA) approval and marketing of the newly approved agent in terms of prescribing information including genotoxicity and

reproductive toxicity, extrinsic factors such as drug–drug interactions and effect of food, and intrinsic factors including organ dysfunction, but is not involved in post-marketing issues such as drug pricing.

2. **D.** Exposure–response analysis describes the probabilities of increases in efficacy and safety with increases in drug dosing, thereby defining the risk–benefit ratio and therapeutic window. These analyses can be conducted during and following all clinical trial phases once the spectrum of adverse effects and preliminary data regarding efficacy can be determined.

3. **D.** The nonclinical pharmacology and toxicology studies provide information used in planning multiple aspects of the clinical trials.

4. **A.** Taking a drug with food may change how well it is absorbed. Concomitant medications may affect the mechanism, metabolism, or intracellular uptake of drugs and therefore may alter the efficacy. For drugs that are excreted by the kidney or liver, impairment of the excretory function usually increases drug exposure.

5. **B.** The recommended Phase 2 dose is selected based on all available pharmacokinetic, pharmacodynamic, safety, tolerability and efficacy data rather than just the MTD. Especially for targeted therapies, the MTD may exceed the dose at which pharmacologic activity has plateaued.

6. **B.** The increment between dose levels in a Phase 1 trial depends on the expected steepness of the dose–toxicity curve. Drugs with a steep dose–toxicity curve, such as cytotoxic drugs, warrant use of a scheme with rapidly reducing increments between cohorts (e.g., modified Fibonacci sequence), while drugs with little or no expected toxicity may be tested using dose increments on a log scale.

7. **B.** For a Phase 1 dose-escalation trial, the decision to escalate to the next dose level should be based on all available pharmacologic, pharmacokinetic, and clinical data rather than just the incidence of dose-limiting toxicities. For example, with a relatively nontoxic targeted therapy that might not cause any dose-limiting toxicities, it may not be necessary to escalate the dose once target saturation is reached.

8. **A.** Population pharmacokinetics analyses may show significant associations between exposure and patient-related factors that may inform a change in the recommended dose for different subgroups of patients.

9. **B.** Patients with cancer may have renal or liver function abnormalities, but that does not preclude their need for a safe and effective treatment. Instead, once the effects of organ function on exposure are determined and safe dosing can be recommended for patients with renal or liver impairment, such patients may be included in trials to test the efficacy of new anticancer drugs.

10. **A.** The pivotal clinical trial provides the basis for labeling the recommended dose in the prescribing information, so it is imperative that the drug dose and schedule are optimized prior to use in the pivotal trial.

SELECTED REFERENCES

Bullock JM, Rahman A, Liu Q. Lessons learned: Dose selection of small molecule-targeted oncology drugs. Clin Cancer Res. 2016;22(11):2630-8. https://doi.org/10.1158/1078-0432.CCR-15-2646

Good Laboratory Practice for Nonclinical Laboratory Studies. 21 C.F.R. Part 58 (1978). https://www.ecfr.gov/current/title-21/chapter-I/subchapter-A/part-58

Le Tourneau C, Lee JJ, Siu LL. Dose escalation methods in phase I cancer clinical trials. J Natl Cancer Inst. 2009;101(10):708–20. https://doi.org/10.1093/jnci/djp079

Office of New Drugs, Center for Drug Evaluation and Research. Good Review Practice: Clinical Review of Investigational New Drug Applications. U.S. Food and Drug Administration; December 2013. Available from: https://www.fda.gov/downloads/Drugs/Guidance ComplianceRegulatory Information/UCM377108.pdf

U.S. Food and Drug Administration. Assessing the Effects of Food on Drugs in INDs and NDAs—Clinical Pharmacology Considerations; June 2022. Available from: https://www.fda.gov/regulatory-information/search-fda-guidance-documents/assessing-effects-food-drugs-inds-and-ndas-clinical-pharmacology-considerations

U.S. Food and Drug Administration. Clinical Drug Interaction Studies—Cytochrome P450 Enzyme- and Transporter-mediated Drug Interactions; January 2020. Available from: https://www.fda.gov/regulatory-information/search-fda-guidance-documents/clinical-drug-interaction-studies-cytochrome-p450-enzyme-and-transporter-mediated-drug-interactions

U.S. Food and Drug Administration. E4 Dose-Response Information to Support Drug Registration; July 1996. Available from: https://www.fda.gov/Drugs/GuidanceComplianceRegulatoryInformation/Guidances/default.htm

U.S. Food and Drug Administration. E14 Clinical Evaluation of QT/QTc Interval Prolongation and Proarrhythmic Potential for Non-antiarrhythmic Drugs Questions and Answers (R3) Guidance for Industry; June 2017. Available from: https://www.fda.gov/Drugs/GuidanceComplianceRegulatory Information/Guidances/default.htm

U.S. Food and Drug Administration. Exposure-Response Relationships—Study Design, Data Analysis, and Regulatory Applications; April 2003. Available from: https://www.fda.gov/regulatory-information/search-fda-guidance-documents/exposure-response-relationships-study-design-data-analysis-and-regulatory-applications

U.S. Food and Drug Administration. Food-Effect Bioavailability and Fed Bioequivalence Studies; December 2002. Available from: https://www.fda.gov/regulatory-information/search-fda-guidance-documents/food-effect-bioavailability-and-fed-bioequivalence-studies

U.S. Food and Drug Administration. Formal Meetings Between the FDA and Sponsors or Applicants of PDUFA Products Guidance for Industry; December 2017. Available from: https://www.fda.gov/Drugs/GuidanceComplianceRegulatoryInformation/Guidances/default.htm

U.S. Food and Drug Administration. Guidances (Drugs). Available from: http://www.fda.gov/Drugs/GuidanceComplianceRegulatoryInformation/Guidances/default.htm

U.S. Food and Drug Administration. Investigational New Drug (IND) Application. Available from: http://www.fda.gov/Drugs/DevelopmentApprovalProcess/HowDrugsareDevelopedandApproved/ApprovalApplications/InvestigationalNewDrugINDApplication/default.htm

U.S. Food and Drug Administration. In Vitro Drug Interaction Studies—Cytochrome P450 Enzyme- and Transporter-mediated Drug Interactions; January 2020. Available from: https://www.fda.gov/regulatory-information/search-fda-guidance-documents/in-vitro-drug-interaction-studies-cytochrome-p450-enzyme-and-transporter-mediated-drug-interactions

U.S. Food and Drug Administration. M3(R2) Nonclinical Safety Studies for the Conduct of Human Clinical Trials and Marketing Authorization for Pharmaceuticals; January 2010. Available from: http://www.fda.gov/Drugs/GuidanceComplianceRegulatoryInformation/Guidances/default.htm

U.S. Food and Drug Administration. M3(R2) Nonclinical Safety Studies for the Conduct of Human Clinical Trials and Marketing Authorization for Pharmaceuticals: Questions and Answers; February 2013. Available from: http://www.fda.gov/Drugs/GuidanceComplianceRegulatoryInformation/Guidances/default.htm

U.S. Food and Drug Administration. New Drug Application (NDA). Available from: https://www.fda.gov/Drugs/DevelopmentApprovalProcess/HowDrugsareDevelopedandApproved/ApprovalApplications/NewDrugApplicationNDA/default.htm

U.S. Food and Drug Administration. Oncology Pharmaceuticals: Reproductive Toxicity Testing and Labeling Recommendations; May 2019. Available from: https://www.fda.gov/regulatory-information/search-fda-guidance-documents/oncology-pharmaceuticals-reproductive-toxicity-testing-and-labeling-recommendations-guidance

U.S. Food and Drug Administration. Pharmacokinetics in Patients with Impaired Hepatic Function: Study Design, Data Analysis, and Impact on Dosing and Labeling; May 2003. Available from: https://www.fda.gov/regulatory-information/search-fda-guidance-documents/pharmacokinetics-patients-impaired-hepatic-function-study-design-data-analysis-and-impact-dosing-and

U.S. Food and Drug Administration. Pharmacokinetics in Patients with Impaired Renal Function—Study Design, Data Analysis, and Impact on Dosing and Labeling; September 2020. Available from: https://www.fda.gov/regulatory-information/search-fda-guidance-documents/pharmacokinetics-patients-impaired-renal-function-study-design-data-analysis-and-impact-dosing-and

U.S. Food and Drug Administration. Population Pharmacokinetics; February 2022. Available from: https://www.fda.gov/regulatory-information/search-fda-guidance-documents/population-pharmacokinetics

U.S. Food and Drug Administration. S5(R3) Detection of Toxicity to Reproduction; May 2021. Available from: https://www.fda.gov/regulatory-information/search-fda-guidance-documents/s5r3-detection-toxicity-reproduction

U.S. Food and Drug Administration. S6(R1) Preclinical Safety Evaluation of Biotechnology-Derived Pharmaceuticals; May 2012. Available from: https://www.fda.gov/regulatory-information/search-fda-guidance-documents/s6r1-preclinical-safety-evaluation-biotechnology-derived-pharmaceuticals

U.S. Food and Drug Administration. S9 Nonclinical Evaluation for Anticancer Pharmaceuticals; March 2010. Available from: https://www.fda.gov/regulatory-information/search-fda-guidance-documents/s9-nonclinical-evaluation-anticancer-pharmaceuticals

U.S. Food and Drug Administration. S9 Nonclinical Evaluation for Anticancer Pharmaceuticals Questions and Answers; June 2018. Available from: https://www.fda.gov/regulatory-information/search-fda-guidance-documents/s9-nonclinical-evaluation-anticancer-pharmaceuticals-questions-and-answers

U.S. Food and Drug Administration. Severely Debilitating or Life-Threatening Hematologic Disorders: Nonclinical Development of Pharmaceuticals; March 2019. Available from: https://www.fda.gov/downloads/Drugs/GuidanceComplianceRegulatoryInformation/Guidances/UCM605393.pdf

Classical Cytotoxic Agents

CHAPTER 5

Alkylating Agents and Drugs Perturbing DNA Structure

ASHKAN EMADI • EDWARD A. SAUSVILLE

INTRODUCTION

The inception of chemotherapy as a therapeutic agent is built on the foundation of biochemical warfare. The synthesis of mustard gas in 1854 and its subsequent use during World War I highlighted its severe skin burns and blisters as well as pulmonary, gastrointestinal, and myelosuppressive toxicities. After swapping out the sulfide group (–S–) in favor of an amine group (:N—), chlormethine (also known as mechlorethamine) became one of the first evaluated chemotherapeutic agents of the modern age. It became the prototype medication for alkylating agents.

Mustard gas   **Mechlorethamine**

   An alkyl (e.g., methyl, ethyl, propyl) is a radical (an atom or a molecule that has an unpaired electron) that is derived from an alkane (e.g., methane, ethane, propane) with one hydrogen radical (H•) missing. Alkyls are highly active radicals that form covalent bonds with different molecules; hence, they are always attached to other molecular fragments when administered as a drug, and form the alkyl radical spontaneously or after metabolism. Alkylating agents such as mechlorethamine are frequently used in combination with other agents. MOPP (a combination of mechlorethamine, vincristine [Oncovin], procarbazine, and prednisone) is one of the first regimens that was used with curative intent in oncology for treatment of Hodgkin lymphoma.

MECHANISM OF ACTION

Alkylating agents directly damage the DNA via DNA intra- and interstrand covalent cross-linking, triggering DNA strand breaks, resulting in abnormal base pairing and inhibiting cell division, ultimately leading to cell death. Generally, they can act during all phases of the cell cycle. Bone marrow suppression, including leukopenia, neutropenia, lymphopenia, anemia, and thrombocytopenia, is a common adverse event of all alkylating agents. Other common adverse events include gonadal toxicity/failure, carcinogenicity, and nausea and vomiting.

All alkylating agents can cause therapy-related myeloid neoplasms (t-MNs), including thera-py-related acute myeloid leukemia (t-AML) and therapy-related myelodysplastic syndromes (t-MDSs), that usually occur 5 to 7 years after treatment and involve abnormalities of chromosome 5 and/or 7.

CLASSIFICATION OF ALKYLATING AGENTS

There are different types of alkylating agents based on their chemical structures:

- *Nitrogen mustard:* These agents can produce aziridine (or ethyleneimine) as active moiety. The clinically used nitrogen mustard chemotherapeutics include mechlorethamine, chlorambucil, melphalan (and its derivative melphalan flufenamide), bendamustine, cyclophosphamide, ifosfamide, and thiotepa.
- *Alkyl sulfonate:* busulfan
  - Currently busulfan is mainly used in combination with other agents as part of conditioning regimens prior to allogeneic hematopoietic stem cell transplantation (alloHSCT). The most frequent serious adverse event of treatment with busulfan at the recommended dose and schedule is prolonged myelosuppression, occurring in 100% of patients.
  - Seizures can occur in patients receiving intravenous (IV) busulfan as well as high-dose oral busulfan at doses generating plasma drug levels similar to IV busulfan. Prophylactic anticonvulsants (e.g., phenytoin) must be initiated prior to treatment with busulfan-containing regimens.
  - High (>1,500 µM × min) busulfan area under the plasma drug concentration-time curve (AUC), which reflects the actual body exposure to drug after administration of a dose of the drug, is reported to be associated with an increased risk of developing hepatic veno-occlusive disease (VOD) or sinusoidal obstruction syndrome (SOS). Based on clinical examination and laboratory findings, the incidence of VOD/SOS is approximately 10% in patients treated with high-dose busulfan in the setting of alloHSCT with approximately 30% to 40% mortality rate.
    - VOD/SOS occurs due to injury of the hepatic sinusoidal endothelial cells with loss of wall integrity resulting in sinusoidal obstruction and development of postsinusoidal portal hypertension. Diagnostic criteria for VOD/SOS post alloHSCT according to Baltimore criteria include "bilirubin ≥2 mg/dL and at least two of the following: painful hepatomegaly, weight gain (>5%), ascites" or histologically proven VOD.
    - Defibrotide, an oligonucleotide mixture with profibrinolytic properties, is indicated for the treatment of adult and pediatric patients with VOD/SOS with renal or pulmonary dysfunction following alloHSCT.
  - Bronchopulmonary dysplasia with pulmonary fibrosis (busulfan lung) is a rare but serious adverse event that can occur following chronic busulfan therapy with the median onset of symptoms being 4 years after therapy.
  - Busulfan can cause severe skin hyperpigmentation.

- *Nitrosourea:* carmustine (BCNU), lomustine (CCNU), and streptozocin
- *Triazine:* procarbazine, dacarbazine, and temozolomide
- *Platinum salts:* cisplatin, carboplatin, oxaliplatin

Most of these alkylating agents are metabolized hepatically with metabolites excreted in the urine; dose adjustment for renal dysfunction and severe hepatic dysfunction may be required.

Platinums are eliminated via the kidneys and require dose adjustment for renal dysfunction. Nephrotoxicity due to cisplatin is associated with renal tubular damage and is dose-dependent and cumulative; noted in approximately 30% of patients treated with a single dose of cisplatin ≥ 50 mg/m^2. For oxaliplatin dosing: if creatinine clearance (CrCl) ≥ 30 mL/min, dosage adjustment is not necessary; if CrCl <30 mL/min, dose should be reduced from 85 mg/m^2 to 65 mg/m^2. *Platinums do NOT require dose adjustment for hepatic dysfunction.*

Nitrogen Mustards

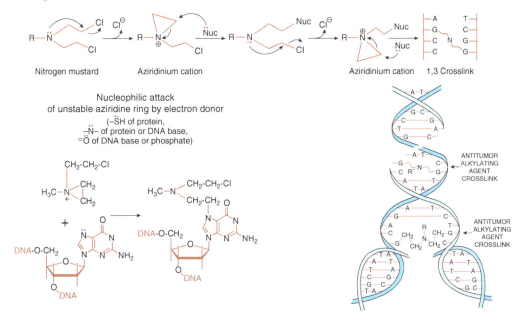

FIGURE 5.1 Mechanism of action of DNA alkylation by nitrogen mustards.
In a nitrogen mustard, the nitrogen atom displaces the chloride to result in a strained, three-membered intermediate cation called aziridinium. This ion easily forms covalent bonds with nucleophiles, represented by Nuc in the figure, such as nitrogens of DNA (e.g., N7 position of guanine) or proteins, oxygen atoms of DNA, or sulfur atoms of proteins. The second chemical transformation of the nitrogen mustard provides another aziridinium ion, which upon reaction with another DNA nucleophile, forms a DNA crosslink.

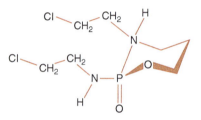

Cyclophosphamide

Ifosfamide

Two mustard moieties
(– CH$_2$ – CH$_2$ – Cl) are
attached to the nitrogen
outside the ring.

One mustard moiety is attached to the
nitrogen outside the ring and another
mustard is attached to the nitrogen on
the ring, which after being released and
metabolized causes neurologic toxicity
specifically seen by ifosfamide,
but not cyclophosphamide.

FIGURE 5.2 Cyclophosphamide and ifosfamide.
Cyclophosphamide (also called Cytoxan) and ifosfamide are prodrugs. To date,
even with the advent of several novel targeted therapies and immunotherapies,
cyclophosphamide combined with other chemotherapeutic agents is used with
curative intent for treatment of many hematologic malignancies as well as solid
tumors. A few examples of chemotherapy regimens include:

- CHOP (cyclophosphamide, hydroxydaunorubicin [doxorubicin], Oncovin
  [vincristine], prednisone) with (for B cell) and without (for T cell) rituximab to
  treat both indolent and aggressive forms of non-Hodgkin lymphoma
- CODOX-M/IVAC (cyclophosphamide, vincristine, doxorubicin and high-dose
  methotrexate [CODOX-M] alternating with ifosfamide, etoposide and high-
  dose cytarabine [IVAC]) for aggressive forms of non-Hodgkin lymphoma,
  AIDS-related and high-risk Burkitt lymphoma
- FCR (fludarabine, cyclophosphamide, rituximab) for chronic lymphocytic
  leukemia (CLL)
- HyperCVAD (cyclophosphamide, vincristine, doxorubicin, dexamethasone
  alternating with high-dose methotrexate and high-dose cytarabine) for acute
  lymphoblastic leukemia (ALL)
- CyBorD (cyclophosphamide [oral], bortezomib, dexamethasone) for multiple
  myeloma and AL amyloidosis
- CEDC (cisplatin, etoposide, doxorubicin, cyclophosphamide) and ICE
  (ifosfamide, carboplatin, etoposide) for neuroblastoma
- Cisplatin, etoposide, cyclophosphamide, and vincristine for retinoblastoma
- AC (doxorubicin, cyclophosphamide), CAF (cyclophosphamide, doxorubicin,
  fluorouracil), CMF (cyclophosphamide, methotrexate, fluorouracil), FEC
  (fluorouracil, epirubicin, cyclophosphamide), TAC (docetaxel [Taxotere],
  doxorubicin, cyclophosphamide), TC (docetaxel and cyclophosphamide) in
  the adjuvant setting for the treatment of nonmetastatic breast cancer or for
  the treatment of metastatic breast cancer

(continued)

FIGURE 5.2 **Cyclophosphamide and ifosfamide.** (***continued***)

Ifosfamide combined with other chemotherapeutic agents is used for treatment of hematologic malignancies and solid tumors including recurrent testicular cancers and germ cell tumors, sarcomas (soft tissue, osteogenic, Ewing sarcoma), head and neck cancer, cervical cancer, and non-Hodgkin lymphoma. A few examples of chemotherapy regimens include:

- TIP (paclitaxel, ifosfamide, mesna, cisplatin) for the treatment of advanced-stage testicular cancer and unresectable and recurrent squamous cell head and neck cancer
- VIP (etoposide [VePesid], ifosfamide, cisplatin) for advanced testicular cancer
- AIM (doxorubicin, ifosfamide, mesna), MAID (mesna, doxorubicin, ifosfamide, dacarbazine) for soft tissue sarcoma
- VDC/IE (vincristine, doxorubicin/dactinomycin, cyclophosphamide alternating with ifosfamide, etoposide) for first-line treatment (primary/neoadjuvant/adjuvant) of Ewing sarcoma

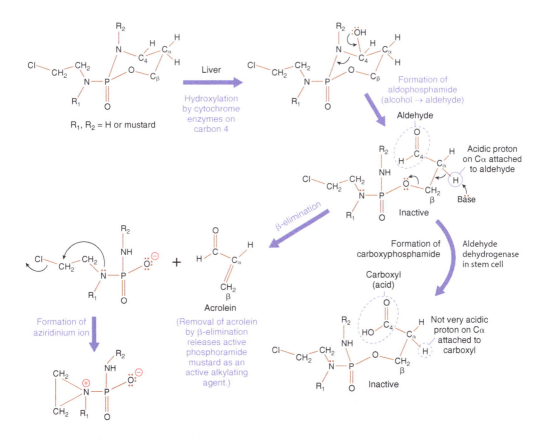

FIGURE 5.3 **Mechanism of cyclophosphamide (and ifosfamide) activation.**

(*continued*)

FIGURE 5.3 **Mechanism of cyclophosphamide (and ifosfamide) activation. (*continued*)**
Cyclophosphamide can be considered one of the first "targeted therapies" due to its dissimilar aldehyde dehydrogenase (ALDH)-dependent activation in different cells. After intravenous or oral administration, cyclophosphamide, in the liver via cytochrome P450 (CYP), is converted to 4-hydroxycyclophosphamide, which stays in equilibrium with aldophosphamide, both of which readily cross the cell membranes by passive diffusion. In cells with high levels of ALDH (e.g., in hematopoietic stem cells), aldophosphamide is irreversibly converted to carboxyphosphamide, which does not decompose to phosphoramide mustard and therefore lacks alkylating capability. In the absence of a high concentration of ALDH (e.g., in lymphocytes), aldophosphamide spontaneously liberates phosphoramide mustard and acrolein (also called propenal). Phosphoramide mustard forms interstrand DNA crosslinks primarily at the guanine sites (Figure 5.1).

Metabolism of ifosfamide defers from cyclophosphamide, resulting in a particular adverse event profile. The first step of metabolism of ifosfamide involves the release of "ring nitrogen mustard" to chloroacetaldehyde (CAA). CAA can penetrate the blood–brain barrier resulting in significant central nervous system (CNS) toxicity manifested by cerebellar ataxia, mental confusion, and complex visual hallucinations. This adverse reaction can be abrogated by administration of methylene blue, which acts as a potent electron acceptor and inhibits the extrahepatic monoamine oxidation of chloroethylamine to CAA. Due to the lack of ring nitrogen mustard, cyclophosphamide does not cause CNS toxicity similar to ifosfamide. Use of aprepitant may enhance the risk of neurotoxicity with ifosfamide via CYP induction.

Post transplantation high-dose cyclophosphamide: The differences between aldehyde dehydrogenase (ALDH) expression in hematopoietic stem cells and lymphocytes has resulted in the wide use of high-dose cyclophosphamide after blood and marrow transplantation to prevent/diminish graft-versus-host disease (GVHD). Alloreactive T cells, but not stem cells, which are activated a few days after allogeneic transplantation, become exquisitely susceptible to killing by high-dose cyclophosphamide. Owing to its stem cell–sparing effects, high-dose cyclophosphamide (typically 50 mg/kg on days 3 and 4 after transplant) has been found to be an effective method for clinical GVHD prophylaxis. The use of high-dose cyclophosphamide during alloHSCT has resulted in significant expansion of donor availability (e.g., haploidentical parents, children and siblings of patients) for patients with hematologic neoplasms such as acute myeloid leukemia (AML) and those with nonmalignant hematologic disorders such as β-thalassemia and sickle cell disease.

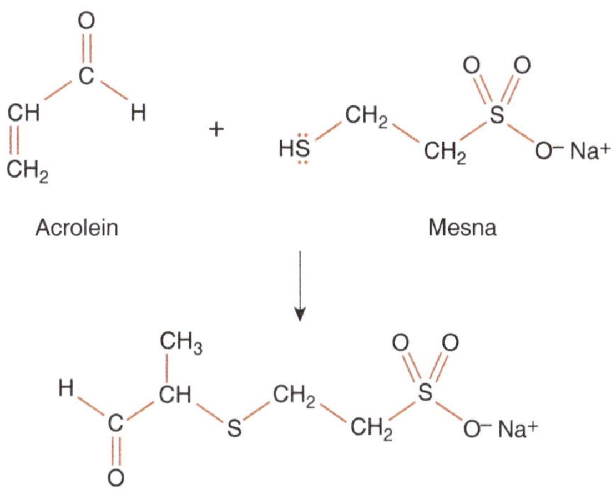

Acrolein   Mesna

Not reactive with urothelial cells

FIGURE 5.4 **What is MESNA? Cyclophosphamide/ifosfamide-induced hemorrhagic cystitis.**

As described in Figure 5.3, the departure of acrolein is absolutely necessary for activation of cyclophosphamide and ifosfamide into active alkylating agents capable of formation of aziridinium ions. Acrolein is the simplest and the strongest electrophilic α,β-unsaturated aldehyde, accounting for its high reactivity with nucleophiles in DNA and proteins. Acrolein reaction with cysteine, lysine, and histidine residues of proteins results in "protein carbonylation" culminating in a change in protein structure and function. Protein carbonyl content is the well-used biomarker of severe oxidative protein damage. Accumulation of acrolein in bladder after administration of moderate- to high-dose of cyclophosphamide and ifosfamide causes hemorrhagic cystitis. Administration of mesna can prevent development of hemorrhagic cystitis because the sulfhydryl group (–SH) in mesna detoxifies the unsaturated aldehyde group in acrolein, resulting in a water-soluble product that is excretable. Use of mesna is a common clinical practice after administration of intermediate-dose to high-dose cyclophosphamide and ifosfamide. Interestingly, the name mesna is the abbreviation of its chemical name: Mercapto Ethane Sulfonate sodium [NAtrium, Na]).

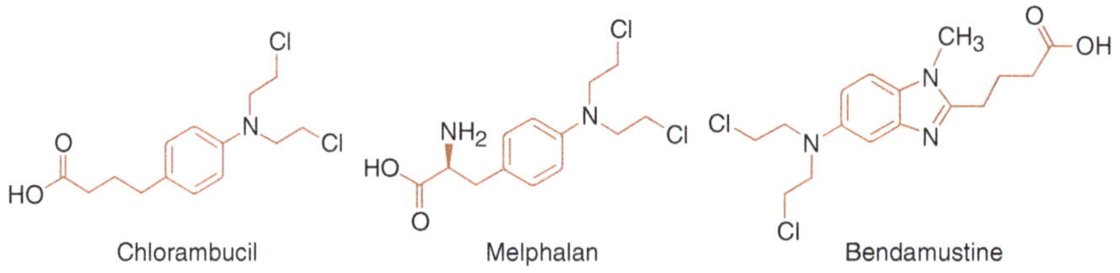

FIGURE 5.5 Other nitrogen mustards.

Chlorambucil is an oral alkylating agent that is rapidly and completely absorbed from the gastrointestinal tract. As a single agent, it was used for treatment of chronic lymphocytic leukemia (CLL); it is not curative but may produce clinically useful palliation. Chlorambucil in combination with obinutuzumab has been approved for the treatment of patients with previously untreated CLL.

Melphalan is a nitrogen mustard attached to the amino acid phenylalanine. Melphalan is transported into cells by amino acid transporters. Plasma cells appear to have a higher tendency to absorb melphalan due its amino acid moiety, which is required for immunoglobulin synthesis. Melphalan is available in both oral and IV formulations. Melphalan is used mainly for the treatment of plasma cell disorders and in conditioning regimens prior to autologous stem cell transplantation for multiple myeloma. Tandem autologous stem cell transplantation relies on an intense approach using melphalan 200 mg/m² for the first transplant and melphalan 140–200 mg/m² plus total body irradiation for the second transplant. Melphalan is incorporated into BEAM (carmustine [BCNU], etoposide, ara-C, melphalan [140 mg/m²]) as one of the most commonly used conditioning regimens for patients with relapsed/refractory lymphoma undergoing autologous stem cell transplantation. Mucositis occurs in 100% of patients following BEAM chemotherapy, requiring IV opioids and sometimes total parenteral nutrition (TPN). Pulmonary infiltrates and fibrosis have been reported in patients after administration of melphalan.

Bendamustine is an intravenous (IV) alkylating agent that was first used clinically in 1963. Bendamustine was used primarily for approximately four decades in East Germany (the former German Democratic Republic) in patients with CLL, non-Hodgkin lymphoma, Hodgkin lymphoma, multiple myeloma, and different subtypes of lung cancer. After German reunification, modern clinical trials tested bendamustine mainly in treating lymphoid malignancies resulting in its FDA approval in the United States in 2008. Bendamustine is approved for treatment of CLL and indolent B-cell non-Hodgkin lymphoma that has progressed during or within 6 months of treatment with rituximab or a rituximab-containing regimen. Bendamustine is also approved in combination with obinutuzumab followed by obinutuzumab monotherapy, for the treatment of patients with follicular lymphoma who relapsed after, or are refractory to, a rituximab-containing regimen. Bendamustine can cause severe myelosuppression (grades 3 and 4) in 98% of patients in the two non-Hodgkin lymphoma clinical trials. Infusion/anaphylactoid reactions to bendamustine have occurred commonly in clinical trials with symptoms including fever, chills, pruritus, and rash. Second primary malignancies including MDS, MPN, AML, bronchial carcinoma, and non-melanoma skin cancer, including basal cell carcinoma and squamous cell carcinoma, have been reported in patients treated with bendamustine. Allopurinol may increase the risk of skin reactions including Stevens-Johnson syndrome with bendamustine.

AML, acute myeloid leukemia; FDA, U.S. Food and Drug Administration; MDS, myelodysplastic syndrome; MPN, myeloproliferative neoplasm.

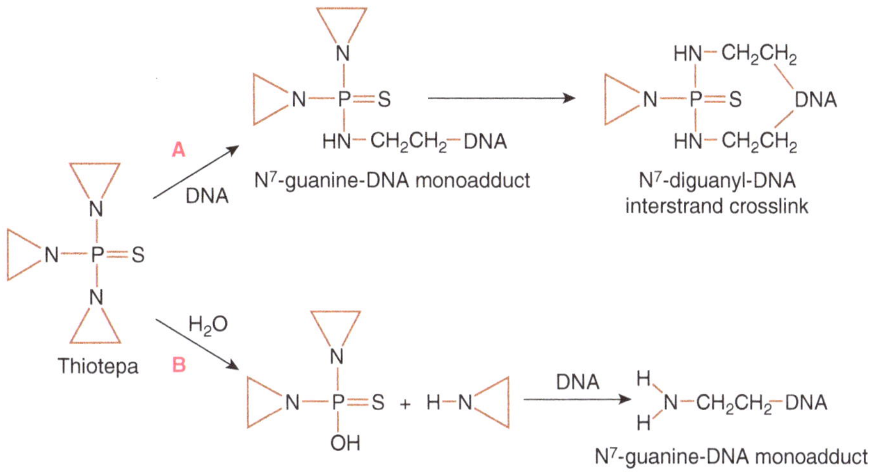

FIGURE 5.6 Ethylenimine, thiotepa.
Thiotepa has three aziridine rings, which are susceptible to nucleophilic attack from DNA resulting in interstrand crosslinking as well as single-base methyl adduction. The unstable aziridine rings are similar to those seen during metabolism of nitrogen mustards. Thiotepa is used to reduce the risk of graft rejection when used in conjunction with high-dose busulfan and cyclophosphamide as a preparative regimen for allogeneic hematopoietic stem cell transplantation for pediatric patients with beta-thalassemia. It is also used for controlling intracavitary effusions secondary to diffuse or localized neoplastic diseases of various serosal cavities and for treatment of superficial papillary carcinoma of the urinary bladder. The MATRix regimen (methotrexate, cytarabine [Ara-C], thiotepa, rituximab) is one of the new standard chemoimmunotherapy for the treatment of patients aged up to 70 years with newly diagnosed primary CNS lymphoma with ~50% complete remission rate. It can cause cutaneous toxicity including skin discoloration, itching, and blistering or peeling skin in the groin, underarms, skin folds, neck and under dressings; hence, the skin should be cleansed (shower or bath) at least twice daily through 48 hours after the last dose of thiotepa. Occlusive dressing should be changed and the covered skin should be cleaned at least twice daily through 48 hours after receiving thiotepa. Patients commonly remain in the hospital and their bed sheets are changed daily for 48 hours after receiving thiotepa.

Nitrosoureas

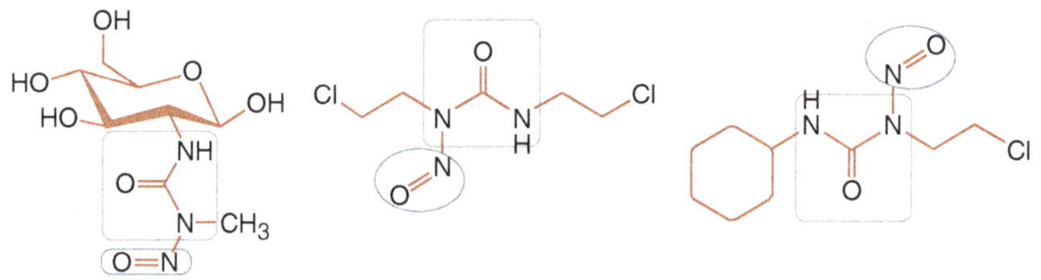

FIGURE 5.7 Nitrosoureas.
Nitroso (circles) ureas (squares) lomustine and carmustine are highly lipid-soluble alkylating agents that allow for penetration of the blood–brain barrier (BBB) and, as such, are used in treating several types of brain cancers, including glioma, glioblastoma multiforme, medulloblastoma, and astrocytoma among other indications. Historically, carmustine was used in chemotherapy regimens for treatment of relapsed or refractory lymphomas.

Nitrosoureas, particularly carmustine, can cause a progressive decline in cognitive function, development of seizures, and coma. Pulmonary toxicity from carmustine is dose related. Patients receiving >1,400 mg/m^2 cumulative dose are at significantly higher risk than those receiving less. Delayed onset pulmonary fibrosis occurring up to 17 years after treatment has been reported in patients who received carmustine in childhood and early adolescence. Carmustine implant (wafer), for intracranial use, is approved for the treatment of newly diagnosed high-grade glioma as an adjunct to surgery and radiation and for the treatment of recurrent glioblastoma as an adjunct to surgery.

Lomustine is given by mouth in capsule form. Pulmonary infiltrates and/or fibrosis occurs with lomustine, and lomustine should be permanently discontinued in patients diagnosed with pulmonary fibrosis. Severe nausea and vomiting usually occur within 3 to 6 hours of taking lomustine. In a Phase 3 clinical trial, addition of lomustine to the backbone of cytarabine and idarubicin for adults age 60 years or older with previously untreated acute myeloid leukemia who were fit to receive intensive chemotherapy and who were without unfavorable cytogenetics, compared with cytarabine and idarubicin alone, resulted in a statistically significant improved 2-year overall survival rate of 56% in the lomustine-containing arm versus 48% in the other arm.

Streptozocin is a naturally occurring compound that is similar to glucose and is transported into the cell by the glucose transport protein GLUT2. Streptozocin is not active orally and should be administered intravenously. It is particularly toxic to the insulin-producing beta cells of the pancreas; hence, it historically is used for the treatment of pancreatic neuroendocrine tumors. Streptozocin can cause hyperglycemia/glucose intolerance, severe pain at injection site, and transaminitis.

Triazines

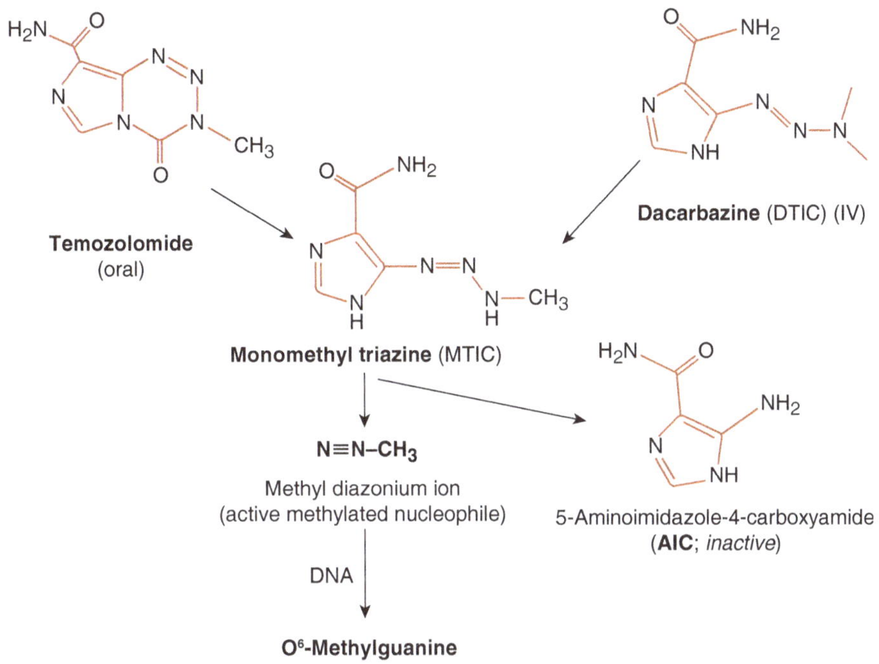

FIGURE 5.8 Triazines (three attached nitrogen atoms) and hydrazines.
Both temozolomide and dacarbazine form monomethyl triazine (MTIC) prior
to becoming the active methylated nucleophile, methyl diazonium ion. In
this setting, both O^6 and N^7 of guanine in DNA act as electron donors with
subsequent methylation (i.e., alkylation of DNA). Procarbazine is a hydrazine
(NH_2–NH_2) alkylating agent.

Procarbazine was approved on July 22, 1969; it is administered orally and
historically was used for treatment of Hodgkin lymphoma. In a cohort of patients
with grade 2 astrocytoma, oligoastrocytoma, or oligodendroglioma who were
younger than 40 years of age and had undergone subtotal resection or biopsy
or who were 40 years of age or older and had undergone biopsy or resection
of any of the tumor, progression-free survival (PFS) and overall survival (OS)
were longer among those who received PCV (procarbazine, CCNU [lomustine],
vincristine) chemotherapy in addition to radiation therapy than among those who
received radiation therapy alone. Procarbazine can cause hemolysis in glucose-
6-phosphate dehydrogenase (G6PD)-deficient patients. It is associated with a
moderate or high emetic potential and it can cause CNS depression. Ethanol
consumption during procarbazine therapy should be avoided, as a disulfiram-
like reaction may occur.

Dacarbazine was approved on May 27, 1975; it is administered intravenously
and historically was used (prior to targeted therapies and immunotherapies) as a
single agent in the treatment of metastatic melanoma. Dacarbazine is still used
as part of the ABVD (Adriamycin, bleomycin, vinblastine, dacarbazine) regimen
to treat Hodgkin lymphoma and as part of the MAID (mesna, Adriamycin,
ifosfamide, dacarbazine) regimen for treating sarcoma. Off-label use of

(continued)

FIGURE 5.8 **Triazines (three attached nitrogen atoms) and hydrazines.** (*continued*) dacarbazine also has been reported for treatment of advanced or metastatic medullary thyroid cancer, advanced pancreatic neuroendocrine tumors, and malignant pheochromocytoma. Dacarbazine can cause flu-like syndrome.

Temozolomide (orally) was originally approved based on response rate on August 11, 1999, for the treatment of adult patients with refractory anaplastic astrocytoma who have experienced disease progression on a drug regimen containing nitrosourea and procarbazine. Temozolomide was subsequently approved for the treatment of adult patients with newly diagnosed glioblastoma multiforme (GBM) concomitantly with radiation therapy and then as maintenance treatment; the addition of concomitant and maintenance temozolomide to radiation therapy showed a statistically significant improvement in overall survival compared to radiotherapy alone (the hazard ratio for death among patients treated with radiotherapy plus temozolomide, as compared with those who received radiotherapy alone, was 0.63 with 95% CI, 0.52 to 0.75; $p < .001$). At 1 year, ~60% of patients who received temozolomide were alive compared with ~50% of patients who did not. Severe lymphopenia occurs in more than 50% of patients receiving temozolomide; hence, prophylaxis against *Pneumocystis jirovecii* to prevent *Pneumocystis* pneumonia (PCP) is warranted. Peripheral edema and drug-related fever occur in approximately 10% of patients receiving temozolomide.

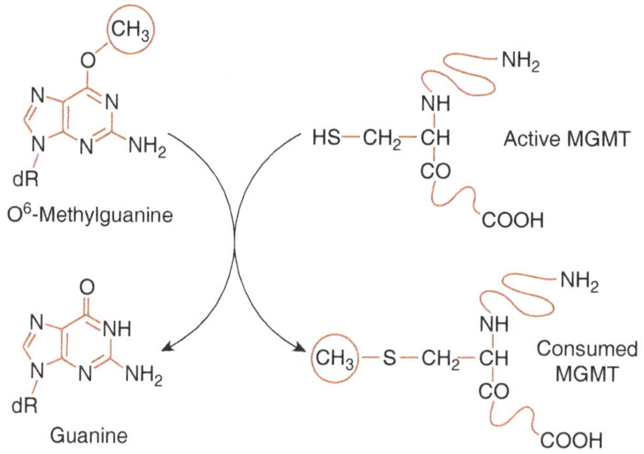

FIGURE 5.9 **Clinical importance of methylguanine methyltransferase.** The DNA repair protein O^6-methylguanine-DNA methyltransferase (MGMT) plays an important role in response to alkylating agents. The enzyme demethylates DNA, and hence undoes the effect of alkylating agents such as temozolomide. Epigenetic silencing through promoter methylation of the MGMT gene impairs this repair process and increases temozolomide-induced cell death. Increased MGMT activity/levels within tumor tissue is associated with temozolomide resistance. Clinical studies have shown MGMT silencing by promoter methylation is associated with temozolomide sensitivity in CNS tumors and longer survival for patients. Determination of MGMT status can be used as the predictive biomarker for response to alkylating agents.

Platinum Compounds

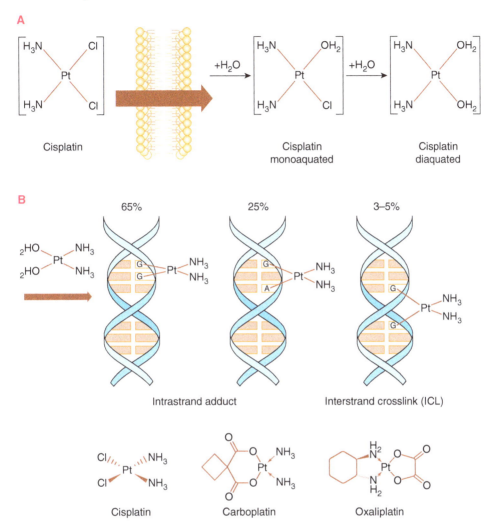

FIGURE 5.10 Platinum compounds.
Platinum agents are grouped with alkylators in that they are alkylating-like, resulting in intrastrand and interstrand crosslinking. They accomplish this crosslinking, however, without addition of alkyl groups. In 1965, the antitumor activity of cisplatin was first discovered during a study on the effect of electric current on bacterial growth, and in the early 1970s cisplatin was developed as a modern chemotherapeutic agent.

Cisplatin. The dose of cisplatin completely varies from one chemotherapy regimen to another. When cisplatin is used concurrently with radiation therapy, it acts as a potent radiation sensitizer. Intravenous (IV) cisplatin based chemotherapy is commonly utilized and is responsible for:

- The high cure rate of seminoma and nonseminomatous testicular germ cell tumors (BEP [bleomycin, etoposide, cisplatin 20 mg/m^2/daily IV days 1–5] and VIP [etoposide, ifosfamide (and mesna), cisplatin 20 mg/m^2/daily IV days 1–5])

(continued)

FIGURE 5.10 Platinum compounds. (*continued*)

- High response and remission rates for advanced ovarian cancer (75 mg/m^2 IV every 3 weeks [in combination with paclitaxel] or 100 mg/m^2 intraperitoneal [IP] on day 2 of a 21-day treatment cycle [in combination with IV cisplatin and IP paclitaxel] for six cycles)
- High response and remission rates for small cell lung cancer (60–80 mg/m^2 on day 1 every 3–4 weeks for four cycles [in combination with etoposide and concurrent/sequential radiation])
- High response rates for locally advanced squamous cell carcinoma of the head and neck particularly in human papillomavirus associated tumors receiving definitive chemoradiation; given either as a radiosensitizer (40 mg/m^2 weekly) or as bolus cisplatin 100 mg/m^2 every 3 weeks
- Neoadjuvant treatment for muscle invasive bladder cancer (MVAC regimen [cisplatin 70 mg/m^2 on day 2 every 28 days in combination with methotrexate, vinblastine, doxorubicin for three cycles] or gemcitabine cisplatin [GC] regimen [70 mg/m^2 on day 1 every 21 days or (split-dose cisplatin) 35 mg/m^2 on days 1 and 8 every 21 days (in combination with gemcitabine) for four cycles])
- Treatment of non-small cell lung cancer (both as adjuvant therapy and for advanced or metastatic disease with different variety of regimens)
- Treatment of esophageal or gastroesophageal junction cancer (pembrolizumab, fluorouracil, cisplatin 80 mg/m^2 on day 1 every 3 weeks for a maximum of six cycles with continuation of pembrolizumab and fluorouracil until disease progression, unacceptable toxicity, or in patients without disease progression for up to 24 months)
- Treatment of squamous cell anal carcinoma (75 mg/m^2 on day 1 every 4 weeks, in combination with continuous infusion fluorouracil)
- Treatment of cervical cancer (different variety of regimens in combination with radiation and fluorouracil, or in combination with paclitaxel and bevacizumab).

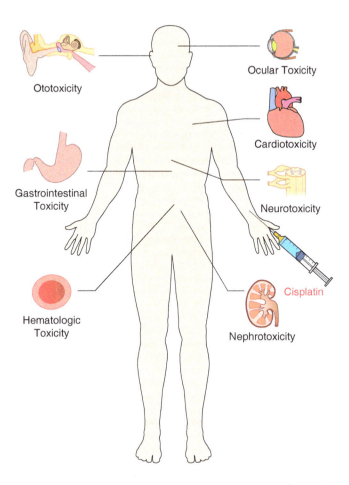

FIGURE 5.11 Cisplatin adverse events.

The observed adverse clinical effects of cisplatin include:

- Ototoxicity (more common in children than adults, presents as tinnitus, high-frequency hearing loss, and decreased ability to hear normal conversational tones)
- Nephrotoxicity (occurs in 25%–35% of patients, dose-related and cumulative; is associated with renal tubular damage presenting as acute renal failure and chronic renal insufficiency). Cisplatin is eliminated via the kidneys and requires dose adjustment for renal dysfunction. Nephrotoxicity and ototoxicity are the result of depleted glutathione with resultant increase in reactive oxidative species.
- Neurotoxicity (presents mainly as peripheral neuropathy, which is dose and duration dependent)
- Gastrointestinal toxicity (nausea and vomiting, which occur in almost 100% of patients). Cisplatin, particularly doses >50 mg/m^2, is considered one of the most emetogenic chemotherapeutics.
- Ocular toxicity (may present as optic neuritis, papilledema, cortical blindness, altered color perception manifesting as a loss of color discrimination, particularly in the blue-yellow area as well as irregular retinal pigmentation of the macular area on funduscopic exam)

(continued)

FIGURE 5.11 Cisplatin adverse events. (*continued*)

- Electrolyte abnormalities including hypomagnesemia, hypocalcemia, hypokalemia
- Myelosuppression including anemia, leukopenia, and thrombocytopenia. Cisplatin (and other platinum compounds) should be administered after taxanes to decrease myelosuppression and enhance efficacy.
- Cisplatin is a vesicant at higher concentrations and an irritant at lower concentrations; hence, extravasation should be avoided.
- Platinum does NOT require dose adjustment for hepatic dysfunction.
- Cisplatin-induced cardiotoxicity is rare with unknown prevalence. Reported cardiac-related adverse events associated with cisplatin include bradycardia, QT interval prolongation, cardiac arrhythmias, and cardiomyopathy with elevated NT-proBNP (N-terminal prohormone brain natriuretic peptide).

Carboplatin. In general, carboplatin has reduced side effects compared with cisplatin. With almost similar efficacy, carboplatin can substitute cisplatin for the treatment of most solid tumors. The Calvert formula is used to calculate the dose of carboplatin; the formula considers the creatinine clearance (CrCl), the desired area under curve (AUC; represents the total drug exposure over time), and the glomerular filtration rate:

$$\text{Total carboplatin dose (mg)} = (\text{target AUC}) (\text{GFR} + 25).$$

Most clinicians cap estimated GFR at a maximum of 125 mL/min to avoid potential carboplatin-related toxicity. The typical AUC for carboplatin ranges from 3 to 7 (mg/mL)·min.

Relative to cisplatin, carboplatin has significantly less nephrotoxicity as well as less severe and more manageable nausea and vomiting. However, compared with cisplatin, carboplatin is more myelosuppressive. For platelet count <50,000/mm^3 or absolute neutrophil count <500/mm^3, carboplatin dose is generally reduced to 75% of the usual dose.

Carboplatin is indicated for treatment of advanced ovarian cancer. However, it is commonly used off-label for treatment of head and neck cancer, breast cancer (advanced or metastatic, neoadjuvant/adjuvant therapy), recurrent or metastatic cervical and endometrial cancers, esophageal and gastric cancers, gestational trophoblastic neoplasia as well as early stage, adjuvant therapy for testicular cancer and conditioning regimen for autologous hematopoietic stem cell transplant for metastatic germ cell tumors, malignant pleural mesothelioma, Merkel cell carcinoma, advanced, atypical or poorly differentiated neuroendocrine tumors, relapsed or refractory Hodgkin and non-Hodgkin lymphomas, small and non-small cell lung cancers, castration-resistant and metastatic prostate cancer, Ewing sarcoma and osteosarcoma, advanced thymic malignancies, anaplastic thyroid carcinoma, cancer of unknown primary.

AUC, area under the curve; CrCl, creatinine clearance; GFR, glomerular filtration rate.

Oxaliplatin. Oxaliplatin is approved for adjuvant treatment of stage III colon cancer (in combination with infusional fluorouracil and leucovorin; FOLFOX regimen) after complete resection of primary tumor as well as for treatment of advanced colorectal cancer (in combination with infusional fluorouracil and leucovorin). Oxaliplatin is commonly used off-label for treatment of many gastrointestinal malignancies including advanced biliary tract cancer, esophageal and gastric cancers, carcinoid neuroendocrine tumors, potentially curable, adjuvant therapy as well as advanced or metastatic pancreatic cancers, advanced or metastatic small bowel adenocarcinoma. Oxaliplatin is also used for treatment of refractory non-Hodgkin lymphomas (combined with gemcitabine; GemOx regimen).

Oxaliplatin should be prepared in dextrose solution with prolonging the infusion time. For oxaliplatin dosing: if CrCl ≥30 mL/min, then no dosage adjustment necessary; if CrCl <30 mL/min, then dose should be reduced from 85 mg/m^2 to 65 mg/m^2.

Clinically significant adverse events related to oxaliplatin include:

- Serious hypersensitivity adverse event, including anaphylaxis, may occur with oxaliplatin administration within minutes of injection and during any cycle.
- Oxaliplatin can cause acute and delayed neuropathy. Cold-sensory neuropathy and cold-induced laryngospasm occur after oxaliplatin and can be dose-limiting toxicities. Supportive care for prevention of oxaliplatin-induced peripheral neuropathy includes avoiding cold temperatures; using scarves and face masks in cold weather; using cotton socks, pot holders, rubber gloves for dish washing; assessing the water temperature in the home; and using moisturizer.
- Severe neutropenia and thrombocytopenia can occur in 40% to 45% of patients receiving oxaliplatin.
- Cough, dyspnea, and hypoxia are frequently observed in patients receiving multiple doses of oxaliplatin. Cessation of the oxaliplatin-containing regimen and initiation of moderate- to high-dose corticosteroid might be helpful.
- Very rare (~0.1–1%) but serious adverse events related to oxaliplatin include posterior reversible encephalopathy syndrome (PRES), pulmonary fibrosis, QT interval prolongation, and ventricular arrhythmias including fatal torsades de pointes and rhabdomyolysis.

Drugs Perturbing DNA Structure

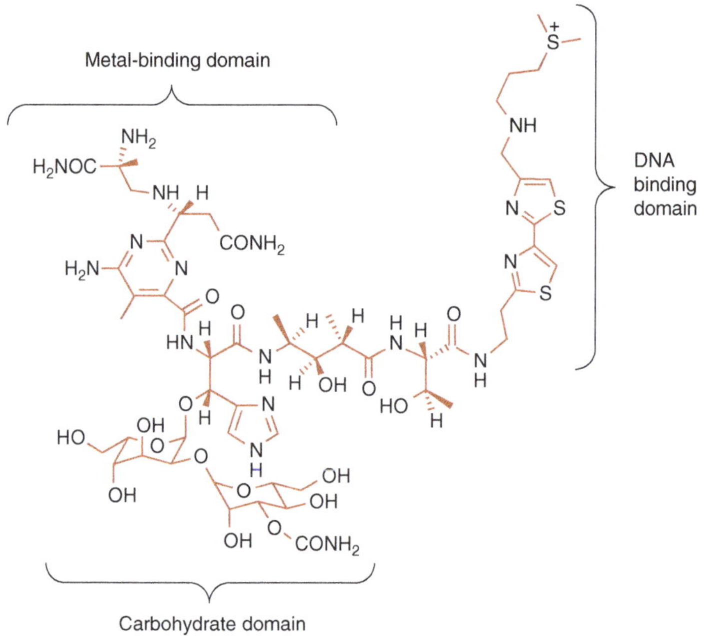

FIGURE 5.12 Bleomycin.

The bleomycins are a group of peptide derivatives isolated from fermentation broth of a bacteria; it therefore is an antitumor antibiotic, functioning in nature as a defense against other bacteria. Bleomycin is a mixture of at least two or more nonribosomally synthesized peptides. One part of the bleomycin molecule can chelate a variety of metal ions and another part of the molecule consists of different members of the bleomycin family of peptides side chains with the ability to bind to DNA. Certain metal complexes with bleomycins, particularly Fe(II)-bleomycin, can react with O_2 while bound to DNA and produce damage to DNA in the form of single and double strand breaks and the loss of bases, particularly thymine bases. The resulting damage to DNA can be difficult to repair and trigger cancer cell death. A major determinant of bleomycin action in cells is a *bleomycin hydrolase*, which degrades bleomycin in mammalian cells.

Because it is a mixture of peptides, bleomycin is dosed according to units of DNA breaking ability. Formulations are available in vials with either 15 or 30 units of metal-free bleomycin, with doses ordered as units. Each unit (U) contains 1.2 to 1.7 mg of polypeptide protein. It is currently used as an intravenous infusion in the potentially curative treatment of germ cell neoplasms in both males and females, and of Hodgkin lymphoma. It also has been injected directly into cutaneous tumors and into malignant pleural effusions, where it causes inflammation and adherence of the pleural surfaces.

Bleomycin is cleared prominently by renal excretion; doses should be reduced in patients with creatinine clearance <60 mL/min. Patients with renal insufficiency have a higher risk of pulmonary toxicity, and are at enhanced risk of mucocutaneous toxicity, as skin cells also have relatively low bleomycin hydrolase activity.

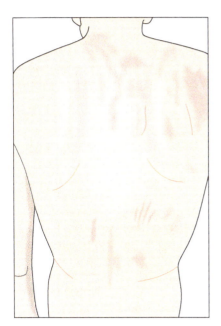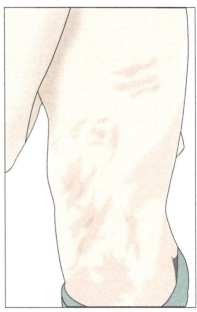

FIGURE 5.13 **Cutaneous toxicity of bleomycin.**
Bleomycin-induced hyperpigmentation or flagellate dermatitis may occur in ~20% of patients treated systematically with bleomycin. The term *flagellate* is originated from the Latin *flagellum*, referring to the whip-like appearance of the dermatitis. Patients present with urticarial rash and generalized pruritus, which improves when the lesions develop into the striking hyperpigmentation-like lesions. Other dermatologic manifestation of bleomycin toxicity include erythema multiforme, violaceous plaques, sclerodermoid and warty hyperkeratotic lesions.

Pulmonary Toxicity of Bleomycin. Adverse effects of systemically injected bleomycin are most prominently related to its damage to pulmonary alveolar epithelial cells, mediated in part by the high O_2 tension present in the lung, along with relatively lower levels of bleomycin hydrolase in the lung. Pulmonary toxicity presents as an interstitial pneumonitis, with cough, dyspnea, and pulmonary infiltrates, which can progress to fatal pulmonary fibrosis. It occurs in 3% to 5% of patients receiving <450 U cumulatively of bleomycin, and in up to 10% of those receiving cumulative doses >450 U.

The incidence of pulmonary toxicity increases with age (>70), prior radiation, and underlying chronic lung disease. Standard protocols for testicular cancer administer 30 U/week for 12 doses, and the incidence of fatal pulmonary reactions in the population of primarily young males is <2%. Although frequently treated when recognized with steroids, efficacy in reversing the changes leading to lung scarring is not clear. Active bleomycin pulmonary toxicity is associated with hypoxemia and decrease in the diffusing capacity of the lungs for carbon monoxide (DLCO). The utility of routine pulmonary function testing with measurement of DLCO to predict the onset of bleomycin toxicity is controversial. Current practice endorses checking pulmonary functions prior to inception of bleomycin-containing chemotherapy regimens, and if unexpectedly abnormal (DLCO <75%) discuss with the patient the increased risk of developing serious

(*continued*)

FIGURE 5.13 **Cutaneous toxicity of bleomycin. (*continued*)**

toxicity and consider alternative treatment strategies. Intercurrent DLCO testing has not clearly been shown to prevent the occurrence of bleomycin lung toxicity, but again a marked change from baseline should be considered as a relative contraindication to bleomycin use.

Of importance, bleomycin exposure during commonly employed regimens for germ cell neoplasms and Hodgkin disease can result in a mechanism-based toxicity with flair of pneumonitis when the patient is exposed to high inspired oxygen tensions as during elective surgery or scuba diving, even without prior clinical lung toxicity during treatment. This in part is due to the intrinsically low levels of bleomycin hydrolase in the lung. Inspired O_2 during surgery should be the minimum to produce O_2 saturation of 92%. Careful discussion should occur with anesthesiologists to alert them to the patient's prior exposure to bleomycin.

Other adverse events encountered with bleomycin include hypersensitivity reactions, and historically "test" doses of the drug were administered. However, with modern premedication algorithms such as corticosteroids and antihistamines the routine value of this practice is not established. Also late Raynaud phenomenon has been reported. Myelosuppression is curiously not a significant feature of bleomycin effects in patients with normal renal function.

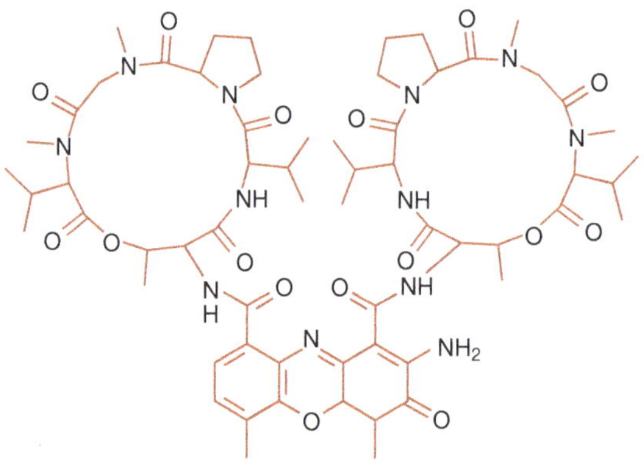

FIGURE 5.14 **Actinomycin D.**

Also an antitumor antibiotic, actinomycin consists of a planar unsaturated ring system that inserts itself or intercalates into the DNA helix, and peptide groups on either side also bind to DNA. It does not have prominent metal-binding capacities. Its principal effect is to decrease RNA synthesis, resulting in cell death after depletion of rapidly turning over mRNAs. At clinically used doses, breaks in DNA of uncertain origin can be detected. Actinomycin is of importance as a component of curative regimens for pediatric sarcomas such as rhabdomyosarcoma and Wilms tumor. It is also used in choriocarcinoma regimens.

Adverse events of actinomycin include prominent nausea, vomiting, cytopenias, and mucositis due to intestinal lining toxicity. It can cause "recall" reactions in radiation ports. It is a prominent vesicant that can cause further damage to soft tissues after extravasation.

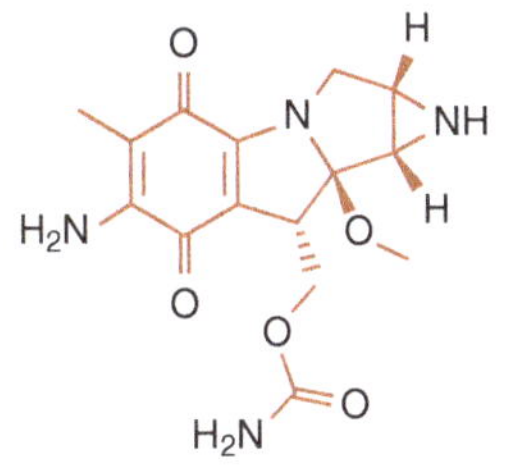

FIGURE 5.15 Mitomycin C.

Mitomycin C, another bacterial product and a benzoquinone, undergoes reduction by a ubiquitously present quinone reductase NQO1 to produce a bi- or trifunctional DNA alkylating agent. Systemically, its use is limited to the potentially curative chemoradiation treatment of anal cancer, along with fluorouracil and radiation. Mitomycin C is also approved for intravesical therapy after transurethral resection of bladder tumor (TURBT) for noninvasive (stage 0) or minimally invasive (stage I) bladder cancers.

Nausea, vomiting, and myelosuppression is common. Patients who receive >50 mg/m^2 experience the increasing incidence of a syndrome resembling hemolytic uremic syndrome (HUS) or thrombotic thrombocytopenic purpura (TTP), with intravascular hemolysis, neurologic features, and renal failure with, however, frequent presence of an interstitial pneumonitis. Plasma exchange and other TTP-directed therapies are not effective. At cumulative doses of >30 mg/m^2, increased incidence of interstitial lung disease and cardiomyopathy alone or in combination are noted. Systemic side effects are not seen with its intravesical use.

CHAPTER SUMMARY

Alkylating agents have been a mainstay of cancer chemotherapy for over 60 years and continue to play formative roles in diverse cytotoxic regimens for a broad spectrum of hematologic and epithelial malignancies as well as cytoreductive regimens for bone marrow transplantation. Several different types of alkylating agents are used in daily oncology clinical practice. These agents exert their cytotoxic effects by directly damaging DNA through intra- and interstrand covalent crosslinking. Although not phase-specific, alkylating agents are cell cycle–dependent and exert their toxicities predominantly on organs with actively cycling cells, such as bone marrow and gastrointestinal mucosal cells. All alkylating agents are capable of inducing t-MDS and t-AML, which are associated with losses of parts or all of chromosome 5 and/or 7, often with complex cytogenetic abnormalities. These myeloid malignancies emerge at a median 5 to 7 years (but as late as 20 years) after alkylating agent therapy, often have complex cytogenetic abnormalities involving multiple chromosomes, exhibit refractoriness to multiple classes of chemotherapeutic agents, and carry a poor prognosis. Understanding the clinical indications and special adverse event profile and the management related to each agent is imperative for hematologists and oncologists.

CLINICAL PEARLS

- To prevent hemorrhagic cystitis, mesna must be used after administration of intermediate-dose to high-dose cyclophosphamide and ifosfamide.
- High-dose ifosfamide can cause encephalopathy, which can be treated/prevented with methylene blue.
- Hypermethylation of the O^6-methylguanine-DNA-methyltransferase (MGMT) gene is associated with improved outcome in glioblastoma and is a predictive biomarker of sensitivity to alkylating agents such as temozolomide.
- Thiotepa is the alkylating agent that can be given intrathecally and management of its potential cutaneous toxicity is important.
- Use of different antiemetic agents after administration of platinum agents, particularly cisplatin, is recommended.

MULTIPLE-CHOICE QUESTIONS

1. A 27-year-old man has been diagnosed with primary mediastinal nonseminomatous germ cell tumors (NSGCTs). His serum alpha fetoprotein (AFP) is 12,500 ng/mL, beta-human chorionic gonadotropin (β-hCG) is 33,000 mIU/mL, and lactate dehydrogenase (LDH) is 2,700 U/L. He is anticipated to undergo postchemotherapy resection of residual mediastinal disease and is at risk of perioperative bleomycin-related lung toxicity. The oncologist elected to treat him with VIP. He received chemotherapy from days 1 to 5: etoposide 75 mg/m^2 IV, ifosfamide 1,200 mg/m^2 IV plus cisplatin 20 mg/m^2 plus mesna (2-mercaptoethane sulfonate sodium [natrium, Na]) 240 mg/m^2 IV bolus on day 1 followed by 1,200 mg/m^2 continuous IV infusion on days 1 to 5. The cycle will be repeated every 3 weeks for four cycles. On day 7, he develops suprapubic pain and hematuria. Which of the following compounds is most likely responsible for this patient's symptoms?

   A. Ifosfamide
   B. Mesna
   C. Cisplatin
   D. Etoposide
   E. Metastatic germ cell tumor to the bladder

2. A 43-year-old man with relapsed diffuse large B-cell lymphoma is admitted for salvage chemoimmunotherapy with R-ICE (rituximab, ifosfamide, carboplatin, etoposide). On the third day of therapy, the patient rapidly progressed from increased sedation and confusion to unresponsiveness. Preliminary lab studies drawn were unrevealing. The treating provider immediately recognized the adverse event and began administration of which therapeutic agent?

   A. Dexamethasone
   B. Dextrose 50%
   C. Vitamin C
   D. Methylene blue
   E. Activated charcoal

3. A 56-year-old woman with glioblastoma multiforme (GBM) is started on temozolo-mide with concurrent brain radiation therapy. She is informed by her oncologist that increased efficacy with temozolomide is seen in patients with GBM with a certain mutational status owing to reduced ability for those cancer cells to have sufficient cel-lular repair. What is this mutational status?

   A. Wild-type IDH1
   B. 1p/19q codeletion
   C. MGMT promotor methylation
   D. NPM1 mutated
   E. FLT3-ITD

4. The above-mentioned 56-year-old woman with GBM is maintained on adjuvant temozolomide following concurrent brain radiation therapy and temozolomide. Ap-proximately 4 months after radiation therapy, she presents to the ED with complaints of increased shortness of breath and dyspnea on exertion. Her vitals on presentation are as follows: blood pressure 98/58 mmHg, heart rate 118/minute, respiratory rate 24/minute, and O_2 saturation 88% on room air. A chest x-ray obtained demonstrates a diffuse bilateral interstitial infiltrate. What is the most likely causative agent?

   A. *Streptococcus pneumoniae*
   B. *Mycoplasma pneumoniae*
   C. *Aspergillus fumigatus*
   D. *Pneumocystis jirovecii*
   E. *Pseudomonas aeruginosa*

5. A 67-year-old man with metastatic colon cancer is being treated with FOLFOX (5-FU, leucovorin, oxaliplatin) and complains of severe numbness/tingling in his ex-tremities during cycle 3 when touching anything cold. What agent is causing these symptoms?

   A. 5-FU
   B. Leucovorin
   C. Oxaliplatin
   D. Ondansetron
   E. Compazine

6. A 58-year-old man with stage IV Hodgkin lymphoma achieves a metabolic complete remission after two cycles of ABVD (doxorubicin, bleomycin, vinblastine, dacarbazine). He comes to clinic 10 days after completion of his fourth cycle of treat-ment complaining of dry cough and dyspnea. Physical examination reveals crackles and crepitations in both lungs. Vital signs show a low-grade fever and mild hypoxia (arterial oxygen saturation is 82% on room air), but otherwise are unremarkable. Chest x-ray studies suggest pneumonia, and bronchoscopy reveals gram-negative rods consistent with *Pseudomonas*. He was adequately treated with broad-spectrum antibiotics, and becomes afebrile but his respiratory status continues to deteriorate. A lung biopsy reveals lung fibrosis. Which of the following statements about his condition is accurate?

A. Synergism between doxorubicin and dacarbazine is causing serious cardiomyopathy.

B. A severe idiosyncratic reaction consisting of hypotension, mental confusion, fever, chills, and wheezing has been reported in ~10% of lymphoma patients treated with bleomycin.

C. Bleomycin-induced pneumonitis/pulmonary fibrosis occurs in 25% of patients with Hodgkin lymphoma and testicular cancer.

D. Bleomycin must be discontinued for pulmonary diffusion capacity for carbon monoxide (DLCO) <25% to 30% of baseline.

E. Severe myelosuppression is commonly seen with ABVD, but treatment should not be held for neutropenia and prophylactic treatment with granulocyte colony-stimulating factor (G-CSF) is required.

7. A 49-year-old man is to undergo palliative treatment for his recurrent head and neck cancer. He receives cisplatin (100 mg/m^2 IV on day 1) and fluorouracil (1,000 mg/m^2 per day, continuous infusion, for 4 days). This is based on the results from Phase 3 trials showing this regimen can produce response rates of ~30%, which is significantly better than with single-agent cisplatin or methotrexate. Which one of the following interventions is recommended before initiation of the chemotherapy regimen?

A. Start beta-blocker to decrease the incidence of fluorouracil-induced coronary vasospasm.

B. Use antireflective coating glasses to reduce glare and reflections on the surface of the lenses, improving patients' vision-correcting ability and decreasing the probability of loss of color discrimination particularly in the blue-yellow axis.

C. Limit the use of hot water on hands and feet with twice daily cool showers or baths to prevent hand-foot syndrome.

D. Use amifostine to prevent cisplatin-induced dysgeusia, an abnormal or impaired sense of taste.

E. Use antiemetic therapy with a combination of an NK1R (neurokinin 1 receptor) antagonist, a 5-HT$_3$ (5-hydroxytryptamine) receptor antagonist, dexamethasone, and olanzapine on day 1, and continue dexamethasone and olanzapine on days 2 to 4.

8. A 26-year-old man, PhD student, presents to his primary care provider with a painless left scrotal mass that he noticed after sexual intercourse. A workup for sexually transmitted infections is negative, and the mass does not improve with empiric antibiotic treatment. The patient undergoes a testicular ultrasound exam, which shows a 2.1-cm hypoechoic lesion in an otherwise normal-appearing left testicular parenchyma, concerning for malignancy. What is the appropriate information to discuss with the patient?

A. Measurement of α-fetoprotein, LDH and β-hCG

B. CT chest, abdomen, and pelvis with and without contrast

C. The five histopathologic subtypes of testicular germ cell tumors are seminomas, embryonal carcinomas, teratomas, yolk sac tumors, and choriocarcinomas.

D. Chemotherapy regimens commonly used for testicular cancers are BEP and VIP

E. All of the above

9. A 63-year-old woman was diagnosed with stage III colon cancer during her sched-
    uled colonoscopy. She underwent a complete resection. She is a full-time endocrinol-
    ogist and an avid marathon runner. She is scheduled to start FOLFOX chemotherapy.
    She asks about evidence for calcium and magnesium supplement infusions during
    her chemotherapy to ameliorate oxaliplatin neuropathy. What do you tell her?

    A. Compared to placebo, it does not meaningfully help decreasing neurotoxicity.
    B. It decreases peripheral neuropathy in 50% of cases.
    C. Magnesium sulfate, but not calcium carbonate, decreases the probability of neu-
        ropathy in 25% of cases.
    D. It helps prevent only sensory, but not motor, neuropathy.
    E. It improves performance status and physical activity.

10. A 29-year-old woman is diagnosed with T-cell acute lymphoblastic leukemia (ALL).
    Her oncologist chooses a pediatric-inspired chemotherapy regimen with curative
    intent for her. Throughout ~3 years of treatment, she will receive several intrathecal
    chemotherapy injections to prevent ALL relapse in the CNS. Which one of the fol-
    lowing chemotherapeutic agents is commonly used for intrathecal administration?

    A. Vincristine plus daunorubicin
    B. Methotrexate, hydrocortisone, and cytarabine
    C. Cyclophosphamide
    D. CCNU alternating with BCNU
    E. Temozolomide monotherapy

ANSWERS TO MULTIPLE-CHOICE QUESTIONS

1. **A.** Ifosfamide. Acrolein (propenal) is a urotoxic metabolite of cyclophosphamide and
    ifosfamide, which can cause hemorrhagic cystitis and hematuria. Via the chemical
    reaction of its sulfhydryl (SH) group with α,β-unsaturated carbonyl-containing com-
    pounds such as acrolein, mesna assists to detoxify urotoxicity of acrolein. Even with
    the use of mesna, the incidence of consistent or severe hematuria was 33% in patients
    who were undergoing bone marrow transplant conditioning with regimens that in-
    cluded high-dose cyclophosphamide.

2. **D.** Methylene blue. Ifosfamide is a prodrug that requires hepatic activation to its
    cytotoxic metabolite ifosfamide mustard and also inactive neurotoxic metabolite
    chloroacetaldehyde (CAA). The CNS toxicities include delirium, confusion, leth-
    argy, drowsiness, disorientation, hallucinations, stupor, personality changes, mutism,
    encephalopathy, muscle twitching and incontinence, seizure, coma, and potentially
    death. The reported incidence of CNS toxicity is approximately 10% to 20% of pa-
    tients treated with ifosfamide. The symptoms usually occur during or shortly after
    drug administration. Usually within 2 to 3 days after stopping the ifosfamide, the
    symptoms spontaneously resolve in most of the patients. Methylene blue is a treat-
    ment for methemoglobinemia and cyanide poisoning and has been recommended
    for treatment of ifosfamide-induced neurotoxicity. No randomized controlled trials

demonstrated the use of methylene blue in ifosfamide neurotoxicity, but a series of case reports strongly suggest its benefit. The potential adverse events of methylene blue include dizziness, hypertension, headache, nausea, vomiting, and blue-green discoloration of the skin, urine, and stool. Methylene blue is contraindicated in subjects with glucose-6-phosphate dehydrogenase (G6PD) deficiency.

3. **C.** MGMT promotor methylation. Methylation of O^6-methylguanine-DNA methyltransferase (MGMT) promotor predicts improved prognosis in high-grade gliomas and GBM, and it is predictive of improved responsiveness to alkylating agent chemotherapy. MGMT promotor methylation has no diagnostic value. Isocitrate dehydrogenase (IDH) mutations confer improved prognosis across all diffuse gliomas of various grades. 1p/19q codeletion testing is required for diffuse gliomas with oligodendroglial component, and it is not routinely performed on GBM specimens. 1p/19q codeletion is associated with some subsets of wild-type IDH astrocytomas and confers a worse prognosis. NPM1 and FLT3 mutations are seen in patients with acute myeloid leukemia.

4. **D.** *Pneumocystis jirovecii*. *Pneumocystis* pneumonia (PCP) prophylaxis is recommended for the following patients: (1) acute lymphocytic leukemia (ALL) patients, (2) those taking a purine analog in combination with cyclophosphamide, (3) those receiving alemtuzumab, temozolomide in conjunction with radiation therapy, and PI3K inhibitors such as idelalisib, (4) allogeneic hematopoietic cell transplant and solid organ transplant recipients, (5) and those receiving a glucocorticoid dose equivalent to ≥20 mg of prednisone daily for 1 month or longer who also have another source of immunocompromise. For patients with GBM receiving temozolomide, PCP prophylaxis is recommended particularly during the concomitant radiation phase of treatment, even for patients who are not taking glucocorticoids. PCP prophylaxis is continued until absolute lymphocyte count is >800/μL.

5. **C.** Oxaliplatin. Two distinct neurologic complications can occur with oxaliplatin: (1) an acute neurosensory effect (happening during or shortly after the first few infusions), (2) a cumulative sensory neuropathy, with distal loss of sensation and dysesthesias. Acute neurotoxicity might be due to chelation of calcium by oxalate (a metabolite of oxaliplatin) with transient activation of peripheral nerve voltage-gated calcium-dependent sodium channels causing hyperexcitability of peripheral nerves. Cumulative sensory neuropathy is dose-dependent, symmetric distal axonal neuropathy without motor involvement. Interestingly, a randomized clinical trial of patients with colon cancer undergoing adjuvant therapy receiving either FOLFOX with IV calcium/magnesium before and after oxaliplatin or placebo before and after oxaliplatin showed that infusion of calcium and magnesium does not reduce cumulative neurotoxicity or significantly reduce oxaliplatin-related acute neuropathy. Oxaliplatin-induced neuropathy can negatively impact the quality of life of cancer patients.

6. **D.** Pulmonary toxicity occurs in 3% to 5% of patients receiving <450 U cumulative dose of bleomycin, and in up to 10% of those receiving cumulative doses >450 U. Current clinical practice recommends to discontinue bleomycin-containing chemotherapy regimens if DLCO decreases to less than 75% from baseline. A rare severe

hypersensitivity idiosyncratic reaction manifesting with hypotension, mental confusion, fever, chills, and wheezing has been reported in ~1% (not 10%) of lymphoma patients treated with bleomycin. Use of empiric G-CSF during treatment with ABVD has not been shown to be necessary or associated with less infectious-related toxicity. A report showed a significantly increased incidence of bleomycin-associated lung toxicity when G-CSF was used with bleomycin-containing chemotherapy in Hodgkin lymphoma, with associated high mortality rate.

7. **E.** Use of different antiemetic agents for the first few days during and after administration of high-dose cisplatin is recommended. Amifostine is a thiophosphate-containing agent that is a scavenger of free radicals generated in tissues exposed to radiation. Amifostine is the only pharmacologic agent with established efficacy in the prevention of xerostomia. Nevertheless, its role in patient management is uncertain, and currently, the routine use of amifostine in patients receiving combined modality chemoradiation is not routinely recommended. There is no evidence to justify the recommendation for the routine use of beta-blocker and of antireflective coating glasses after administration of chemotherapy.

8. **E.** BEP and VIP are two common chemotherapy regimens that are often used for testicular cancers.

9. **A.** The Phase 3 N08CB/Alliance trial looked at over 353 patients with colon cancer undergoing adjuvant therapy with FOLFOX. Patients were randomized to either FOLFOX with IV calcium/magnesium before and after oxaliplatin, placebo before and after oxaliplatin, or IV calcium/magnesium before and placebo after oxaliplatin. The study results showed that infusion of calcium and magnesium does not reduce cumulative neurotoxicity or significantly reduce oxaliplatin-related acute neuropathy.

10. **B.** Intrathecal (IT) chemotherapy can be administered via lumbar puncture (LP) or via direct administration into the ventricles via a subcutaneous access device such as an Ommaya reservoir. The chemotherapeutic drugs that are commonly used for IT administration include methotrexate, cytarabine, and nonpreservative steroids. Thiotepa, topotecan, etoposide are cytotoxic chemotherapy that have been used intrathecally. Rituximab, trastuzumab, and interferon alfa-2b are biologic/immunologic agents that have been administered intrathecally. Toxicity following IT chemotherapy may include nausea or vomiting, arachnoiditis (headache, back pain, nuchal rigidity, fever), and chronic leukoencephalopathy (confusion, somnolence, ataxia, seizures). The headache usually is constant, worsens within 15 minutes of standing, and is relieved within 15 minutes of lying down. Bed rest and analgesics are primary treatments. Caffeine and sodium benzoate significantly improve the symptoms of post-LP headache when given at a dose of 500 mg in 1,000 mL normal saline over 1 hour.

SELECTED REFERENCES

André T, Boni C, Mounedji-Boudiaf L, et al. Oxaliplatin, fluorouracil, and leucovorin as adjuvant treatment for colon cancer. N Engl J Med. 2004;350(23):2343–51. https://doi.org/10.1056/NEJMoa032709

Bayraktar UD, Bashir Q, Qazilbash M, et al. Fifty years of melphalan use in hematopoietic stem cell transplantation. Biol Blood Marrow Transplant. 2013;19(3):344–56. https://doi.org/10.1016/j.bbmt.2012.08.011

Buckner JC, Shaw EG, Pugh SL, et al. Radiation plus procarbazine, CCNU, and vincristine in low-grade glioma. N Engl J Med. 2016;374(14):1344–55. https://doi.org/10.1056/NEJMoa1500925

Devita VT Jr, Serpick AA, Carbone PP. Combination chemotherapy in the treatment of advanced Hodgkin's disease. Ann Intern Med. 1970;73(6):881–95. https://doi.org/10.7326/0003-4819-73-6-881

Emadi A, Jones RJ, Brodsky RA. Cyclophosphamide and cancer: Golden anniversary. Nat Rev Clin Oncol. 2009;6(11):638–47. https://doi.org/10.1038/nrclinonc.2009.146

Evens AM, Cilley J, Ortiz T, et al. G-CSF is not necessary to maintain over 99% dose-intensity with ABVD in the treatment of Hodgkin lymphoma: Low toxicity and excellent outcomes in a 10-year analysis. Br J Haematol. 2007;137(6):545–52. https://doi.org/10.1111/j.1365-2141.2007.06598.x

Ferreri AJM, Cwynarski K, Pulczynski E, et al. Chemoimmunotherapy with methotrexate, cytarabine, thiotepa, and rituximab (Matrix regimen) in patients with primary CNS lymphoma: Results of the first randomisation of the International Extranodal Lymphoma Study Group-32 (IELSG32) phase 2 trial. Lancet Haematol. 2016;3(5):e217–27. https://doi.org/10.1016/S2352-3026(16)00036-3

Loprinzi CL, Qin R, Dakhil SR, et al. Phase III randomized, placebo-controlled, double-blind study of intravenous calcium and magnesium to prevent oxaliplatin-induced sensory neurotoxicity (N08CB/Alliance). J Clin Oncol. 2014;32(10):997–1005. https://doi.org/10.1200/JCO.2013.52.0536

Pigneux A, Béné MC, Salmi LR, et al. Improved survival by adding lomustine to conventional chemotherapy for elderly patients with AML without unfavorable cytogenetics: Results of the LAM-SA 2007 FILO Trial. J Clin Oncol. 2018;36(32):3203–10. https://doi.org/10.1200/JCO.2018.78.7366

Reddy H, Duffy A, Holtzman NG, Emadi A. The role of β-elimination for the clinical activity of hypomethylating agents and cyclophosphamide analogues. Am J Cancer Ther Pharmacol. 2016;3(1):1–8. https://www.ncbi.nlm.nih.gov/pmc/articles/PMC6217992

Shepherd JD, Pringle LE, Barnett MJ, et al. Mesna versus hyperhydration for the prevention of cyclophosphamide-induced hemorrhagic cystitis in bone marrow transplantation. J Clin Oncol. 1991;9(11):2016–20. https://doi.org/10.1200/JCO.1991.9.11.2016

Sleijfer S. Bleomycin-induced pneumonitis. Chest. 2001;120(2):617–24. https://doi.org/10.1378/chest.120.2.617

Stupp R, Mason WP, van den Bent MJ, et al. Radiotherapy plus concomitant and adjuvant temozolomide for glioblastoma. N Engl J Med. 2005;352(10):987–96. https://doi.org/10.1056/NEJMoa043330

Watson RA, De La Peña H, Tsakok MT, et al. Development of a best-practice clinical guideline for the use of bleomycin in the treatment of germ cell tumours in the UK. Br J Cancer. 2018;119(9):1044–51. https://doi.org/10.1038/s41416-018-0300-x

CHAPTER 6

Pyrimidine- and Purine-Based Antimetabolites, Hydroxyurea, and Asparaginases

ASHKAN EMADI • JUDITH E. KARP

INTRODUCTION

Chemotherapeutic antimetabolites are structurally similar to normal metabolites (e.g., "fluoro"pyrimidine or "thio"purine) but functionally disruptive to their normal work culminating in interruption of replication and growth of cancer cells. This occurs through substrate competition for enzyme-binding sites or incorporation directly into DNA or RNA. Antimetabolites are cell cycle–dependent and late G1/S phase–specific, with major effects on the processes involved in DNA replication.

The major classes of antimetabolites are pyrimidine analogs, purine analogs, and antifolates. Pyrimidine and purine analogs are nucleic acids that mimic normal subunits of DNA but are modified slightly by substitution of a hydrogen with a halogen or an oxygen with a sulfur or arabinose sugar with ribose/deoxyribose, etc. The so-called hypomethylating agents (HMAs) azacitidine and decitabine are cytosine analogs that target the enzyme DNA methyltransferase (DNMT) and are discussed in Chapter 10 (Epigenetic Modulators). Antifolates target DNA enzymatic pathways that include dihydrofolate reductase and thymidylate synthase, which are involved in DNA synthesis, and are discussed in Chapter 7 (Antifolate Antimetabolites).

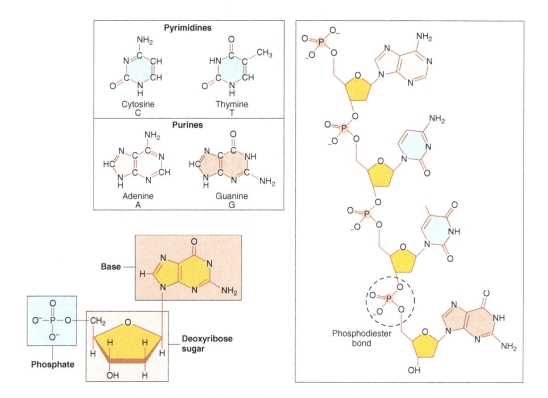

FIGURE 6.1 **Normal DNA structure consists of phosphate, deoxyribose, and base.**
Bases can be either pyrimidines or purines. Modifications to pyrimidine and purine structure form deoxyribonucleotide or ribonucleotide analogs that can be incorporated into DNA and inhibit enzymes involved in DNA replication such as DNA polymerase.

EMADI CLASSIFICATION OF ANTIMETABOLITES: A SUREFIRE HIT WITH ONCOLOGISTS

1. Halogen-decorated purines and pyrimidines (e.g., cladribine, fludarabine, clofarabine, 5-FU)
2. Substitution of oxygen with sulphur (e.g., mercaptopurine, thioguanine, azathioprine)
3. Substitution of –CH with nitrogen (e.g., azacitidine, decitabine)
4. Fake sugars (e.g., cytarabine, gemcitabine, nelarabine)
5. Fake folic acids (e.g., methotrexate, pralatrexate, pemetrexed)
6. Interference of plasma amino acid levels (e.g., asparaginase, crisantaspase)
7. Inhibition of R→D (ribose→deoxyribose) conversion (e.g., hydroxyurea)

PYRIMIDINE ANALOGS

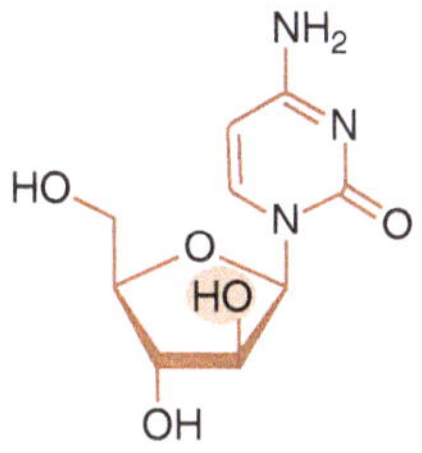

Cytarabine (Ara-C, Cytosine Arabinoside)

- Cytarabine was first synthesized in 1959 and since then it has been the most universally used chemotherapeutic agent in the treatment of acute myeloid leukemia (AML). Structurally, its arabinose sugar moiety is epimeric at the $2'$-position with ribose (highlighted OH).

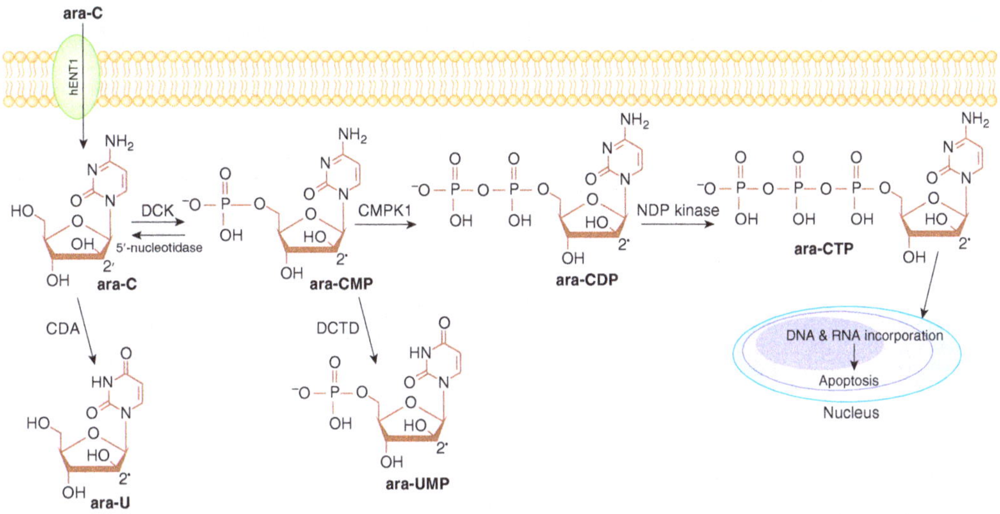

FIGURE 6.2 Genes involved in metabolic pathways and transporters of cytarabine. After entering the cells via its transporter hENT1, ara-C is phosphorylated in a stepwise manner at the $5'$ position of arabinose. Phosphorylation is mediated initially by DCK to convert ara-C to (ara-CMP), then by CMPK1 to ara-CDP, and finally by NDPK to the active metabolite, ara-CTP. Intracellular concentration of ara-CTP is directly correlated with the therapeutic effect of ara-C. Deaminase enzymes (CDA and DCTD) can convert and inactivate ara-C and ara-CMP to ara-U and ara-UMP, respectively. Inactivation of ara-C can also occur through ara-CMP dephosphorylation by $5'$-nucleotidase back to ara-C.

The most important parameters in sensitivity or resistance to ara-C include conversion to nucleotides by kinases, inactivation by removing amine group by deaminases, half-life of active form ara-CTP, and the magnitude of its incorporation into DNA.

ara-C, cytarabine; ara-CDP, ara-C diphosphate; ara-CMP, ara-C monophosphate; ara-CTP, ara-C triphosphate; ara-U, uracil arabinoside; ara-UMP, ara-uridine monophosphate; CDA, cytidine deaminase; CMPK1, cytidine/uridine monophosphate kinase 1; DCK, deoxycytidine kinase; DCTD, deoxycytidylate deaminase; hENT, human equilibrative nucleoside transporter; NDP, nucleoside diphosphate; NDPK, nucleoside diphosphate kinase.

- Mechanisms of antineoplastic activity of cytarabine include negatively affecting DNA synthesis in the following ways: (1) prevention of the transformation of cytidylate to 2'-deoxycytidylate, (2) inhibition of DNA polymerase A and B for replication and repair, and (3) incorporation into DNA to inhibit template function and chain elongation.
- Cytarabine is given via intravenous (IV) administration. It also be given intrathecally (50–100 mg per injection) for prevention or treatment of central nervous system leukemia (both acute lymphoblastic leukemia [ALL] and AML) and lymphoma.

Depocyte is cytarabine liposome injection and is used for the intrathecal (IT) treatment of lymphomatous meningitis and acute leukemia-related central nervous system (CNS) disease.

- Approximately 75% of each administered dose of cytarabine is excreted in urine. Dose adjustment in renal impairment is mandatory, especially in the setting of high-dose ara-C (HiDAC).
- Adverse events of cytarabine reported at all doses include myelosuppression, gastrointestinal toxicities (nausea/vomiting, mucositis, diarrhea), elevation in transaminases and intrahepatic cholestasis, cytarabine syndrome (fever, myalgia, bone pain, chest pain, rash), pancreatitis, and maculopapular rash.
- Adverse events of high doses (>1 g/m^2 per dose) of cytarabine (HiDAC) include
  - Central nervous system (CNS)
    - *Acute cerebellar toxicity*
      - Occurs in ~10% of patients receiving HiDAC
      - Usually occurs between 3 and 8 days after initiation of HiDAC
      - Can manifest as dysarthria, dysdiadochokinesia, dysmetria, ataxia, and nystagmus, usually with concomitant cerebral dysfunction
      - Diagnosis is clinical. CT scan, MRI and cerebrospinal fluid examination are nearly always normal. An EEG shows slow wave activity.
      - If moderate to severe cerebellar toxicity occurs, it is recommended that cytarabine should be discontinued and never used again. There is no effective therapy for the cerebellar toxicity due to HiDAC other than discontinuation of the drug and supportive measures.
      - The major risk factor is *renal insufficiency*. A review of medical records of 101 consecutive patients showed that if HiDAC was given during renal insufficiency (defined as serum creatinine ≥1.5 mg/dL or an increase in serum creatinine >0.5 mg/dL), any degree of neurotoxicity during administration of HiDAC was 62% and severe neurotoxicity was 42%, compared with 8% and 3%, respectively (*p* <.001), if HiDAC

was administered during normal renal function. Administration of HiDAC with creatinine clearance (CrCl) <60 mL/min resulted in 76% neurotoxicity compared with 8% in patients with CrCl >60 mL/min (p <.001).

- Personality changes, encephalopathy, seizures, coma
- Gastrointestinal (GI)
  - Oral mucosa, esophageal, gastric, and rectal ulcers
  - Abdominal pain and diarrhea
  - Pancreatitis and peritonitis
- Ocular
  - Keratitis (inflammation of the cornea)
    - Corneal deposits presenting as photophobia, foreign body sensation, mild-to-moderate vision loss
    - For moderate- and high-dose cytarabine regimens, *prophylaxis with ophthalmic corticosteroids* must be given throughout cytarabine treatment and up to 72 hours posttreatment.
  - Hemorrhagic conjunctivitis
- Pulmonary
  - Pulmonary edema
  - Sudden respiratory distress syndrome: severe dyspnea with a rapid onset and refractory hypoxia with diffuse pulmonary infiltrates, leading to respiratory failure

A few examples of cytarabine-containing chemotherapy regimens include:
- 7+3 (usually administered as a continuous IV infusion of 100–200 mg/m^2/day for 7 days combined with an anthracycline for 3 days) for remission induction regimen for AML
- HiDAC (1,500–3,000 mg/m^2/dose every 12 hours on days 1, 3, and 5 for 3–4 cycles) for consolidation therapy used in AML and ALL
- CLAG (±M) (cladribine, ara-C, G-CSF, ±mitoxantrone) for salvage therapy (as well as frontline therapy) for AML and ALL
- FLAG (±Ida) (fludarabine, ara-C, G-CSF, ±idarubicin) for salvage therapy (as well as frontline therapy) for AML and ALL
- HAM (±pegA) (HiDAC, mitoxantrone, ±pegasparaginase) for salvage therapy for AML, ALL, and mixed phenotype acute leukemia (MPAL)
- DHAP (±R) (dexamethasone, HiDAC, cisplatin, ±rituximab) for salvage therapy of relapsed or refractory non-Hodgkin lymphoma and Hodgkin lymphoma

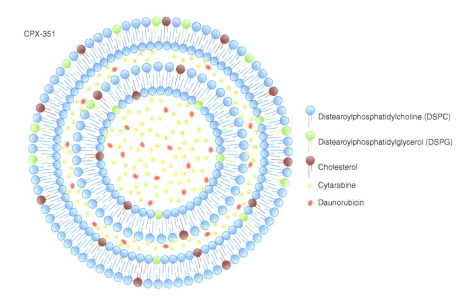

FIGURE 6.3 CPX-351 (VYXEOS): liposomal encapsulation of cytarabine plus daunorubicin.

CPX-351 is a bilamellar liposome composed of PC:PG: cholesterol in a 7:2:1 ratio. The cytarabine:daunorubicin ratio is fixed at 5:1 molar, for a final dose of 100 mg and 44 mg, respectively. The liposomal delivery system yields an increased concentration in bone marrow relative to plasma with preferential delivery to leukemic cells. After cellular internalization, the encapsulated drugs are released in the nucleus with a T½ of 24 hours.

CPX-351 is approved for adults with secondary AML arising from MDS/AML or from prior cytotoxic therapy (t-AML) based on significantly longer median overall survival (9.6 months) relative to traditional "7+3" (6 months). Toxicities are similar to those of cytarabine and daunorubicin individually (febrile neutropenia, infection, rash, oral and gastrointestinal mucositis, hepatic dysfunction, hypertension, and decreased left ventricular ejection fraction). Myelosuppression may be prolonged relative to giving cytarabine and daunorubicin in nonliposomal combinations.

AML, acute myeloid leukemia; PC, phosphatidylcholine; PG, phosphatidylglycerol; MDS, myelodysplasia.

Fluoropyrimidine: 5-Fluorouracil (5-FU)

- 5-FU was approved by the U.S. Food and Drug Administration (FDA) in 1962 for the treatment of colorectal cancer (CRC) and since then has been an essential drug that is widely used to treat many solid tumors of digestive origin including colorectal, anal, pancreatic, esophageal, gastric, and ampullary tumors as well as other epithelial tumors such as breast, cervix, and head and neck cancers.

- Treatment modalities that incorporate 5-FU (dose, timing, and administration) vary according to the origin of the tumor.

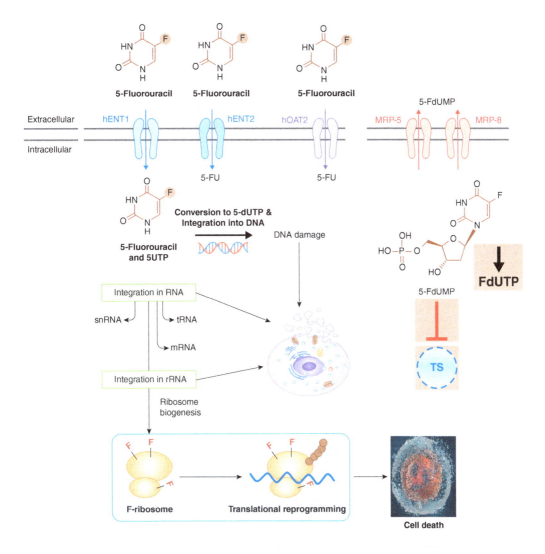

FIGURE 6.4 Complex mode of action of 5-FU.

Intracellular entrance of 5-FU is mediated by hENT1 and hENT2 as well as by hOAT2. Efflux of 5-FdUMP, the active metabolite of 5-FU, occurs via MRP-5 and MRP-8.

As an analog of uracil and thymine, mechanisms of antineoplastic activity of 5-FU include inhibition of both RNA and DNA (major mechanism) synthesis. 5-FdUMP binds to TS, which normally catalyzes the conversion of dUMP to dTMP. The resultant 5-FdTMP is triphosphorylated and incorporated into DNA, subsequently causing single-strand breaks and termination of DNA replication. The "thymineless death" is the phenomenon by which cancer cells die when they are deprived of dTTP.

(continued)

FIGURE 6.4 Complex mode of action of 5-FU. (*continued*)

The binding of 5-FdUMP to TS is stabilized by leucovorin, the reduced form of folate. See Chapter **7**, for further discussion of folic acid metabolism and TS and their roles in the conversion of dUMP to dTMP.

dTTP, deoxythymidine triphosphate; dTMP, deoxythymidine monophosphate; dUMP, deoxyuridine monophosphate; FdTMP, fluorodeoxythymidine monophosphate; FdUMP, fluorodeoxyuridine monophosphate; FdUTP, fluorodeoxyuridine triphosphate; 5-FU, 5-fluorouracil; hENT, human equilibrative nucleoside transporter; hOAT, human organic anion transporter; mRNA, messenger RNA; MRP, multidrug resistance protein; rRNA, ribosomal RNA; snRNA, small nuclear RNA; tRNA, transfer RNA; TS, thymidylate synthase; UTP, uridine triphosphate.

- 5-FU is administered intravenously; it is renally excreted, requiring dose modification for reduced glomerular filtration rate (GFR).
- Dihydropyrimidine dehydrogenase (DPD) is the initial and rate-limiting enzyme in 5-FU metabolism; subjects who are DPD intermediate or poor metabolizers are at risk of developing severe, life-threatening, or fatal 5-FU-associated toxicity.
- Adverse events of 5-FU include myelosuppression, GI toxicities (nausea, vomiting, diarrhea, oral mucositis, and anorexia), hepatotoxicity (elevation in transaminases, hyperbilirubinemia), cardiotoxicity (coronary vasospasm, QT prolongation), cerebellar toxicity (rare).

A few examples of 5-FU-containing chemotherapy regimens include:
- Gastrointestinal cancers: multiple regimens for newly diagnosed and refractory CRC including FOLFOX (leucovorin, 5-FU, oxaliplatin), FOLFIRI (leucovorin, 5-FU, irinotecan), FLOT (5-FU, leucovorin, oxaliplatin, docetaxel), FOLFIRINOX (FOL = leucovorin calcium [folinic acid], F = 5-FU, IRIN = irinotecan hydrochloride, OX = oxaliplatin) for metastatic pancreatic adenocarcinoma, and ECF (epirubicin, cisplatin, 5-FU) for gastric cancer and cancer of the esophagogastric junction
- Breast cancer (metastatic): FEC (5-FU, epirubicin, cyclophosphamide) and FEC-T (FCE followed by docetaxel [aka Taxotere]) for neoadjuvant and adjuvant, CAF (cyclophosphamide, doxorubicin, 5-FU), and CMF (cyclophosphamide, methotrexate, 5-FU)
- Ovarian cancer: 5-FU+leucovorin with taxane or oxaliplatin
- Head and neck cancer: combined with radiation and cisplatin

Fluoropyrimidine Prodrugs: Capecitabine and Tegafur

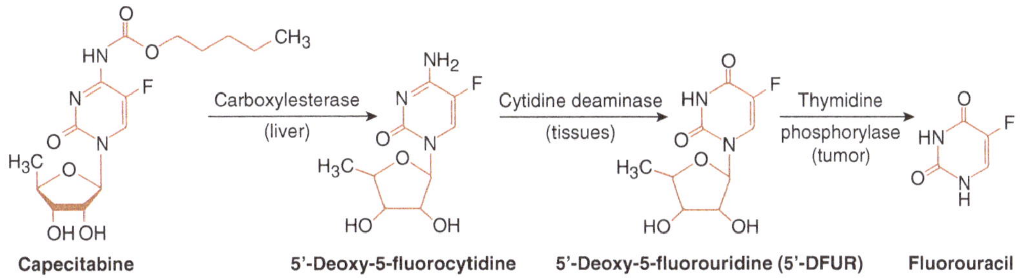

FIGURE 6.5 **Capecitabine (Xeloda) metabolic activation to fluorouracil.**
Capecitabine is an oral fluoropyrimidine that acts as continuous infusion 5-FU and hypothetically produces 5-FU at higher concentrations at the tumor tissue. Capecitabine is activated to 5-FU via a three-step enzymatic pathway.

After absorption in the gut, in the liver, and by the action of carboxyl esterase, the ester is removed from the amine and capecitabine is converted to 5'-DFCR. The amine (NH$_2$) group of cytosine moiety of 5'-DFCR is removed and substituted by oxygen to form a carbonyl group (hence uracil moiety) and 5'-DFUR as the product. The final step requires thymidine phosphorylase, an enzyme that is significantly more active in tumor than normal tissue, to convert 5'-DFUR to 5-FU.

5'-DFCR, 5'-deoxy-5-fluorocytidine; 5'-DFUR, 5'-deoxy-5-fluorouridine; 5-FU, 5-fluorouracil.

- Capecitabine should be taken with water within 30 minutes after a meal. Food can reduce both the rate and extent of absorption of capecitabine. The usual dose of capecitabine as monotherapy or in combination is 1,000–1,250 mg/m^2 twice daily orally for 2 to 3 weeks depending on the indication and the regimen.
- The dose of capecitabine should be reduced by 25% in patients with moderate renal impairment.
- The common and/or serious adverse events of capecitabine that requires attention include:
  - Coagulopathy that may result in bleeding and death. Patients receiving concomitant capecitabine and oral coumarin-derivative anticoagulants such as warfarin must have their anticoagulant response (international normalized ratio or prothrombin time) monitored frequently in order to fine-tune the anticoagulant dose accordingly.
  - Diarrhea that may be severe causing life-threatening dehydration. Capecitabine administration should be interrupted immediately until diarrhea resolves or decreases to grade 1. Standard antidiarrheal treatments are often recommended
  - Cardiotoxicity is common in patients with a prior history of coronary artery disease.
  - Increased risk of severe or fatal adverse events in patients with low or absent dihydropyrimidine dehydrogenase (DPD) activity. No capecitabine dose has been proved safe in patients with absent DPD activity.
  - Severe mucocutaneous reactions, Steven-Johnson syndrome (SJS) and toxic epidermal necrolysis (TEN), have been reported after exposure to capecitabine; in such conditions capecitabine should be permanently discontinued. Capecitabine may induce *hand-and-foot syndrome* or *palmar-plantar erythrodysesthesia*. Hand-foot syndrome can manifest as redness, swelling, and pain on the palms of the hands and/or the soles of the feet with occasional blisters and cracked, flaking, or peeling skin with severe pain and difficulty walking or using hands. Patients who

experience hand-foot syndrome should avoid sources of heat, including hot water, saunas, sitting in the sun, or sitting in front of a sunny window and cool showers or bath or ice packs are recommended. For treatment of hand-foot syndrome, topical anti-inflammatory medications including corticosteroid creams as well as topical pain relievers, such as lidocaine and topical moisturizing exfoliant including urea, salicylic acid, or ammonium lactate, can be useful.

- Hyperbilirubinemia
- Neutropenia and/or thrombocytopenia

A few examples of capecitabine-containing chemotherapy regimens include:
- Gastrointestinal cancers: multiple regimens for newly diagnosed and refractory CRC including CAPOX or XELOX (capecitabine, oxaliplatin); capecitabine-based chemoradiation regimens for the preoperative treatment of patients with locally advanced rectal cancer.
- Breast cancer: capecitabine is used as monotherapy or in combination with docetaxel.

- **Tegafur** is a formulated oral agent consisting of a combination of the prodrug tegafur (tetrahydrofuranyl-5-FU) and uracil in a 1:4 molar ratio. The high concentration of uracil can reversibly inhibit the DPD, thereby inhibiting first-pass DPD-mediated hepatic metabolism of 5-FU and permitting administration of 5-FU as the orally bioavailable prodrug tegafur.
- Tegafur is bioactivated to 5-FU by liver microsomal cytochrome P450 enzymes.
- Tegafur is not approved by the U.S. FDA; however, it is widely used in other countries for treatment of CRC.

Gemcitabine

- Gemcitabine mimics cytosine and is transported into cells and phosphorylated to its triphosphate form to inhibit DNA synthesis by acting as a competitive inhibitor of DNA polymerase and by inhibition of ribonucleotide reductase (RNR; targets M1 subunit).
- Gemcitabine is usually administered at 1,000 mg/m^2 IV over 30 minutes; it can also be administered via intravesical instillation for early stage bladder cancer.
- Gemcitabine is activated intracellularly by deoxycytidine kinase (DCK) to become phosphorylated; it may be given at fixed dose rate (FDR; e.g., 10 mg/m^2/min) to avoid DCK saturation.
- Adverse events of gemcitabine include:
  - Myelosuppression (mainly neutropenia)
  - Edema
  - Fever
  - Hepatotoxicity (primarily elevated transaminases but can elevate bilirubin too)
  - Flu-like syndrome, including chills, cough, headache, rhinitis, myalgia, and fatigue
  - Erythematous pruritic maculopapular rash
  - Rare (and often serious) adverse event: pneumonitis, hemolytic uremic syndrome (HUS)/thrombotic thrombocytopenic purpura (TTP)

A few examples of gemcitabine-containing chemotherapy regimens include:

- Monotherapy for pancreatic cancer (adjuvant and metastatic)
- Gemcitabine + 5-FU + leucovorin: pancreatic cancer
- Gemcitabine + Abraxane (paclitaxel protein-bound particles for injectable suspension, albumin-bound) for metastatic adenocarcinoma of the pancreas as first-line treatment
- Gemcitabine + paclitaxel for metastatic breast cancer
- Gemcitabine + docetaxel for different sarcomas
- Gemcitabine + carboplatin for refractory or relapsed ovarian cancer and mesothelioma
- Gemcitabine + cisplatin for NSCLC, bladder, cervical, head and neck, and hepatobiliary cancers
- Gemcitabine + oxaliplatin for refractory or relapsed Hodgkin lymphoma
- Testicular germ cell tumor

PURINE ANALOGS

Fludarabine

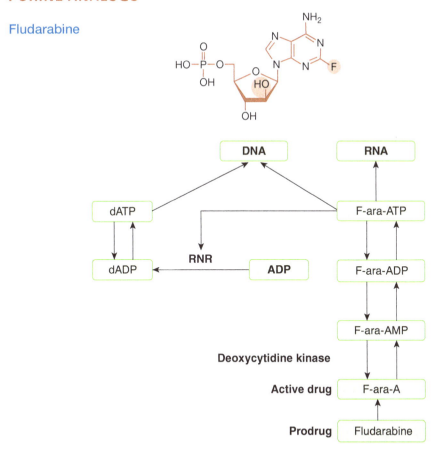

FIGURE 6.6 Metabolism of fludarabine and its antineoplastic mechanism of action. Fludarabine is a fluorinated nucleotide analog of the antiviral agent vidarabine (adenine arabinoside or ara-A). Fludarabine is rapidly dephosphorylated in

(continued)

FIGURE 6.6 **Metabolism of fludarabine and its antineoplastic mechanism of action.** (*continued*)

plasma to 2-fluoro-ara-adenine (F-ara-A), and then stepwise phosphorylated intracellularly by deoxycytidine kinase to the active triphosphate, 2-fluoro-ara-ATP (F-ara-ATP).

F-ara-ATP mimics adenosine triphosphate and works in the following ways: It is incorporated into DNA to cause DNA strand breaks, inhibits DNA polymerase, inhibits ribonucleotide reductase (RNR targets M1 subunit), inhibits DNA primase and ligase I, and effectively acts as a DNA chain terminator at the 3′-end of DNA.

Fludarabine is administered parenterally as a phosphate salt and it is recommended to administer it over ~30 minutes.

Oral fludarabine has similar toxicities as IV but greater frequency of diarrhea.

ADP, adenosine diphosphate; AMP, adenosine monophosphate; ara, arabinoside; ATP, adenosine triphosphate; dADP, deoxyadenosine diphosphate; dATP, deoxyadenosine triphosphate; RNR, ribonucleotide reductase.

- Adverse events of fludarabine include:
  ○ Myelosuppression (mainly lymphopenia); *Pneumocystis jirovecii* pneumonia (PJP) prophylaxis until CD4 count >200 cells/μL is recommended.
  ○ Dose-dependent neurotoxicity
  ○ Elevated transaminases
  ○ Rash
  ○ Edema (in up to 20% of patients)
  ○ Life-threatening (and sometimes fatal) autoimmune conditions including hemolytic anemia, autoimmune thrombocytopenia, Evans syndrome, and acquired hemophilia
  ○ It is not recommended to use fludarabine in combination with pentostatin as the combination carries an unacceptable high incidence of fatal pulmonary toxicities.

A few examples of fludarabine-containing chemotherapy regimens include:
- FCR (fludarabine, cyclophosphamide, rituximab) for chronic lymphocytic leukemia (CLL)
- FLAG-Ida AML (fludarabine, cytarabine, filgrastim, idarubicin); fludarabine potentiates activation of cytarabine evidenced by comparison of ara-CTP pharmacokinetics in circulating AML cells, which demonstrated that the area under the curve (AUC) of ara-CTP increased significantly by approximately two folds after fludarabine infusion
- allogeneic hematopoietic stem cell transplant conditioning (with busulfan or cyclophosphamide)
- conditioning regimen before CAR-T and other cellular therapies (fludarabine [Flu] 25 mg/m^2 daily x 5 [days -6 to -2]) in combination with cyclophosphamide (Cy; 50 mg/kg x 2 [days -5 and -4] – See also Chapter 18
  A comprehensive multivariable analysis of 132 factors, including clinical and treatment characteristics, serum biomarkers, and CAR-T cell manufacturing and pharmacokinetic data was performed to identify biomarkers associated with complete remission CR and progression-free

survival PFS after anti-CD19 CAR-T cell therapy in patients with aggressive B-cell non-Hodgkin lymphoma who received either low- or high-intensity Cy/Flu lymphodepletion.

Lower pre-lymphodepletion serum LDH and greater increase in serum monocyte chemoattract protein-1 (MCP-1) concentration in response to lymphodepletion were associated with better probability of achieving a CR and better PFS.

Patients receiving high-intensity lymphodepletion had a higher probability of achieving a favorable cytokine profile, defined as day 0 MCP-1 and peak IL-7 concentrations above their respective medians, compared with those receiving low-intensity lymphodepletion.

- Waldenstrom macroglobulinemia (with rituximab)

Cladribine

Cladribine is a prodrug that requires intracellular phosphorylation by deoxycytidine kinase for activation.

Cladribine mimics adenosine and works in the following ways: (a) incorporated into DNA to cause DNA strand breaks, (b) inhibits DNA polymerase, (c) inhibits ribonucleotide reductase RNR M1 subunit, (d) triggers apoptosis in non-dividing cells, and (e) hypomethylates properties by inhibition of methyl group transfer of S-adenosyl methionine (SAM) depletion of memory B cells.

Cladribine is 50% renally cleared. It requires dose reduction in renal impairment.

In regimens using high-dose cytarabine combined with cladribine, ara-C infusion should be started 2 hours after cladribine completion.

- Important of adverse events of cladribine include:
  - Myelosuppression (prolonged neutropenia, anemia, and thrombocytopenia); PCP prophylaxis until CD4 count >200 cells/μL is recommended.
  - Crosses the blood–brain barrier and can cause dose-dependent neurotoxicity
  - Nephrotoxicity
  - Fever and rash

A few examples of cladribine-containing chemotherapy regimens include:
- CLAG±M (cladribine, cytarabine, filgrastim with or without mitoxantrone) for AML
- Hairy cell leukemia
- Langerhans cell histiocytosis and Erdheim-Chester disease
- Multiple sclerosis

Clofarabine

Clofarabine is essentially a hybrid of cladribine and fludarabine. It is intracellularly phosphorylated by deoxycytidine kinase (dCK) to the 5′-monophosphate for activation, the rate-limiting step in activation of this prodrug. Of note, dCK has a wide-ranging substrate specificity, with a much higher activity to deoxycytidine than to deoxyadenosine and deoxyguanosine; however, clofarabine is reported to be a better substrate of dCK than deoxycytidine. As a second-generation halogen-decorated purine analog, it was designed to be resistant to adenosine deaminase. Clofarabine increases intracellular concentrations of cytarabine triphosphate to potentiate cytarabine cytotoxicity.

Clofarabine mimics adenosine and works in the following ways: (a) incorporated into DNA to cause DNA strand breaks, (b) inhibits DNA polymerase, (c) inhibits ribonucleotide reductase (RNR M1 subunit), (d) induces cellular apoptosis via induction of mitochondrial damage, and (e) at low doses, it has hypomethylating activity.

Clofarabine (52 mg/m^2 daily for 5 days IV) received accelerated approval by the FDA in 2004 for the treatment of pediatric patients 1 to 21 years old with relapsed or refractory ALL after at least two prior regimens. The composite CR rate was ~20% with ~10 weeks' duration of CR. Although clofarabine has been investigated for treatment of younger and older patients with AML as monotherapy or in combination with other agents, it has NOT been approved for AML treatment.

- Important adverse events of clofarabine include:
  - Severe myelosuppression resulting in prolonged neutropenia, anemia, and thrombocytopenia causing febrile neutropenia and sepsis in more than 80% of patients; PCP prophylaxis until CD4 count >200 cells/μL is recommended.
  - Dermatologic toxicities including palmar-plantar erythrodysesthesia (~15%), pruritus (~45%), skin rash (~40%), and rare but serious and fatal cases of Stevens-Johnson syndrome and toxic epidermal necrolysis.
  - Capillary leak syndrome/systemic inflammatory response syndrome (rare but serious) manifests with tachypnea, tachycardia, pulmonary edema, hypotension; prophylactic steroids for prevention sometimes is used. Clofarabine should be discontinued if hypotension develops during the 5 days of administration.
  - Nephrotoxicity (increased serum creatinine in 50% of patients); for CrCl 30 to 60 mL/min, the dose should be reduced by 50%.

Nelarabine

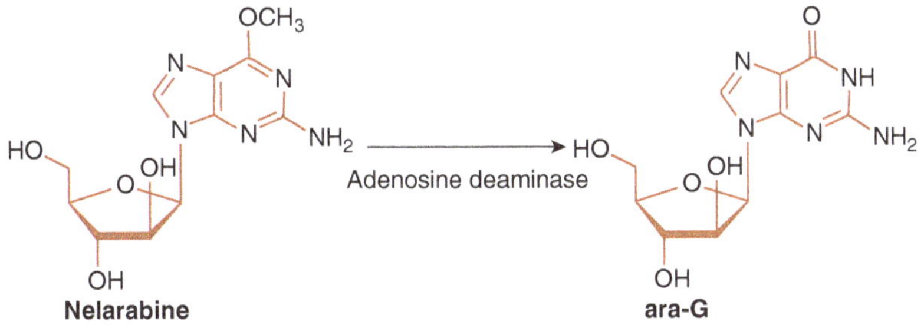

FIGURE 6.7 **Nelarabine (a prodrug) activation to guanosine arabinoside (ara-G).** Nelarabine is a prodrug that is demethylated by ADA to ara-G, which accumulates in higher concentrations in T-cells compared to B-cells. Intracellularly, it is monophosphorylated by dGk and dCK, and subsequently converted to the active 5′-triphosphate, ara-GTP.

Nelarabine mimics guanosine and works in the following ways: (a) it is incorporated into DNA to inhibit DNA primer extension leading to inhibition of DNA synthesis and inducing apoptosis, and (b) it inhibits RNR.

ADA, adenosine deaminase; ara-G, guanosine arabinoside; dCK, deoxycytidine kinase; dGK, deoxyguanosine kinase; RNR, ribonucleotide reductase.

- Important adverse events of nelarabine include:
  - Myelosuppression
  - Hepatotoxicity (elevated transaminases)
  - Fever
  - Dose-limiting toxicity: severe neurotoxicities include CNS toxicities such as severe somnolence, convulsions, and peripheral neuropathy ranging from numbness and paresthesias to motor weakness and paralysis. Adverse reactions associated with demyelination, and ascending peripheral neuropathies similar in appearance to Guillain-Barré syndrome may also occur. Full recovery from these adverse reactions has not always occurred with cessation of therapy with nelarabine. Nelarabine must be discontinued for neurologic adverse reactions of NCI Common Toxicity Criteria for Adverse Events (CTCAE) Grade 2 or greater.

A few examples of nelarabine-containing chemotherapy regimens include:
- Monotherapy (a 1,500 mg/m^2 IV over 2 hours on days 1, 3, and 5 repeated every 21 days) for relapsed or refractory T-cell acute lymphoblastic leukemia T-ALL and T-cell lymphoblastic lymphoma T-LBL in pediatric and adult patients
- Children's Oncology Group reported the results of AALL0434, a phase III RCT testing nelarabine in newly diagnosed T-ALL. The trial enrolled 1,562 evaluable patients with T-ALL age 1–31 years who received the augmented Berlin-Frankfurt-Muenster (ABFM) regimen with a 2×2 pseudo-factorial randomization to receive escalating-dose methotrexate without leucovorin rescue plus pegaspargase or high-dose methotrexate with leucovorin rescue.

After induction, intermediate- and high-risk patients were also randomly assigned to receive or not receive six 5-day courses of nelarabine incorporated into aBFM. The 5-year disease-free survival (DFS) rates for patients receiving nelarabine ($N = 323$) and no nelarabine ($N = 336$) were ~88%, and ~82% respectively ($P = 0.029$). Patients treated with escalating-dose methotrexate without leucovorin rescue plus pegaspargase plus nelarabine had a 5-year DFS of 91% ($N = 147$). Of note, nelarabine is NOT approved for frontline treatment of T-ALL/T-LBL.

Pentostatin

Pentostatin mimics adenosine and is a potent inhibitor of ADA with subsequent accumulation of dATP, which causes: (a) inhibition of RNR resulting in decreased formation of other deoxyribonucleotides such as dCTP and dGTP to slow DNA synthesis and alter DNA replication and repair, and (b) inhibition of adenosyl homocysteine hydrolase, resulting in decreased cellular S-adenosyl methionine (SAM) preventing cellular methylation reactions needed for cell proliferation.

In general, pentostatin is well-tolerated. Adverse events include myelosuppression, elevated transaminases, nausea, and renal toxicity; it is primarily renally eliminated (40%–80%) and requires dose reduction in renal impairment. Pentostatin may cause CNS toxicity.

A few examples of pentostatin-containing chemotherapy regimens include:
- Monotherapy (4 mg/m^2 once every 2 weeks) for treatment of untreated and interferon alfa-refractory hairy cell leukemia in patients with active disease (clinically significant anemia, neutropenia, thrombocytopenia, or disease-related symptoms)
- In combination with cyclophosphamide and rituximab for CLL
- Monotherapy (4 mg/m^2 once weekly for 3 weeks, then 4 mg/m^2 once every 2 weeks for 6 weeks, then 4 mg/m^2 once a month for a maximum of 6 months) for treatment of cutaneous T-cell lymphoma or mycosis fungoides/Sezary syndrome
- For treatment of steroid-refractory GvHD
- For treatment of refractory T-cell large granular lymphocytic (LGL) syndrome
- With or without alemtuzumab, for treatment of refractory T-cell prolymphocytic leukemia

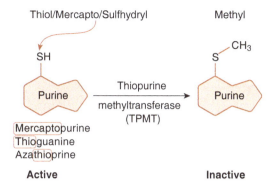

FIGURE 6.8 Polymorphism in thiopurine methyltransferase (TPMT).
Substituting oxygen with sulfur has been one strategy to generate fake nucleic acids, which possess antineoplastic activity. These agents are called thiopurine or thiopyrimidine. TPMT is a cytoplasmic enzyme that methylates (i.e., adds CH_3 group) aromatic compounds such as the thiopurine drugs 6-MP, 6-thioguanine, and azathioprine and inactivates them. The thiopurine drugs are used to treat ALL or organ transplant patients. TPMT is also discussed in Chapter 2.

The *TPMT* gene is highly polymorphic. Checking the TPMT genetic polymorphism represents one of the first examples in which testing for a genetic variant of a drug-metabolizing enzyme has entered standard clinical practice. Genetic polymorphisms in TPMT result in trimodal distribution of TPMT activity in the population: low (0.3%), intermediate (11.1%), and high (88.6%). Patients with low TPMT activity are at increased risk for thiopurine-induced myelotoxicity including severe neutropenia and thrombocytopenia as well as severe mucositis. The dose of thiopurine drugs in patients with low and intermediate TPMT activity needs to be reduced and a CBC needs to be checked frequently.

6-MP and thioguanine are available as oral tablets or suspensions. 6-MP is also metabolized to inactive metabolite by xanthine oxidase; hence, 6-MP requires significant dose reductions (by 75%) if given concomitantly with xanthine oxidase inhibitors such as allopurinol or febuxostat that are commonly used for the treatment/prevention of hyperuricemia.

ALL, acute lymphoblastic leukemia; CBC. complete blood count; 6-MP, 6-mercaptopurine; TPMT, thiopurine methyltransferase.

RIBONUCLEOTIDE REDUCTASE INHIBITION

Ribonucleotide reductase is a critical enzyme in the intracellular metabolism of pyrimidines and purines responsible for reducing ribose to deoxyribose and making deoxyribonucleotides for eventual incorporation into newly synthesized DNA. Inhibition of ribonucleotide reductase leads to decreased formation of deoxynueotides with resultant cell cycle arrest in mid-to-late G1 phase, impeding entry into S phase with consequent impairment of DNA replication and repair.

Deoxyribonucleotide triphosphates (dNTP) are required for DNA synthesis and de novo pathway for dNTP synthesis is through the reduction of the C2′-OH bond of ribonucleotides to deoxyribonucleotides.

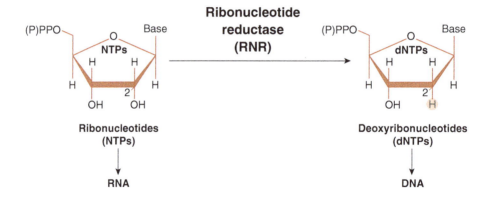

FIGURE 6.9 Ribonucleotide reductase (RNR) is responsible for synthesizing deoxyribonucleotides, which is the sugar building block of DNA.

dNTP, deoxyribonucleoside triphosphate; NTP, nucleoside triphosphate.

HYDROXYUREA

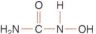

- Hydroxyurea (also known as hydroxycarbamide) was first synthesized in 1869 by two German medicinal chemists and received its initial approval in 1967 as an anticancer drug for noncurative treatment of multiple solid tumors and hematologic neoplasms.
- The mechanism of antineoplastic action of hydroxyurea is inhibition of ribonucleotide reductase (RNR), particularly RNR-M2 subunit, which is responsible for converting ribonucleotides to deoxyribonucleotides (Figure 6.9) exerting its major impact prior to DNA synthesis.
- Its modern uses in oncology include:
  - Control of hyperleukocytosis in the setting of acute leukemias and accelerated/blast phase of chronic myeloid leukemia. Doses are titrated to changes in peripheral white blood cell (WBC) count.
  - Cytoreductive therapy in Philadelphia chromosome-negative myeloproliferative neoplasms (primarily essential thrombocythemia [ET] and polycythemia vera [PV]). Hydroxyurea was shown to be superior to anagrelide for the control of ET.
  - Control of leukocytosis or splenomegaly in systemic mastocytosis with an associated hematologic neoplasm (SM-AHN).
  - Radiosensitization for head and neck cancers by maintaining cells in the radiation-sensitive G1 phase and interfering with D-A repair.
- In addition to RNR inhibition, hydroxyurea has diverse set of mechanisms (Figure 6.10). FDA-approved hydroxyurea (oral tablet/capsule) for the treatment of sickle cell disease (SCD) in 1998, and since then hydroxyurea remains a vital drug in the pharmacologic treatment of SCD. For SCD, the initial dose is 15 mg/kg once daily with blood counts monitoring every 2 weeks; and if blood counts in acceptable range, increase by 5 mg/kg/day every 8–12 weeks until the maximum tolerated dose of 35 mg/kg/day.

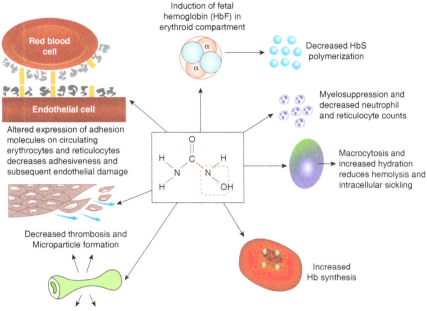

FIGURE 6.10 Effects and mechanisms of action of hydroxyurea in sickle cell disease.

In sickle cell disease, hydroxyurea increases HbF via intermittent cytotoxic suppression of erythroid progenitors that affect the kinetics of erythropoiesis, leading to recruitment of erythroid progenitors with increased HbF levels. Free radical formation, iron chelation, activation of soluble guanylyl cyclase, and direct nitric oxide production are among other mechanisms of hydroxyurea in the management of sickle cell disease.

Hb, hemoglobin; HbF, hemoglobin F.

- Common adverse events of hydroxyurea include macrocytosis, myelosuppression (primarily leukopenia), nausea, dermatologic disorders with long-term therapy (hyperpigmentation, maculopapular eruption, dry skin, foot ulcer), and mucocutaneous vasculitis with high doses.

ASPARAGINASE

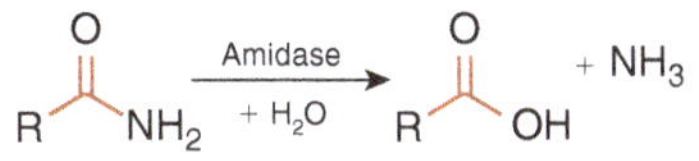

FIGURE 6.11 Asparaginase is an amidohydrolase enzyme.

Asparaginases are enzymes that catalyze the conversion of amides to carboxylic acid and ammonia; hence, they are amidohydrolases.

Two "amide-containing" amino acids in humans are Gln and Asn. Asparaginases convert Asn and Gln to aspartate and glutamate, respectively, decreasing plasma concentrations of Asn and Gln.

(continued)

FIGURE 6.11 **Asparaginase is an amidohydrolase enzyme. (*continued*)**

Bacteria, including *Escherichia coli (E. coli), Dickeya dadantii* (also called *Erwinia chrysanthemi), Helicobacter pylori, Pectobacterium carotovorum, Mycobacterium bovis, Streptomyces griseus, Acinetobacter, Proteus vulgaris, Serratia marcescens, Vibrio succinogenes, Nocardia spp., Wolinella succinogenes, Bacillus subtilis, Pseudomonas* strains have been the sources for L-asparaginase extraction. Although not clinically available, L-asparaginase has been isolated from guinea pigs as well as from humans.

The Km of the *E. coli*-derived asparaginase and *Erwinia* asparaginase for Asn are 1.15×10^{-5} M and $5.8–8.0 \times 10^{-5}$ M, respectively, which suggests the higher affinity of the *E. coli* enzyme for Asn. *Erwinia* asparaginase Km $1.7–6.7 \times 10^{-3}$ M appears to have greater glutaminase activity than *E. coli* asparaginase (Km $3.5–6.25 \times 10^{-3}$ M) for deamidation of Gln.

Of note, in vitro studies demonstrated that Gln depletion induced a dose-dependent reduction in cell proliferation in epithelial solid tumor cell lines including HCT116 p53+/+, HCT116 p53-/-, MDA-MD-231, MDA-MB-453, MCF7, TK10, A549, and T47D.

Asn, asparagine; Gln, glutamine.

Question: What is the unit for asparaginase activity? How is it measured?

Answer: One unit (U) or international unit (IU) of asparaginase is defined as the amount of enzyme that catalyzes the formation of 1.0 micromole (µM) of aspartate per minute at 25°C. Aspartate can be detected colorometrically ($\lambda = 570$ nm) or by fluorescence (Ex/Em = 535/590 nm) using a coupled enzymatic reaction.

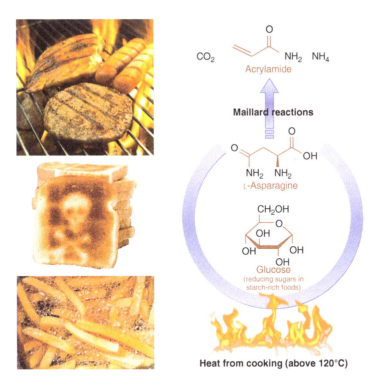

FIGURE 6.12 Asparaginase in medicine and in food industry.
Different asparaginases are approved by the FDA as *a component of a multi-agent chemotherapeutic regimen for treatment of pediatric and adult patients with ALL*.

The Maillard reaction occurs in high (140°C–165°C) temperatures between amino acids and sugars e.g., in starchy food; it produces a distinctive flavor in browned food such as baked potatoes, seared steaks, French fries, cookies, biscuits and breads, and so on. This reaction is the basis for many of the flavoring food recipes. At high temperatures, acrylamide can form. Acrylamide is considered the a potential carcinogen.

In addition to its medicinal use, L-asparaginase has been used in reducing the formation of acrylamide in food industry (e.g., Acrylaway® and PreventASe®).

ALL, acute lymphoblastic leukemia; FDA, U.S. Food and Drug Administration.

Question: What are the clinically available asparaginases?

Answer:

From E. coli: L-asparaginase is a tetrameric enzyme that is produced endogenously by *E. coli* and consists of identical 34.5 kDa subunits. Clinically used/available *E. coli*-derived asparaginases include:
- short-acting L-asparaginase (not commercially available anymore in the United States)
- pegaspargase (Oncaspar): currently the most commonly used product as a component of a multi-agent chemotherapeutic regimen for treatment of pediatric and adult patients with first-line ALL.

○ Pegaspargase was used in the seminal and paradigm-shifting clinical trial CALGB-10403. In this trial, 295 patients (age range 17–39 years) with Philadelphia chromosome-negative ALL were enrolled in a pediatric-inspired regimen. Overall treatment-related mortality was 3%. Median event-free survival (EFS) was ~78 months (95% CI, 41.8 to not reached), more than double the historical control of 30 months (95% CI, 22–38 months); 3-year EFS was 59% (95% CI, 54–65%). Median overall survival (OS) was not reached. Estimated 3-year OS was 73% (95% CI, 68–78%). Pretreatment risk factors associated with worse treatment outcomes included obesity and the presence of the Philadelphia-like gene expression signature.

- Calaspargase pegol–mknl (Asparlas) is approved as a component of a multi-agent chemotherapeutic regimen for the treatment of ALL in pediatric and young adult patients age 1 month to 21 years. In this asparaginase, the linker between the enzyme (L-asparaginase) and monomethoxypolyethylene glycol (mPEG) is a succinimidyl carbonate (SC), which is a chemically stable carbamate bond between the mPEG moiety and the lysine groups of the protein.

From Erwinia chrysanthemi (also called **Crisantaspase***; due to several biochemical and clinical differences between asparaginases with different bacterial sources and hopefully to remove confusion, asparaginase produced by* Erwinia chrysanthemi *is known as crisantaspase):*

- Erwinaze: not available anymore due to manufacturing issues
- Asparaginase *Erwinia chrysanthemi* (recombinant-rywn; Rylaze) is approved as a component of a multi-agent chemotherapeutic regimen for the treatment of ALL and LBL in adult and pediatric patients 1 month or older who have developed hypersensitivity to *E. coli*-derived asparaginase.
- Pegcrisantaspase (PegC; recombinant pegylated crisantaspase that has been used in pediatric patients with ALL and currently under investigation [with promising results] in combination with venetoclax in early-phase clinical trials for patients with relapsed/refractory AML [NCT04666649])
- A PASylated (proline/alanine/serine) *Erwinia* asparaginase is currently in the pre-clinical pipeline, potentially providing hope for a long-acting *Erwinia* asparaginase in the future without hypersensitivity to PEG-driven antibodies.

Glutamine

FIGURE 6.13 Glutamine.
Gln is the most abundant amino acid in the intracellular compartment, with tissue concentrations of ~20 mM, depending on the tissue. Gln is also the most abundant amino acid in human plasma, with concentrations ranging from 300 to 900 µM.

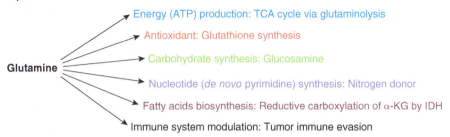

Glutamine
- Energy (ATP) production: TCA cycle via glutaminolysis
- Antioxidant: Glutathione synthesis
- Carbohydrate synthesis: Glucosamine
- Nucleotide (*de novo* pyrimidine) synthesis: Nitrogen donor
- Fatty acids biosynthesis: Reductive carboxylation of α-KG by IDH
- Immune system modulation: Tumor immune evasion

Interference with Gln metabolism has been shown to overcome resistance to Bcl-2 inhibition in AML and other cell types.

The synergistic anti-AML activity of the combination of the Bcl-2 inhibitor Ven and PegC in complex karyotype AML has been reported with very promising preclinical activity. The mechanism of the Ven–PegC regimen is mediated through depletion of Gln induced by PegC, which would not only inhibit proliferation of AML cells but also enhance the antiapoptotic activity of Ven-mediated antagonism of Bcl-2 in myeloblasts by decreasing the expression of proteins such as MCL-1, whose translation is dependent on eukaryotic translation initiation factor 4E (eIF4E)- eIF4E-binding protein (4EBP1) interaction. The inhibition of 4E-BP1 phosphorylation results in decreased mRNA translation and protein synthesis selectively in AML cells.

AML, acute myeloid leukemia; Gln, glutamine; mRNA, messenger RNA; PegC, pegcrisantaspase; Ven, venetoclax.

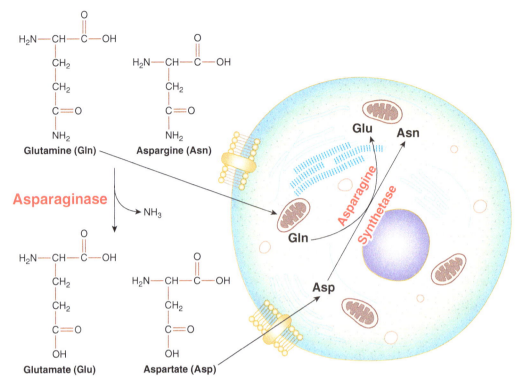

Blood

FIGURE 6.14 Asparaginases, as amidohydrolases, possess both asparaginase and glutaminase activity and deplete plasma asparagine and glutamine.
When Asn levels are low, ASNS catalyzes transamination of Gln to aspartate, resulting in production of glutamate and Asn. ALL cells generally exhibit little to no detectable ASNS expression, which makes ALL cells auxotrophs for Asn and renders them particularly sensitive to Asn depletion.

ALL, acute lymphoblastic leukemia; Asn, asparagine; ASNS, asparagine synthetase; Gln, glutamine.

TABLE 6.1 Recommendation on Dosing, Monitoring, and Management of Asparaginase Administration

ASDPARAGINASE-RELATED ISSUE	DOSING/MONITORING/MANAGEMENT
Dosing strategies	• Pegaspargase (2,000–2,500 IU/m^2 intravenously [IV]) capped at one vial (3,750 IU) for all non clinical trial adult patients • Rylaze: Two regimens can be used to replace a long-acting asparaginase product: (1) 25 mg/m^2 intramuscularly (IM) every 48 hours × six doses, (2) 25 mg/m^2 IM on Monday morning and Wednesday morning and 50 mg/m^2 on Friday afternoon × 2 weeks (six doses)

(continued)

TABLE 6.1 Recommendation on Dosing, Monitoring, and Management of Asparaginase Administration (*continued*)

ASDPARAGINASE-RELATED ISSUE	DOSING/MONITORING/MANAGEMENT
Hypersensitivity reactions	• Premedication with acetaminophen, hydrocortisone, and diphenhydramine to decrease the probability of hypersensitivity reactions • Permanent discontinuation of pegaspargase and switching to crisantaspase (Rylaze, asparaginase *Erwinia chrysanthemi*) for patients who experience a grade 3 or higher severe hypersensitivity reaction
Hepatotoxicity	• Monitor aspartate aminotransferase (AST), alanine aminotransferase (ALT), total bilirubin, and direct bilirubin at baseline and weekly for at least 4 weeks after each pegaspargase dose. • If direct bilirubin >3 mg/dL or liver function tests (LFTs) >3 × the upper limit of normal (ULN), administer vitamin B complex one tablet by mouth (PO) twice daily and L-carnitine 50 mg/kg/day IV (or PO) in six divided doses daily. • Patients with asparaginase/crisantaspase-induced hyperbilirubinemia or transaminitis may receive asparaginase/crisantaspase in subsequent cycles of treatment if the bilirubin/AST/ALT return to normal range and potential clinical benefit outweighs risk.
Pancreatitis	• Monitor amylase and lipase at baseline, 2–3 days after administration of asparaginase/crisantaspase, then weekly for at least 4 weeks after each asparaginase/crisantaspase dose. • Permanently discontinue asparaginase/crisantaspase in patients who develop clinical pancreatitis (e.g., severe abdominal pain) with amylase/lipase elevation >3 × ULN for >3 days and/or develop pancreatic pseudocyst. It is recommended that these patients not receive any other asparaginase/crisantaspase products.
Hemorrhage	• Monitor fibrinogen at baseline and 2–3 times weekly for at least 4 weeks after the initial dose of asparaginase/crisantaspase and up to three times per week as needed for at least 4 weeks for each subsequent dose. If fibrinogen <80 mg/dL, replete with 1 unit of cryoprecipitate. Administration of cryoprecipitate is somewhat controversial due to increased risk of thrombosis. • Withhold subsequent asparaginase/crisantaspase doses for >grade 2 hemorrhage in conjunction with hypofibrinogenemia until toxicity <grade 1 as defined by Common Terminology Criteria for Adverse Events (CTCAE).

(continued)

TABLE 6.1 Recommendation on Dosing, Monitoring, and Management of Asparaginase Administration (*continued*)

ASDPARAGINASE-RELATED ISSUE	DOSING/MONITORING/MANAGEMENT
Thromboprophylaxis	• Administration of enoxaparin to all patients for at least 4 weeks after each pegaspargase dose: enoxaparin 40 mg subcutaneously (SQ) daily for patients <80 kg; enoxaparin 60 mg SQ daily for patients >80 kg. Patients must meet the following criteria: not already receiving therapeutic anticoagulation; platelet count >30,000/μL; absence of significant bleeding; creatinine clearance >30 mL/min. • Monitor antithrombin III level at baseline and twice weekly for at least 4 weeks after each asparaginase/crisantaspase dose (or until two sequential levels normalize to >50%). Replete antithrombin III when level is ≤50%. • Antithrombin III dose = ([80% − current antithrombin III level %] × body weight in kg)/1.4.

CHAPTER SUMMARY

This chapter addresses the clinical pharmacology of purine and pyrimidine antimetabolites that are commonly used for treatment of hematologic neoplasms and some solid tumors. The mechanism of action of each agent as well as their common or clinically important adverse events along with FDA-approved indications and commonly off-label administered regimens are described. Hydroxyurea, as one of the first developed chemotherapeutics with probably the simplest chemical structure, is still in clinical use benefiting subjects with sickle cell disease and as a universally used cytoreductive agent for treatment of acute leukemias and myeloproliferative neoplasms. This chapter comprehensively discusses hydroxyurea. Targeting amino acid metabolisms has been exploited for treatment of hematologic and solid malignancies. This chapter comprehensively and uniquely discusses different asparaginase products, their mechanism of action, FDA-approved indications and some novel combinations of asparaginases and crisantaspases for treatment of non-ALL cancers. The chapter also provides some guideline on dosing of asparaginases as well as monitoring and management of potential asparaginase/crisantaspase-related adverse events of interest.

CLINICAL PEARLS

- Antimetabolites are toxic to all cell types that are active in cell cycle and undergoing DNA synthesis. As such, normal oral and gastrointestinal mucosa, skin, and liver are susceptible to the cytotoxic effects of these drugs.
- 5-FU/capecitabine can induce a severe palmar-plantar erythrodysesthesia (hand-foot syndrome) associated with painful erythroderma and blistering. This can also occur with cytarabine and gemcitabine.
- Nelarabine can cause severe, and often irreversible, neurologic toxicities including sensory, motor, autonomic, and CNS adverse events.

- CNS toxicity associated with high-dose cytarabine can be severe and irreversible. Cerebellar testing including a handwriting sample and finger-nose examination is mandatory prior to each administration of high-dose cytarabine infusion and drug should be discontinued for any early signs of cerebellar dysfunction. Daily (and more frequently if clinically indicated) monitoring of kidney function is absolutely necessary during the administration of high-dose cytarabine.
- In chemotherapy regimens that combine cytarabine with cladribine or fludarabine or clofarabine, it is recommended that cytarabine be administered approximately 2–4 hours after these antimetabolites. These halogen-containing antimetabolites induce the intracellular expression of deoxycytidine kinase and, in theory, can enhance the cytotoxic effect of cytarabine.
- Prophylaxis against PJP is recommended after administration of T-cell toxic halogen-containing antimetabolites.

MULTIPLE-CHOICE QUESTIONS

1. A 44-year-old woman with leukocytosis/lymphocytosis and cervical lymphadenopathy (LAD) was diagnosed with chronic lymphocytic leukemia (CLL). Her CLL has 13q deletion and mutated immunoglobulin heavy-chain gene rearrangement CLL. She received six cycles of FCR (fludarabine, cyclophosphamide, and rituximab) and achieved complete remission with complete resolution of lymphadenopathy and splenomegaly along with normalization of WBC and platelet counts. However, the patient reports severe fatigue and mild dyspnea on exertion. CBC shows hemoglobin 4.8 g/dL. What is the most likely reason for her profound anemia?

    A. Autoimmune hemolytic anemia
    B. Minimal residual disease in bone marrow
    C. Fludarabine-induced GI microperforation
    D. Cyclophosphamide-induced myelodysplasia
    E. Rituximab-induced hemagglutination

2. A 48-year-old hematologic oncologist is receiving 7-day administration of cladribine (0.1 mg/kg/day by continuous IV infusion) for his recently diagnosed hairy cell leukemia. His fatigue and splenomegaly are already improved after day 4. On day 6, he develops fever of 101.1°F. He is hemodynamically stable and he complains of no specific symptoms. Examination is unremarkable. Chest x-ray is negative. CBC shows WBC count 2,200/μL, absolute neutrophil count (ANC) 1,050/μL, hemoglobin 8.9 g/dL, and platelet count 74,000/μL. Blood and urine cultures are pending. What is the most likely etiology of his fever?

    A. Zoster reactivation
    B. PCP pneumonia
    C. Cladribine-induced fever
    D. Neutropenic fever
    E. Splenic infarction

3. A 54-year-old man with history of pT3N1M0 colon adenocarcinoma is undergoing adjuvant chemotherapy with FOLFOX. The second day of chemo, he is admitted to the ED with severe chest pain. Echocardiographs before surgery (top) and in the ED (bottom) are shown. What it the most likely cause of this condition?

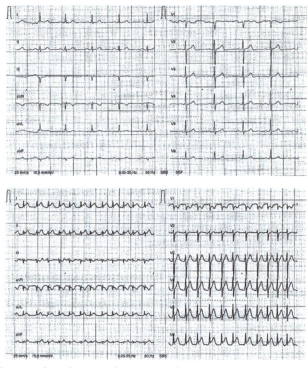

A. Oxaliplatin-induced sympathetic stimulation
B. 5-FU–induced coronary vasospasm
C. Hypersensitivity reaction to leucovorin
D. Rapid infusion of oxaliplatin

4. A 59-year-old man is receiving capecitabine (1,500 mg orally twice daily, 2 weeks on, 1 week off) as adjuvant chemotherapy for his high-risk stage II colon cancer (T4N0M0, microsatellite stable). Ten days after the first dose of capecitabine, he is admitted for severe nausea/vomiting, mucositis, diarrhea, acute kidney injury (AKI), and coronary vasospasm. He is not dihydropyrimidine dehydrogenase deficient. His son is telling you that he wanted to defeat cancer to the last cell. With that aim in mind, he was taking capecitabine at 3,000 mg orally twice daily three times a week. In the next few days, his clinical situation is deteriorating. Your fellow is seeking an antidote. Which of the following agents has shown efficacy in this setting?

A. IV leucovorin
B. Dexrazoxane (Zinecard)
C. Uridine triacetate
D. Glucarpidase
E. Anti-fluoropyrimidine antibody

5. A middle-aged man with diagnosis of AML with inv(16) has achieved complete remission with induction therapy. Consolidation therapy with high-dose cytarabine (HiDAC), 3,000 mg/m^2, twice daily on days 1 to 6 was started for him. The patient lives in the Ohio River Valley. He has not taken his acyclovir prophylaxis due to musculoskeletal pain. Also, due to significant insurance copay, he has not taken his posaconazole for history of fungal pneumonia. Laboratory tests at the beginning of treatment were normal, except for a creatinine of 1.7 mg/dL. Three days after admission, the patient complained of minimal gait disturbance. The next day, he developed ataxia, nystagmus, and dysarthria. What is the most likely diagnosis?

   A. Cytarabine-induced cerebellar toxicity
   B. CNS tumor lysis of resistant AML stem cells
   C. *Histoplasma* meningitis
   D. Herpes simplex virus encephalitis
   E. CNS leukemia with core binding factor cytogenetic abnormality

6. JM is a 22-year-old man with T-cell acute lymphoblastic leukemia (ALL), who has been treated based on a pediatric-inspired protocol and has achieved complete remission with minimal residual disease negativity after induction therapy. In the interim maintenance phase of the protocol, during infusion of L-asparaginase, he develops a localized and transient erythematous rash on his chest and abdominal areas. Which one of the following is true?

   A. Development of anti-asparaginase IgG without clinical hypersensitivity may lead to a reduction in clinical effect.
   B. The risk of infusion reaction is higher when L-asparaginase is infused with vincristine and prednisone.
   C. Pegylated asparaginase (pegaspargase) is the most immunogenic formulation of asparaginase.
   D. The rate of infusion reaction is higher with intramuscular injection compared with IV injection.

7. Which one of the following sequential chemotherapy administrations does NOT increase the efficacy of the regimen by synergism between the chemotherapeutic components of each regimen?

   A. High-dose methotrexate before high-dose cytarabine in even courses of hyper-CVAD regimen
   B. Cytarabine starting 2 hours after cladribine in CLAG-M
   C. Cytarabine 4 hours after fludarabine in FLAG-Ida
   D. Asparaginase after methotrexate in pediatric-inspired protocol for treatment of ALL
   E. Oxaliplatin before 5-FU (bolus and continuous) in FOLFOX

8. A 27-year-old woman with Philadelphia chromosome-negative B-cell acute lymphoblastic leukemia (ALL) is receiving her second dose of pegaspargase during consolidation course of the pediatric-inspired protocol CALGB10403. She achieved minimal residual disease (MRD) negative complete remission (CR) after the induction. Approximately 20 minutes after start of pegaspargase *fluoropyrimidine* or *thiopurine* infusion, she becomes

severely short of breath with generalized rash. Physical exam showed oxygen saturation of 84% on room air, stridor, and bilateral wheezing. Rapid response team is called. After administration of IV H1 and H2 blockers and 250 mg of methylprednisolone, she started recovering and intubation was not needed. The patient and family are concerned about future administration of pegaspargase, but they do not want to decrease the probability of cure. What is the best course of action moving forward?

A. Future pegaspargase administration should be intramuscular.
B. Due to severe and life-threatening anaphylactic reaction, all asparaginase products are contraindicated for future use. This will not result in statistically significant inferior clinical outcome.
C. Replace pegaspargase with crisantaspase.
D. Replace pegaspargase with calaspargase pegol-mknl.

9. For patients with lymphoproliferative neoplasms receiving definitive chemotherapy with curative intent, for which agent is therapeutic drug monitoring (TDM) indicated and shown to improve clinical outcomes in randomized clinical trials?

A. Asparaginase
B. Cyclophosphamide
C. Blinatumomab
D. Fludarabine (when combined with venetoclax)

10. A 55-year-old man is treated with capecitabine for his colon cancer. He develops numbness in his palms and soles, which are followed by symmetrical tender redness of the fat pads of his proximal phalanges. He asks about this situation. Which of the following statements accurately address his question?

A. Genetic testing for polymorphism for dihydropyrimidine dehydrogenase (DPD) and thymidylate synthase (TS) is standard of care and can avoid this adverse event.
B. Fluctuation in plasma level of capecitabine is more frequently associated with the incidence of acral erythema.
C. His symptoms are not dose related.
D. He may lose his fingerprints.

ANSWERS TO MULTIPLE-CHOICE QUESTIONS

1. **A.** Autoimmune cytopenia, particularly autoimmune hemolytic anemia and autoimmune thrombocytopenia, are observed in 5% to 10% of patients with CLL. Fludarabine can induce autoimmune hemolytic anemia (AIHA), which is not common but can be severe and fatal, particularly if a patient is re-treated with fludarabine after a prior episode of AIHA. This may be due to fludarabine-induced release of a suppressed autoantibody to a native red blood cell antigen. GI microperforation is not a side effect specific to fludarabine. Rituximab is the first-line treatment for cold AIHA and second-line treatment for warm AIHA. It does not induce hemagglutination.

2. **C.** Cladribine-induced fever. Fever is a common drug-related side effect of cladribine and may occur after the dose is given. The patient is still receiving cladribine on the day he spikes a fever, so the cause is most likely drug-related. Zoster reactivation presents

with a painful unilateral vesicular eruption. Fever may accompany the reactivation but is rare, thus making option A unlikely. Patients receiving purine analog therapy (i.e., cladribine, fludarabine) and T-cell depleting therapy are particularly at high risk for developing PCP. For cancer patients, the time frame to develop PCP is at least a few weeks after starting chemotherapy treatment, which makes option B incorrect. In order to meet the definition of febrile neutropenia per National Comprehensive Cancer Network (NCCN) guidelines, the absolute neutrophil count (ANC) must be <500 neutrophils/μL or <1,000 neutrophils/μL and a predicted decline to <500/μL over the next 48 hours. The patient currently does not meet the definition of neutropenia. Splenic infarction may present with a fever, but affected patients are also symptomatic with symptoms such as acute upper-quadrant pain and tenderness, nausea, or vomiting. The patient did not complain of any of these specific clinical symptoms.

3. **B.** 5-FU (5-fluorouracil) and capecitabine are associated with cardiotoxicity that presents as chest pain, acute coronary syndrome/myocardial infarction, or death. Cardiotoxicity tends to occur during the first cycle of administration with symptoms initiating 12 hours following infusion but can occur any time up to 1 to 2 days after infusion. It is proposed that coronary vasospasm leads to 5-FU–related myocardial ischemia. The coronary vasospasm may have echocardiogram findings that suggest coronary occlusion such as ST-segment elevation, other ST-T abnormalities, and troponin elevation. Only case reports have been published about oxaliplatin echocardiogram changes making options A and D unlikely. Hypersensitivity to leucovorin is rare. Case reports have described patients commonly presenting with flushing, hives, headaches, body pain, and elevated blood pressure. Chest pain is possible, but a very uncommon presentation.

4. **C.** Uridine triacetate (Vistogard) is a pyrimidine analog that was FDA approved in 2015 for the emergency treatment of adult and pediatric patients following 5-fluorouracil (5-FU) or capecitabine overdose regardless of the presence of symptoms. It is also approved for patients who exhibit early-onset, severe, or life-threatening toxicity affecting the cardiac or central nervous system, and/or early-onset, unusually severe adverse reactions within 96 hours following the end of 5-FU or capecitabine administration. The adult dosing is 10 g (1 packet) orally every 6 hours for 20 doses. The reaction below shows conversion of uridine triacetate:

Leucovorin is used to prevent the toxicities of high-dose methotrexate. Dexrazoxane is used for both prevention of cardiotoxicity from anthracycline-based chemotherapy and for prevention of tissue injury after anthracycline extravasation. Glucarpidase is a recombinant bacterial enzyme that is a rescue agent for patients with toxic plasma methotrexate concentrations in patients with delayed methotrexate excretion and impaired renal function.

5.   **A.** Major side effects associated with high-dose cytarabine include acute cerebellar toxicity that can present with symptoms such as ataxia and dysarthria. Renal insufficiency defined as serum creatinine ≥1.5 mg/dL or an increase in serum creatinine >0.5 mg/dL is a risk factor for high-dose cytarabine-induced neurotoxicity. As such, patients with renal dysfunction prior to starting therapy should have their cytarabine doses reduced. All patients receiving high-dose cytarabine are at a risk for cerebellar toxicity, regardless of renal function, so it is imperative to perform cerebellar assessments daily while on therapy. Immunocompromised patients who live in the Ohio and Mississippi River valleys are at risk for developing *Histoplasma* infection. At the beginning of consolidation, the absolute neutrophil count (ANC) is normal, which makes the likelihood of fungal infection like *Histoplasma* unlikely. Herpes simplex virus (HSV) encephalitis often presents with a rapid onset of fever, headache, seizures, impaired consciousness, and focal neurologic signs. His symptoms are not consistent with HSV encephalitis.

6.   **A.** Development of anti-asparaginase IgG without clinical hypersensitivity may lead to a reduction in clinical effect. If IgG anti-l-asparaginase antibodies develop, they can lead to reduced efficacy of l-asparaginase. Repeated exposure to asparaginase products increases the risk of developintramuscularng neutralizing anti-asparaginase antibodies that may not produce clinical symptoms of allergic reaction but may reduce overall efficacy by inhibiting enzymatic activity. This is called "silent hypersensitivity" or "deactivation." The risk of infusion reaction would be lower when l-asparaginase is infused with vincristine and prednisone, since prednisone (or any steroid) will mask the infusion reaction. Pegaspargase is polyethylene glycol covalently linked to the asparaginase structure. This formulation decreases immunogenicity and prolongs the half-life. The use of intramuscular injection of l-asparaginase is well tolerated and does not appear to result in increased hypersensitivity reaction.

7.   **E.** Oxaliplatin before 5-FU (bolus and continuous) in FOLFOX does not increase the effect of 5-FU. The active form of ara-C is the triphosphorylated derivative ara-CTP, which is a nucleotide that inhibits DNA polymerase. Upon entry of ara-C into the cell, the initial phosphorylation is by deoxycytidine kinase to ara-C monophosphate (ara-CMP). Synergistic killing of human leukemic cells is seen when methotrexate is given before cytarabine. Methotrexate at high doses leads to decrease in deoxycytidine triphosphate (dCTP) pools and less inhibition of deoxycytidine kinase. Drugs that lower dCTP are expected to produce greater quantities of ara-CMP and lead to higher quantities of the cytotoxic ara-CTP. Thus, methotrexate administration prior to cytarabine allows for enhanced intracellular phosphorylation of cytarabine and increased killing of cells. Administering cladribine before cytarabine decreases all concentrations of deoxynucleotide triphosphates (dNTPs). This, in turn, increases the activity of deoxycytidine kinase and results in accumulation of ara-CMP and ultimately ara-CTP in leukemic cells. Infusion of fludarabine before ara-C augments the rate of ara-CTP synthesis in circulating AML blasts during therapy. Methotrexate is

transported into the cell via the human-reduced folate carrier, folate receptor system, and pH-sensitive transporter. Once intracellular, methotrexate is polyglutamated to increase the potency of dihydrofolate reductase (DHFR) inhibition. Since asparaginase deletes glutamine and asparagine supply within the cell, asparaginase must be given *after* methotrexate. Otherwise, glutamine supply is depleted prior to methotrexate administration and DHFR inhibition is compromised.

8. **C.** Development of hypersensitivity reaction to *E. coli*-derived asparaginase should preclude the future use of both IV and intramuscular administration of *E. coli*-derived asparaginase. Crisantaspase (asparaginase *Erwinia chrysanthemi* (recombinant)-rywn) is approved and indicated for the exact indication to be administered as a component of a multiagent chemotherapeutic regimen for the treatment ALL and lymphoblastic lymphoma in adult and pediatric patients 1 month or older who have developed hypersensitivity to *E. coli*-derived asparaginase.

9. **A.** Comparison of fixed dose (FD) versus individualized dose of *E. coli*-derived asparaginase in treatment of ALL and performing TDM based on nadir serum asparaginase activity (NSAA) resulted in a superior 5-year event-free survival (90% vs. 82% for FD; $p = .04$) in favor of individualized dosing. NSAA <0.1 IU/mL despite dose adjustment or when coupled with *E. coli*-derived asparaginase antibody positivity is called "silent inactivation" and switching to is recommended.

10. **D.** Fingerprints, also called dermatoglyphics, are characterized by the pattern of ridges and furrows on the fingertips. Capecitabine can cause loss of fingerprints, which is also called adermatoglyphia. Hand-foot syndrome always precedes the onset of fingerprint loss. Adermatoglyphia can occur as early as 2 weeks to as late as 4 years after starting capecitabine. Ramifications include inability to process government documents or obtain a driver's license, or inability to access telephone, computer, or other device that requires fingerprint identification scanning. Adermatoglyphia can be reversible for some individuals but not all. Genetic testing for polymorphism for DPD and thymidylate synthase is NOT standard of care.

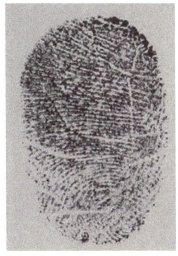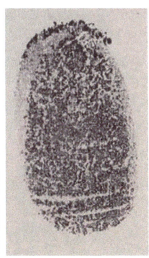

A   Before treatment   B   After treatment

SELECTED REFERENCES

Avramis VI. Asparaginases: A successful class of drugs against leukemias and lymphomas. J Pediatr Hematol Oncol. 2011;33(8):573–9. https://doi.org/10.1097/MPH.0b013e31823313be

Bade NA, Lu C, Patzke CL, et al. Optimizing pegylated asparaginase use: An institutional guideline for dosing, monitoring, and management. J Oncol Pharm Pract. 2020;26(1):74–92. https://doi.org/10.1177/1078155219838316

Chabner B, Longo D. Cancer Chemotherapy, Immunotherapy, and Biotherapy: Principles and Practice, 5th ed. Philadelphia: Wolters Kluwer; 2011.

Cheson BD, Vena DA, Foss FM, Sorensen JM. Neurotoxicity of purine analogs: A review. J Clin Oncol. 1994;12(10):2216–28. https://doi.org/10.1200/JCO.1994.12.10.2216

Damon LE, Mass R, Linker CA. The association between high-dose cytarabine neurotoxicity and renal insufficiency. J Clin Oncol. 1989;7(10):1563–8. https://doi.org/10.1200/JCO.1989.7.10.1563

Dillman RO, Davis RB, Green MR, et al. A comparative study of two different doses of cytarabine for acute myeloid leukemia: A phase III trial of cancer and leukemia group B. Blood. 1991;15;78(10):2520–6. https://doi.org/10.1182/blood.V78.10.2520.bloodjournal78102520

Emadi A. Exploiting AML vulnerability: Glutamine dependency. Blood. 2015;126(11):1269–70. https://doi.org/10.1182/blood-2015-07-659508

Emadi A, Jun SA, Tsukamoto T, et al. Inhibition of glutaminase selectively suppresses the growth of primary AML cells with IDH mutations. Exp Hematol. 2014;42(4):247–51. https://doi.org/10.1016/j.exphem.2013.12.001

Emadi A, Kapadia B, Bollino D, et al. Venetoclax and pegcrisantaspase for complex karyotype acute myeloid leukemia. Leukemia. 2021;35(7):1907–24. https://doi.org/10.1038/s41375-020-01080-6

Emadi A, Karp JE. The clinically relevant pharmacogenomic changes in acute myelogenous leukemia. Pharmacogenomics. 2012;13(11):1257–69. https://doi.org/10.2217/pgs.12.102

Emadi A, Law JY, Strovel ET, et al. Asparaginase Erwinia chrysanthemi effectively depletes plasma glutamine in adult patients with relapsed/refractory acute myeloid leukemia. Cancer Chemother Pharmacol. 2018;81(1):217–22. https://doi.org/10.1007/s00280-017-3459-6

Emadi A, Zokaee H, Sausville EA. Asparaginase in the treatment of non-ALL hematologic malignancies. Cancer Chemother Pharmacol. 2014;73(5):875–83. https://doi.org/10.1007/s00280-014-2402-3

Gandhi V, Estey E, Keating MJ, Plunkett W. Fludarabine potentiates metabolism of cytarabine in patients with acute myelogenous leukemia during therapy. J Clin Oncol. 1993;11(1):116–24. https://doi.org/10.1200/JCO.1993.11.1.116

Heidelberger C, Chaudhuri NK, Danneberg P, et al. Fluorinated pyrimidines, a new class of tumour-inhibitory compounds. Nature. 1957;179(4561):663–6. https://doi.org/10.1038/179663a0

Hirayama AV, Gauthier J, Hay KA, et al. The response to lymphodepletion impacts PFS in patients with aggressive non-Hodgkin lymphoma treated with CD19 CAR T cells. Blood. 2019;133(17):1876–87. https://doi.org/10.1182/blood-2018-11-887067

Ho PP, Milikin EB, Bobbitt JL, et al. Crystalline L-asparaginase from Escherichia coli B. I. Purification and chemical characterization. J Biol Chem. 1970;245(14):3708–15. https://doi.org/10.1016/S0021-9258(18)62984-9

Jacque N, Ronchetti AM, Larrue C, et al. Targeting glutaminolysis has antileukemic activity in acute myeloid leukemia and synergizes with BCL-2 inhibition. Blood. 2015;126(11):1346–56. https://doi.org/10.1182/blood-2015-01-621870

Kapadia B, Shetty AC, Bollino D, et al. Translatome changes in acute myeloid leukemia cells postexposure to pegcrisantaspase and venetoclax. Exp Hematol. 2022;108:55–63. https://doi.org/10.1016/j.exphem.2022.01.006

Kashanian SM, Holtzman NG, Patzke CL, et al. Venous thromboembolism incidence and risk factors in adults with acute lymphoblastic leukemia treated with and without pegylated E. coli asparaginase-containing regimens. Cancer Chemother Pharmacol. 2021;87(6):817–26. https://doi.org/10.1007/s00280-021-04252-y

Lancet JE, Uy GL, Cortes JE, et al. CPX-351 (cytarabine and daunorubicin) liposome for injection versus conventional cytarabine plus daunorubicin in older patients with newly diagnosed secondary acute myeloid leukemia. J Clin Oncol. 2018;36(26):2684–92. https://doi.org/10.1200/JCO.2017.77.6112

Mayer LD, Tardi P, Louie AC. CPX-351: A nanoscale liposomal co-formulation of daunorubicin and cytarabine with unique biodistribution and tumor cell uptake properties. Int J Nanomedicine. 2019;14:3819–30. https://doi.org/10.2147/IJN.S139450

Moola ZB, Scawen MD, Atkinson T, Nicholls DJ. *Erwinia chrysanthemi* L-asparaginase: Epitope mapping and production of antigenically modified enzymes. Biochem J. 1994;302(3):921–7. https://doi.org/10.1042/bj3020921

Patzke CL, Duffy AP, Duong VH, et al. Comparison of high-dose cytarabine, mitoxantrone, pegaspargase (HAM-pegA) to high-dose cytarabine, mitoxantrone, cladribine, and filgrastim (CLAG-M) as first-line salvage cytotoxic chemotherapy for relapsed/refractory acute myeloid leukemia. J Clin Med. 2020;9(2):536. https://doi.org/10.3390/jcm9020536

Patzke CL, Emadi A. High dose cytarabine, mitoxantrone, pegasapargase (HAM-pegA) in combination with dasatinib for the first-line treatment of Philadelphia chromosome positive mixed phenotype acute leukemia. Am J Leuk Res. 2020;4(1):1020.

Phillips RM, Saleem MU, Williams A, Morgan J. Kinetic analysis of the glutaminase activity of L-asparaginases derived from Erwinia chrysanthemi (Erwinase®) and Escherichia coli (Kidrolase). Mol Cancer Ther. 2013;12(11 Suppl):C154. https://doi.org/10.1158/1535-7163.TARG-13-C154

Preisler H, Davis RB, Kirshner J, et al. Comparison of three remission induction regimens and two postinduction strategies for the treatment of acute nonlymphocytic leukemia: A cancer and leukemia group B study. Blood. 1987;69(5):1441–9. https://doi.org/10.1182/blood.V69.5.1441.1441

Rigouin C, Nguyen HA, Schalk AM, Lavie A. Discovery of human-like L-asparaginases with potential clinical use by directed evolution. Sci Rep. 2017;7(1):10224. https://doi.org/10.1038/s41598-017-10758-4

Stock W, Luger SM, Advani AS, et al. A pediatric regimen for older adolescents and young adults with acute lymphoblastic leukemia: Results of CALGB 10403. Blood. 2019;133(14):1548–59. https://doi.org/10.1182/blood-2018-10-881961

Weiss RB, Freiman J, Kweder SL, et al. Hemolytic anemia after fludarabine therapy for chronic lymphocytic leukemia. J Clin Oncol. 1998;16(5):1885–9. https://doi.org/10.1200/JCO.1998.16.5.1885

Yates J, Glidewell O, Wiernik P, et al. Cytosine arabinoside with daunorubicin or driamycin for therapy of acute myelocytic leukemia: A CALGB study. Blood. 1982;60(2):454–62. https://doi.org/10.1182/blood.V60.2.454.bloodjournal602454

CHAPTER 7

Antifolate Antimetabolites

JUSTIN LAWSON

INTRODUCTION

Folate (in the form of folic acid or tetrahydrofolate) is an essential nutrient recognized during the mid-20th century as a vitamin in the B complex (specifically vitamin B_9). Deficiency of folate is associated with macrocytic (megaloblastic) anemia. The biochemical basis for this was defined also in the mid-20th century as related to the necessity of reduced folate derivatives for the synthesis of nucleic acid precursors, including thymine nucleoside and purine precursors, as well as participating in other reactions in metabolism to move one-carbon (1-C) units critical to metabolism of certain amino acids such as serine and glycine. Understanding of this biochemistry actually suggests ways of interfering with folate metabolism in a way that should cause inhibition of malignant cell growth. Indeed, the use of certain antifolate agents such as methotrexate was historically associated with the first transient dramatic responses of pediatric acute lymphoblastic leukemia (ALL) to drug therapy and encouraged the development of further advances in chemotherapy so that now this disease is in the majority of cases a curable neoplasm. Likewise, single-agent methotrexate led to the first cures of a solid tumor by chemotherapy in the case of choriocarcinoma.

ROLE OF FOLIC ACID IN METABOLISM

Folic acid is an essential nutrient that acts as a supplier of methyl groups to synthesize purines, pyrimidines, and certain amino acids. When able to donate methyl groups, folic acid exists as a reduced, methylene folate known as 5,10-methylenetetrahydrofolate (Me-THF).

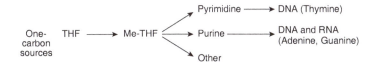

FIGURE 7.1 Folic acid use in cell physiology.

Me, methylene; THF, tetrahydrofolate.

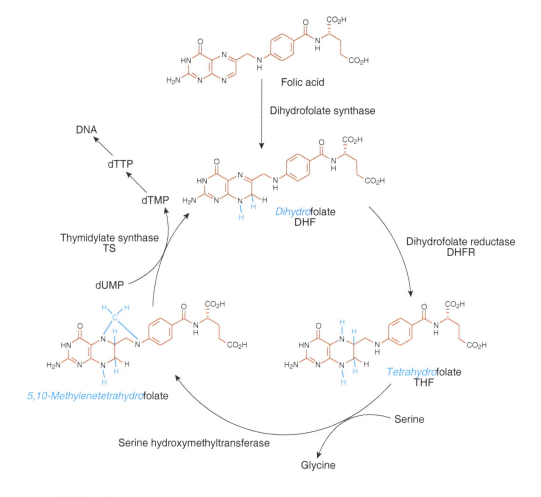

FIGURE 7.2 Folic acid structure.

Folic acid has three subunits: a pteridine ring, a para-aminobenzoic acid, and a glutamic acid. Folic acid's name originates from the Latin word *folium* meaning *leaf*. Extract of yeast and liver that contained folic acid was used to treat anemia in pregnant textile workers in Bombay, India, in 1930.

Since 1992 the U.S. Public Health Service has recommended that all women of childbearing age should consume 0.4 mg daily of folic acid. Perinatal supplementation of folic acid (4 mg daily) significantly reduces neural tube defects including spina bifida and anencephaly in fetuses. Of note, since 1998 in the United States, all grains have been fortified with 0.14 mg/100 g of grain.

FIGURE 7.3 Folic acid cycle as relevant for conversion of deoxyuridine monophosphate (dUMP) to deoxythymidine monophosphate (dTMP).

(continued)

FIGURE 7.3 Folic acid cycle as relevant for conversion of deoxyuridine monophosphate (dUMP) to deoxythymidine monophosphate (dTMP). (*continued*)

Mammals are deficient for *de novo* folate synthesis and thus rely on folate uptake from the extracellular environment. Folic acid from the diet is reduced to dihydrofolate (DHF) via dihydrofolate synthase, then to tetrahydrofolate (THF) via dihydrofolate reductase (DHFR). Serine hydroxymethyltransferase converts serine to glycine and donates the resulting methyl group to THF to create methylenetetrahydrofolate (Me-THF), a molecule that serves as a source for a methyl group in several cellular reactions. Me-THF gives up its carbon and is oxidized to DHF via thymidylate synthase (TS) in the process of synthesizing dTMP from dUMP. DHF is reduced back to THF via DHFR, resetting the cycle to continue facilitation of methyl donations for dTMP, and ultimately DNA synthesis.

dTTP, deoxythymidine triphosphate.

ANTIFOLATES AND THEIR MECHANISM OF ACTION

TABLE 7.1 Antifolate Medications, Oncologic Use, and Differences in Structures as Compared to Folic Acid

DRUG	TARGET	COMMON ONCOLOGIC USES	CHEMICAL STRUCTURE
Methotrexate (MTX)	DHFR	High dose: ALL, NHL, primary CNS lymphoma, osteosarcoma Low dose: various malignancies including breast, CTCL, ALL maintenance, as a DMARD in rheumatologic disorders	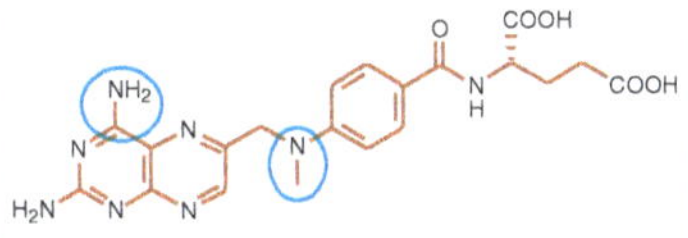 Methotrexate (MTX)

(continued)

TABLE 7.1 Antifolate Medications, Oncologic Use, and Differences in Structures as Compared to Folic Acid (*continued*)

DRUG	TARGET	COMMON ONCOLOGIC USES	CHEMICAL STRUCTURE
Pemetrexed (PMX) The recommended dose of PMX for most of its indications in patients with a CrCl ≥45 mL/min is 500 mg/m² given intravenously over 10 minutes	DHFR, TS, GARFT, AIRCARFT	• In combination with pembrolizumab and platinum chemotherapy, for the initial treatment of patients with metastatic nonsquamous NSCLC, with no EGFR or ALK genomic tumor aberrations • In combination with cisplatin for the initial treatment of patients with locally advanced or metastatic, nonsquamous NSCLC • As a single agent for the *maintenance* treatment of patients with locally advanced or metastatic, nonsquamous NSCLC whose disease has not progressed after four cycles of platinum-based first-line chemotherapy • Initial treatment, in combination with cisplatin, of patients with malignant pleural mesothelioma whose disease is unresectable or who are otherwise not candidates for curative surgery	 Pemetrexed (PMX) • *Not indicated* for the treatment of patients with *squamous cell* NSCLC

(continued)

TABLE 7.1 Antifolate Medications, Oncologic Use, and Differences in Structures as Compared to Folic Acid (*continued*)

DRUG	TARGET	COMMON ONCOLOGIC USES	CHEMICAL STRUCTURE
Pralatrexate (PDX)	DHFR	Relapsed or refractory PTCL	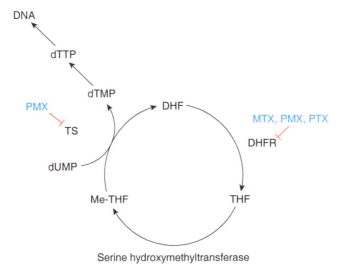Pralatrexate (PDX)

AIRCARFT, aminoimidazole carboxamide ribonucleotide formyltransferase; ALK, anaplastic lymphoma kinase; ALL, acute lymphoblastic leukemia; CNS, central nervous system; CrCl, creatinine clearance; CTCL, cutaneous T-cell lymphoma; DHFR, dihydrofolate reductase; DMARD, disease-modifying antirheumatic drugs; EGFR, epidermal growth factor receptor; GARFT, glycinamide ribonucleotide formyltransferase; NHL, non-Hodgkin lymphoma; NSCLC, non-small cell lung cancer; PTCL, peripheral T-cell lymphoma; TS, thymidylate synthase.

FIGURE 7.4 Antifolate mechanism of action.

First-generation antifolate drugs are exemplified by methotrexate (MTX). It acts primarily by inhibiting dihydrofolate reductase (DHFR), the enzyme responsible for reducing DHF and producing one-carbon recipients. Second-generation antifolate drugs are exemplified by pemetrexed (PMX). In addition to DHFR, PMX also inhibits thymidylate synthase (TS) and glycinamide ribonucleotide formyltransferase (GARFT), resulting in a distinct (from MTX) spectrum of antifolate activity, more directly affecting pyrimidine and purine precursors.

The predecessor of MTX was another analog of folic acid named aminopterin, which was one of the first chemotherapy agents that produced remissions in children with acute lymphoblastic leukemia. MTX was the first agent that cured a metastatic cancer (choriocarcinoma) in 1956.

DHF, dihydrofolate; dTMP, deoxythymidine monophosphate; dTTP, deoxythymidine triphosphate; dUMP, deoxyuridine monophosphate; Me-THF, methylenetetrahydrofolate; PTX, paclitaxel; THF, tetrahydrofolate.

FOLATE TRANSPORTERS

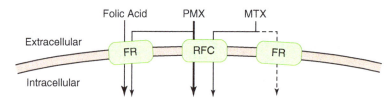

FIGURE 7.5 Relative affinities of folate receptor (FR) and reduced folate carrier (RFC).

Folate is a polar (negatively charged) molecule and does not passively diffuse across cell membranes, except at high concentrations. Therefore, folate requires a transporter to facilitate movement through the cell membrane.

Folate receptors (FRα, FRβ, and FRγ) are cysteine-rich cell-surface glycoproteins that bind folate with high affinity to facilitate cellular uptake of folate. FRα possesses a globular structure stabilized by eight disulfide bonds and contains a deep open folate-binding pocket of residues that are conserved in all receptor subtypes. The wide-ranging interactions between the receptor and the ligand elucidate the high folate-binding affinity of folate receptors.

Folate receptors, especially FRα, are overexpressed in several cancers to encounter the high folate demand of rapidly dividing cells. Pemetrexed (PMX) has similar affinity to folic acid for these receptors. The dependency of many tumors on folate supply has been exploited via development of anti-FRα antibodies as well as folate-conjugated drugs and toxins.

The RFC (also called SLC19A1) is the major transporter of folate, dihydrofolate, tetrahydrofolate, methotrexate (MTX) and PMX to different tissues at their neutral pH. The human RFC gene is located on chromosome 21q22.3. Children and adolescents with Down syndrome (trisomy 21) are at higher risk for development of MTX-associated side effects including severe mucositis and stomatitis, infections, bone marrow suppression, and hepato-, nephro-, and neurotoxicity. PMX has roughly twice the affinity for RFC compared to MTX.

INTRACELLULAR METABOLISM OF FOLATE AND ANTIFOLATES

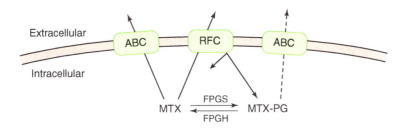

FIGURE 7.6 **Polyglutamate "trapping" of methotrexate (MTX).**
Once in the cell, folate can be polyglutamated with multiple glutamate groups via the enzyme folylpolyglutamyl synthetase (FPGS) to form polyglutamylated folates (F-PG). Polyglutamation also occurs for certain antifolate drugs, for example, MTX + (Glutamate)$_n$ → MTX-PG.

The polyglutamate addition to these molecules makes the modified target significantly more polar, reducing its affinity for folate transporters, effectively "trapping" the antifolate drugs within cells, thereby providing a large intracellular reservoir of drug and enhancing its cytotoxic activity. Various efflux proteins, including various subtypes of ATP binding cassette (ABC) efflux protein, may remove MTX and MTX-PG from within the cell, but in vitro data suggest that MTX-PG has significantly reduced binding affinity compared to MTX.

ATP, adenosine triphosphate; FPGH, folylpolyglutamyl hydrolase; RFC, reduced folate carrier.

ABSORPTION AND ELIMINATION OF ANTIFOLATES

At doses of ≤25 mg/m^2, adequate MTX absorption may be achieved by oral doses. Higher doses require parenteral (intravenous [IV] or intramuscular) administration for complete absorption.

MTX, PMX, and PDX are all eliminated primarily via renal excretion predominantly by glomerular filtration and tubular secretion.

- IMPORTANT: Dose reduction is required with renal dysfunction and administration may not be possible in renal failure.
- Additionally, MTX, PMX, and PDX all interact with drugs affecting renal blood flow or tubular function (e.g., nonsteroidal anti-inflammatory agents [NSAIDs; aspirin]) ultimately reducing renal elimination and increasing overall drug exposure.

MTX binds to albumin within the blood, and toxicity may be enhanced by other albumin binders (e.g., sulfonamides, phenytoin).

High doses of MTX (>500 mg/m^2) can affect liver function. This typically manifests as a transient elevation of liver enzymes in almost all patients that resolves within a few days, although this effect may persist in some patients. Long-term exposure to low doses of MTX can also lead to liver damage.

Tumor cells may also have altered polyglutamylation and cellular transport mechanisms compared to normal cells. When administered at doses >500 mg/m^2, MTX can enter cells by passive diffusion, not requiring folate cell membrane transport; this strategy is used in treatment of sarcomas, lymphomas, and ALL.

ANTIFOLATE ADVERSE EVENTS

TABLE 7.2 Antifolate Toxicities and Supportive Agents

DRUG	TOXICITIES / DRUG INTERACTIONS	SUPPORTIVE CARE AND RESCUE
Methotrexate (MTX)	● Mucositis, nausea/vomiting, hepatotoxicity, impaired fertility, diarrhea, modest cytopenias ● MTX can accumulate in third spaces, which can slow renal elimination rates and increase exposure, thereby increasing toxicity. Special attention must be made for pleural or pericardial effusion, ascites, or severe leg edema ● Bactrim (trimethoprim/sulfamethoxazole) increases MTX-related myelosuppression, mucositis, nephrotoxicity	
High-dose MTX (HDMTX)	● Acute kidney injury (AKI), neurotoxicity	● Urine alkalization (urine pH >7.0) prevents AKI ● Glucarpidase rescues from severe AKI ● Leucovorin prevents other life-threatening toxicities ● Penicillins, proton pump inhibitors (PPIs), nonsteroidal anti-inflammatory drugs (NSAIDs), and probenecid all reduce active renal secretion of MTX and should be avoided until MTX is cleared.
Pemetrexed (PMX)	● Rash ● Diarrhea ● Cytopenias ● Conjunctivitis and increased lacrimation	● Dexamethasone (4 mg orally, twice daily the day before, the day of, and the day after PMX administration) to prevent rash ● Folic acid (400 mcg to 1,000 mcg orally, once daily, beginning 7 days prior to the first dose of PMX and continue until 21 days after the last dose of PMX) to attenuate PMX- and PDX-related cytopenias but does not reduce the anticancer efficacy of these agents ● Vitamin B_{12} (1 mg intramuscularly, 1 week prior to the first dose of PMX and every three cycles) to attenuate PMX-related cytopenias but does not reduce the anticancer efficacy of these agents

(continued)

TABLE 7.2 Antifolate Toxicities and Supportive Agents (*continued*)

DRUG	TOXICITIES / DRUG INTERACTIONS	SUPPORTIVE CARE AND RESCUE
Pralatrexate (PDX)	• Mucositis • Nausea • Cytopenias • Diarrhea	• Folic acid and vitamin B_{12} to prevent cytopenias • Leucovorin may reduce incidence of mucositis

TOXICITY AND RESCUE WITH HIGH-DOSE METHOTREXATE REGIMENS

TABLE 7.3 Tetrahydrofolate Compared to Leucovorin Structure

TETRAHYDROFOLATE	LEUCOVORIN
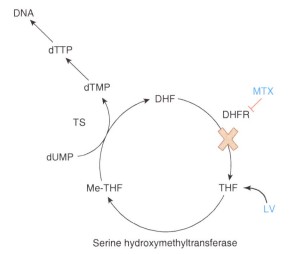	

Serine hydroxymethyltransferase

FIGURE 7.7 Mechanism of leucovorin (LV) "rescue" in high-dose methotrexate (HDMTX).
LV is a 5-formyl derivative of tetrahydrofolate (THF) that enters the cell via a reduced folate carrier (RFC) and is converted intracellularly to Me-THF independent of dihydrofolate reductase (DHFR). By bypassing MTX's primary mechanism of DHFR inhibition, LV acts as a "rescue" agent for cells exposed to high doses of MTX. As with MTX, low doses of LV are readily bioavailable, but doses >25 mg saturate intestinal absorption and require IV administration to ensure adequate drug exposure.

(*continued*)

FIGURE 7.7 Mechanism of leucovorin (LV) "rescue" in high-dose methotrexate (HDMTX). (*continued*)

Administration of LV after high-dose MTX administration is absolutely required to prevent fatal MTX toxicities. LV is typically administered 12 to 24 hours after MTX administration to allow for maximal cytotoxic anticancer activity before DHFR "rescue" of normal cells. The dose of LV must be titrated based on MTX levels to ensure appropriate toxicity rescue and will be continued until MTX levels in the blood have been reduced to safer levels.

DHF, dihydrofolate; dTMP, deoxythymidine monophosphate; dTTP, deoxythymidine triphosphate; dUMP, deoxyuridine monophosphate; IV, intravenous; Me-THF, methylenetetrahydrofolate; MTX, methotrexate; TS, thymidylate synthase.

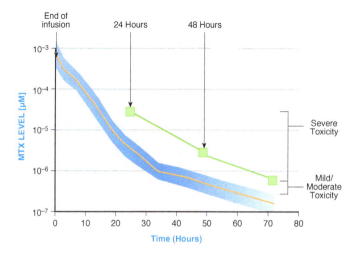

FIGURE 7.8 A nomogram for the expected time-dependent clearance of methotrexate (MTX) after completion of high-dose MTX infusion. Patients generally need to be on leucovorin rescue (and often in-patient) until serum MTX level is <0.05 µM (= 50 nM).

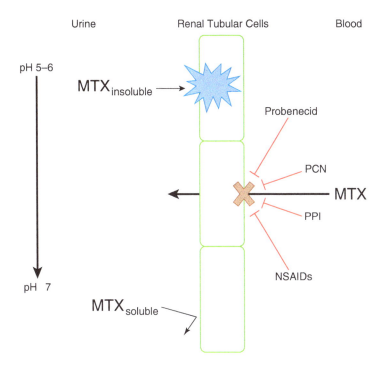

FIGURE 7.9 **Urinary excretion of high-dose methotrexate and effect of medications and urine pH.**

Acute kidney injury is another directly preventable toxicity of high-dose methotrexate (MTX) therapy. Administration strategies to prevent this toxicity include hyperhydration and alkalization of urine with intravenous (IV) solutions containing sodium bicarbonate. MTX, is a di (i.e., 2)-carboxylic acid and its metabolites are poorly soluble at an acidic pH. To prevent crystallization within the renal tubules during elimination, alkalization of urine pH to >7 significantly increases MTX solubility and therefore prevents precipitation and deposition of MTX into the renal tubules. Due to this increased risk of kidney injury, high-dose MTX must never be given in a patient with urine pH of <7. Strategies to alkalinize the urine usually should include IV sodium bicarbonate with oral (PO) bicarbonate and/or IV/PO acetazolamide for additional supplementation should the patient have compromised fluid status or difficulty achieving urine pH >7 with IV sodium bicarbonate alone. Several medications also affect active secretion of MTX into the urine and should be avoided during high-dose MTX clearance; these include penicillins (PCN), nonsteroidal anti-inflammatory drugs (NSAIDs), probenecid, and proton pump inhibitors (PPIs).

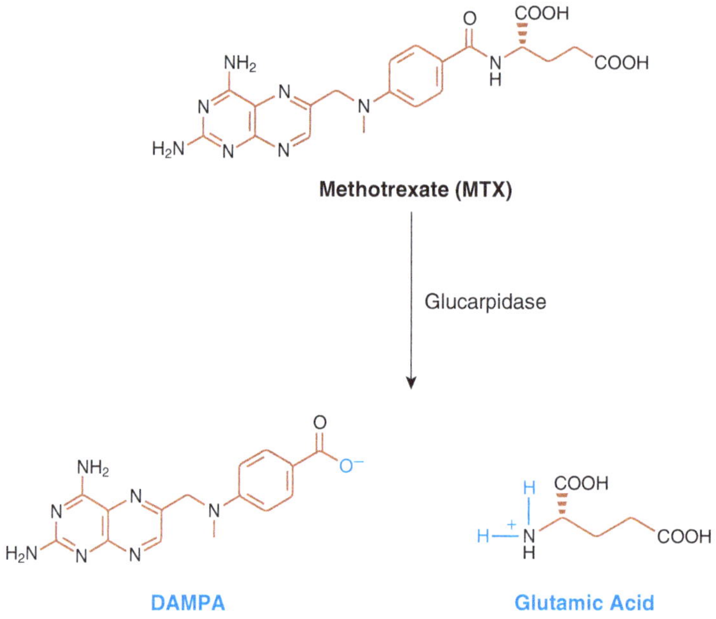

FIGURE 7.10 Mechanism of methotrexate breakdown by glucarpidase.
In circumstances of kidney injury that occur despite appropriate precautions of hydration and urine alkalization, leucovorin rescue will NOT be of benefit because leucovorin acts intracellularly and renal toxicity is a mechanism of extracellular methotrexate crystallization within the renal tubules. Rescue can be achieved with glucarpidase, a recombinant carboxypeptidase that enzymatically and rapidly cleaves MTX to form the amino acid glutamate and soluble 2,4-diamino-N^{10}-methylpteroic acid (DAMPA). It is important to note that depending on the MTX assay being used to monitor blood levels, DAMPA may provide a false positive until eliminated from the body. As glucarpidase will also act on extracellular leucovorin, leucovorin should not be administered within 2 hours before or after glucarpidase administration.

TOXICITY AND SUPPORTIVE CARE FOR PEMETREXED AND PRALATREXATE

As mentioned previously, pemetrexed and pralatrexate were developed after methotrexate in an effort to expand the spectrum of activity and enhance its pharmacokinetic profile. Pemetrexed has additional activity in inhibiting thymidylate synthase and increased affinity for folate receptors responsible for transport into the cancer cell. Pralatrexate has a high affinity for reduced folate carrier-1 and folypolyglutamyl synthase, enhancing the intracellular concentrations as well as its binding affinity to dihydrofolate reductase. Perhaps as a result of these differences, there are additional considerations with respect to the toxicity and supportive care of these agents compared to methotrexate.

Both pemetrexed and pralatrexate require regular intramuscular vitamin B_{12} injections and daily oral folic acid supplementation to prevent significant cytopenias while on therapy. Initial studies with pemetrexed showed unpredictable, significant cytopenias in some patients. Eventually, the link was made between these high-grade cytopenias and patients with high homocysteine levels indicative of a folate deficiency. The early trials were then amended to include regular vitamin B_{12} and folate supplement and, as a result, the rates of grade 3 or higher hematologic toxicities were significantly reduced, leading to the recommendation in the pemetrexed package insert. Ideally, these therapies should start before the patient receives chemotherapy, but some data suggest that same-day initiation of vitamin B_{12} and folic acid supplementation with pemetrexed is as effective as starting therapy 1 week prior.

In addition to cytopenias, pemetrexed has been associated with severe, and sometimes fatal, *bullous and blistering dermatologic toxicities*. The underlying mechanism for these toxicities is not well understood, but has been demonstrated to be prevented with administration of prophylactic corticosteroids. Based on these observations, dexamethasone should be administered for 3 days, starting the day before receiving the pemetrexed to prevent significant dermatologic toxicities.

As with methotrexate, pralatrexate has been associated with significant mucositis, which may necessitate dose interruptions, delays, or reductions. Recent small studies have shown that administration of oral leucovorin 24 hours after pralatrexate have been shown to reduce the incidence of ≥grade 2 mucositis. As when used with high-dose methotrexate, leucovorin acts as a rescue agent for healthy cells when administered after 24 hours, offering a supportive care option for patients receiving pralatrexate without compromising the initial cytotoxic effect on malignant cells.

CHAPTER SUMMARY

Antifolates are a subclass of antimetabolites that cause their cytotoxic effects by preventing the de novo formation of precursors of nucleic acid synthesis, especially thymidine, a nucleic acid essential for the creation of new DNA. The mechanisms vary depending on the drug, but primarily include inhibition of de novo synthesis of deoxythymidine monophosphate (dTMP) from deoxyuridine monophosphate (dUMP). As these medications prevent the synthesis of DNA, they are active during the S phase of the cell cycle. Toxicity of antifolates may be mitigated by rescue strategies with folic acid analog leucovorin, avoidance of drugs that interact with drug elimination processes, and in the case of methotrexate administration under the correct clinical contexts, use of a recombinant drug metabolizing enzyme. Additionally, the newer antifolates have additional supportive care strategies necessary to prevent their unique toxicities.

CLINICAL PEARLS

- High-dose methotrexate (HDMTX), with curative intent, is commonly used for treatment of patients with ALL, primary central nervous system lymphoma, and osteosarcoma. Urine alkalinization is mandatory before administration of HD-MTX. Physical examination for pleural and pericardial effusion must happen every day during administration of HDMTX and until MTX is cleared from serum.
- Due to nephrotoxicity of MTX, special attention must be given during evaluation of potential cerebellar toxicity of high-dose cytarabine (HiDAC) when used in combination with HDMTX (e.g., even cycles of hyper-CVAD); see Chapter 6.
- The genes for MTX transporters are located on chromosome 21. Closely monitor and treat/prevent the toxicity of MTX in patients with Down syndrome with leucovorin.
- MTX is one of the most commonly used chemotherapeutic agents for intrathecal (IT) administration. It is recommended that patients with ALL not take Bactrim (trimethoprim/sulfamethoxazole) for *Pneumocystis jirovecii* pneumonia prophylaxis on days when they receive IT MTX.
- Pemetrexed and pralatrexate require vitamin supplementation with vitamin B_{12} and folic acid. Additional supportive care is also required for prevention of dermatologic toxicities (PMX) and mucositis (PDX).
- Pemetrexed is NOT indicated for treatment of squamous non-small cell lung cancer.

MULTIPLE-CHOICE QUESTIONS

1. What is the primary mechanism of the antifolate drugs?

    A. Bind to exogenous folate, preventing its use in synthesis of the pyrimidine thymidine
    B. Are incorporated into DNA in place of folate, prevent DNA elongation in the S phase
    C. Inhibit dihydrofolate reductase, preventing folic acid from being reduced to a form that assists with synthesis of the pyrimidine thymidine
    D. Inhibit elongation of microtubules during mitosis by competitively inhibiting folate cofactor binding

2. CL is a 58-year-old woman recently diagnosed with metastatic non-small cell adenocarcinoma of the lung. The chemotherapy plan, per her oncologist, is to treat with four to six cycles of carboplatin, pemetrexed, and pembrolizumab. Which of the following medication is recommended for the prevention of toxicity during pemetrexed therapy to prevent cytopenias?

    A. A regular vitamin B_{12} injection and daily low-dose folic acid supplementation
    B. Urine alkalization until pemetrexed levels have been cleared
    C. Leucovorin administered for 48 hours after each dose of pemetrexed
    D. Injection of granulocyte colony-stimulating factor (G-CSF)

3. CL is scheduled to begin treatment with carboplatin/pemetrexed/pembrolizumab in two days. She has been reviewing the medications sent to her portfolio electronic medical record, for starting chemotherapy and has called you, asking why she was prescribed to take dexamethasone starting the day before she is scheduled to receive chemotherapy. Which adverse effect of pemetrexed does dexamethasone help prevent?

   A. Diarrhea
   B. Thrombocytopenia
   C. Mucositis
   D. Rash

4. BH is an 18-year-old man presenting with pain and swelling in his right leg that he noted after playing paintball. An x-ray study of the affected leg showed a concerning lesion requiring further testing. Additional tests (bone scan, MRI, and biopsy of the lesion) confirmed nonmetastatic osteosarcoma in the right proximal tibia. The patient was started on a standard regimen of cisplatin, doxorubicin, and high-dose methotrexate. Past medical history includes depression, headaches, attention deficit hyperactivity disorder (ADHD), and seasonal allergies. BH has no known drug allergies. Which of BH's home medications should be discontinued before he receives high-dose methotrexate?

   A. Escitalopram 20 mg orally daily
   B. Ibuprofen 400 mg orally twice a day as needed for headaches
   C. Methylphenidate 10 mg twice a day in the morning and afternoon
   D. Loratadine 20 mg orally daily

5. BH is currently being treated with cisplatin, doxorubicin, and high-dose methotrexate. He is 2 days post-methotrexate and 3 weeks post-cisplatin and doxorubicin, reporting dysphagia and nausea that might be related to his methotrexate therapy. Complete blood count and comprehensive metabolic panel (CMP) are within normal limits, including normal creatinine. Urine output is also normal with a random urine pH of 7.5. Which of the following is essential to moderate the development of methotrexate-related toxicities?

   A. A monthly vitamin B_{12} injection and daily low-dose folic acid supplementation
   B. Immediate IV glucarpidase administration
   C. Leucovorin administered starting 24 to 48 hours post-methotrexate
   D. Reduction of sodium bicarbonate infusion, titrating to a urine pH of 6 to 7

6. Three days after receiving methotrexate, BH is complaining of significant nausea, vomiting, and mucositis, and his urine output has decreased significantly. Comprehensive metabolic panel (CMP) shows that BH's serum creatinine increased to 3.6 mg/dL. Urine pH was found to be 7.5 and the patient had been receiving a continuous sodium bicarbonate infusion to maintain his urine pH at appropriate levels. A serum methotrexate level after 48 hours was found to be very high at 21 μmol/L. What is the most appropriate treatment for BH's new acute kidney injury?

   A. Immediate hemodialysis
   B. Immediate and simultaneous IV glucarpidase and IV leucovorin administration
   C. Immediate glucarpidase administration followed by scheduled IV leucovorin 2 hours later
   D. Immediate and simultaneous IV furosemide and IV leucovorin administration

7. JR is a 68-year-old woman with acute lymphoblastic leukemia who is hospitalized to receive the cytarabine/methotrexate cycle of hyper-CVAD. Forty-eight hours after starting chemotherapy, she develops a fever of 38.7°C with a blood pressure of 79/55 mmHg. Which antibiotic would be *least* appropriate given the patient's high-dose methotrexate?

   A. Meropenem
   B. Cefepime
   C. Piperacillin/tazobactam
   D. Ceftazidime

8. Which of the following is most likely to enhance a cell's toxicity to methotrexate?

   A. Reduced expression of reduced folate carrier (RFC) protein on the cell membrane
   B. Increased expression of ATP (adenosine triphosphate) binding cassette (ABC) efflux protein on the cell membrane
   C. Increased expression of dihydrofolate reductase (DHFR)
   D. Increased expression of folylpolyglutamyl synthetase (FPGS)

ANSWERS TO MULTIPLE-CHOICE QUESTIONS

1. **C.** Antifolates primarily work by inhibiting dihydrofolate reductase, preventing folic acid from being reduced to tetrahydrofolate, which eventually is modified to provide the methyl group used to convert uridine to thymidine.

2. **A.** A regular vitamin B_{12} injection and daily low-dose folic acid supplementation are indicated to prevent cytopenias associated with pemetrexed. Urine alkalization is appropriate for high-dose methotrexate monitoring, not pemetrexed, and leucovorin and G-CSF are not indicated at all in treatment with pemetrexed.

3. **D.** Dermatologic toxicities associated with pemetrexed are prevented by administration of dexamethasone starting the day before pemetrexed administration.

4. **B.** Nonsteroidal anti-inflammatory drugs (NSAIDs) such as ibuprofen are associated with reduction in active secretion of methotrexate and they pose a risk of acute kidney injury as well. As a result, their use is contraindicated when administering high-dose methotrexate (HDMTX).

5. **C.** High-dose methotrexate is ALWAYS administered with leucovorin as a rescue agent to start 24 to 48 hours after receiving the methotrexate. Glucarpidase is indicated in the treatment of acute kidney injury associated with high methotrexate levels, not prevention of toxicities. Vitamin B_{12} injection and daily low-dose folic acid supplementation are a prevention strategy for pemetrexed and pralatrexate. Urine pH should be maintained >7 when receiving high-dose methotrexate.

6. **C.** Patient is suffering from acute kidney injury related to MTX crystallization in the renal tubules. A decrease in urine output and significant increase in serum creatinine and documented MTX level are indications for immediate glucarpidase administration. Leucovorin can also serve as a substrate for glucarpidase and should, therefore, always be administered at least 2 hours before or after glucarpidase.

7. **C.** High-dose methotrexate toxicities are exacerbated when administered with medications that also use similar pathways for active secretion. Piperacillin/tazobactam is a penicillin antibiotic that uses such pathways and should be avoided until the patient's methotrexate has cleared.

8. **D.** Increased FPGS expression would increase trapped intracellular MTX and, therefore, increase toxicity. All other answers would decrease methotrexate uptake, increase MTX efflux, or serve as a mechanism of resistance to standard doses of MTX.

SELECTED REFERENCES

Allegra CJ, Chabner BA, Drake JC, et al. Enhanced inhibition of thymidylate synthase by methotrexate polyglutamates. J Biol Chem. 1985;260(17):9720–6. https://doi.org/10.1016/S0021-9258(17)39298-0

Chabner BA, Allegra CJ, Curt GA, et al. Polyglutamation of methotrexate. Is methotrexate a prodrug? J Clin Invest. 1985;76(3):907–12. https://doi.org/10.1172/JCI112088

Green JM. Glucarpidase to combat toxic levels of methotrexate in patients. Ther Clin Risk Manag. 2012;8:403–13. https://doi.org/10.2147/TCRM.S30135

Howard SC, McCormick J, Pui CH, et al. Preventing and managing toxicities of high-dose methotrexate. Oncologist. 2016;21(12):1471–82. https://doi.org/10.1634/theoncologist.2015-0164

Kamen B. Folate and antifolate pharmacology. Semin Oncol. 1997;24(5 Suppl 18):S18–30.

Mahmood K, Emadi A. 1-C metabolism-serine, glycine, folates-in acute myeloid leukemia. Pharmaceuticals (Basel). 2021;14(3):190. https://doi.org/10.3390/ph14030190

Visentin M, Zhao R, Goldman ID. The antifolates. Hematol Oncol Clin North Am. 2012;26(3):629–48, ix. https://doi.org/10.1016/j.hoc.2012.02.002

Walling J. From methotrexate to pemetrexed and beyond. A review of the pharmacodynamic and clinical properties of antifolates. Investig New Drugs. 2006;24(1):37–77. https://doi.org/10.1007/s10637-005-4541-1

Wibowo AS, Singh M, Reeder KM, et al. Structures of human folate receptors reveal biological trafficking states and diversity in folate and antifolate recognition. Proc Natl Acad Sci U S A. 2013;110(38):15180–8. https://doi.org/10.1073/pnas.1308827110

Widemann BC, Adamson PC. Understanding and managing methotrexate nephrotoxicity. Oncologist. 2006;11(6):694–703. https://doi.org/10.1634/theoncologist.11-6-694

Wright NJ, Fedor JG, Zhang H, et al. Methotrexate recognition by the human reduced folate carrier SLC19A1. Nature. 2022;609(7929):1056–62. https://doi.org/10.1038/s41586-022-05168-0

CHAPTER 8

Antimitotics

EDWARD A. SAUSVILLE ● **ASHKAN EMADI**

INTRODUCTION

Mitosis is the part of the cell cycle when replicated DNA condenses into chromosomes, each of which is composed of a DNA helix with one template DNA strand and one newly synthesized DNA strand during the prior S phase (see Figure 8.1). The parental and progeny chromosomes, known as "sister chromatids," are still joined at the centromere.

Microtubules are protein structures that link each centromere to a centrosome; tubular structures form spontaneously under appropriate guanosine triphosphate (GTP), cellular signals from tubulin heterodimers, and Mg^{2+} concentrations. Tubulin heterodimers are formed by the noncovalent association of alpha(α)-tubulin and beta(β)-tubulin subunits (see Figure 8.2), which cause sister chromatid movement away from the centromere and into newly formed progeny cells (see Figure 8.3).

During the mid-20th century, screening programs looking for drugs that would block cancer cell growth revealed that numerous "natural products" often used as a defense mechanism by their producing organisms against invading organisms in their microenvironments could disrupt the process of mitosis in cancer cells, and a few of these have proved clinically useful. Microtubule-directed agents include those for which the drug's core structure was isolated from or synthesized from precursors in plants (vinca alkaloids, taxanes), marine organisms (eribulin), and bacteria (epothilones). These agents disrupt chromosome movement during mitosis. This chapter describes mitosis and how clinically useful drugs directed at mitosis act, along with features of drug effects to consider when using them in patients. In addition to the classic effects with disruption of the mitotic apparatus, microtubule-directed drugs at lower concentrations can have "mitosis-independent" effects on cell signaling, vesicular function, and protein transport between intracellular compartments.

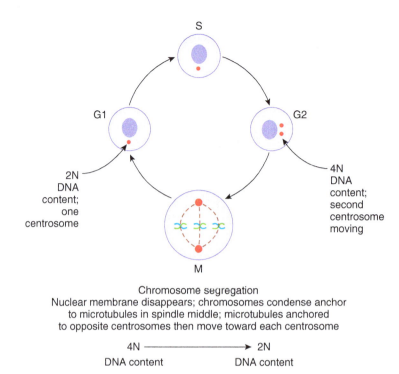

FIGURE 8.1 Cell cycle and temporally related "chromosome cycle."
G1 cells have 2N DNA content in diploid chromosomes; after the S phase,
G2 cells acquire a duplicate centrosome and have 4N DNA content in sister
chromatids. After mitosis, progeny cells have 2N DNA content, and sister
chromatids are now daughter chromosomes.

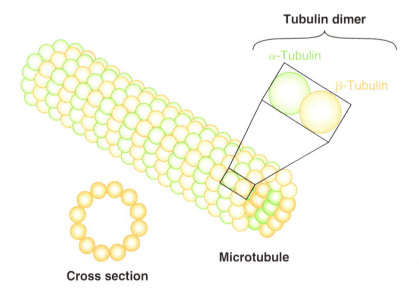

FIGURE 8.2 Microtubule structure.

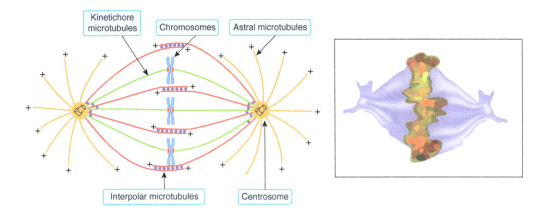

FIGURE 8.3 Microtubules structures with chromosomal assembly.
As G2 transitions to M phase, tubulin heterodimers polymerize noncovalently to form microtubules, which anchor to centrosomes and metaphase chromosomes. The centromere of each progeny chromosome or "sister chromatid" is linked to a centrosome at the opposite poles of the mitotic spindle apparatus by kinetochore microtubules. Centrosomes are connected and stabilized via interpolar microtubules. Centrosomes or spindles are connected to the cell cortex (a structure at the inner face of the cell membrane) via astral microtubules in order to assist them to orient themselves correctly and control the plane of cell division. Cleavage of the centromere sends a set of progeny chromosomes to each of two progeny cells.

VINCA ALKALOIDS

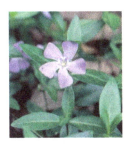
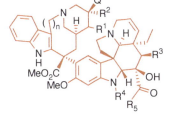
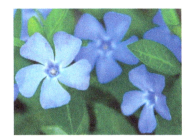

Name	n	Q	R^1	R^2	R^3	R^4	R^5	Therapeutic indication
Vinblastine	2	OH	H	Et	OAc	Me	OMe	Hodgkin lymphoma and bladder cancer
Vinorelbine	1	$Q=R^1 =\varnothing$ (alkene)		Et	OAc	Me	OMe	Osteosarcoma, NSCLC and SCLC
Vincristine	2	OH	H	Et	OAc	CHO	OMe	Several lymphoid malignancies (e.g., ALL, NHL)

FIGURE 8.4 Complex chemical structures of vinca alkaloids; isolated originally from periwinkle.

(continued)

FIGURE 8.4 Complex chemical structures of vinca alkaloids; isolated originally from periwinkle. (*continued*)

The core vinca polycyclic ring system is produced in periwinkle plants, shown above to either side of the core structure. Vinca alkaloids approved for use in clinical practice include vincristine, vinblastine, and vinorelbine. Among these agents, vincristine (also called Oncovin) is the most neurotoxic agent, vinblastine is the most myelotoxic agent, and vinorelbine causes both neurotoxicity and myelotoxicity. Vinca alkaloids are excreted from tumor cells by the multidrug resistance P-glycoprotein; therefore, long infusion regimens may be used to counter efflux mechanisms, but many regimens use vincas infused over relatively short durations.

Vincristine sulfate liposome injection (Marqibo) was originally approved for treatment of adult patients with Philadelphia chromosome-negative ALL who relapsed or whose disease progressed after two or more anti-leukemia therapies. The drug subsequently was withdrawn from the market after inability to conduct a postmarking clinical trial to verify the clinical benefit of the drug, mainly due to difficulty with patient recruitment.

ALL, acute lymphoblastic leukemia.

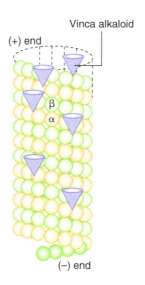

FIGURE 8.5 Vinca alkaloid as microtubule polymer destabilizers.

Vinca alkaloids bind to the β-tubulin subunit of the tubulin heterodimer at the (+) ends and along the sides of microtubules, resulting in destabilization of microtubule polymer and preventing microtubule assembly. Therefore, exposure to these agents results in cell cycle arrest in the early M phase. The arrested cells are susceptible to apoptosis induced by sensing an abnormal mitotic spindle or by attempting mitosis that aberrantly misdistributes chromosomes asymmetrically.

Current practice does not include a short intravenous bolus of vincas to avoid mistaken administration into the CSF through the intrathecal route, which causes lethal neurotoxicity.

(*continued*)

FIGURE 8.5 **Vinca alkaloid as microtubule polymer destabilizers. (*continued*)**

Vincas are cleared by hepatic metabolism; therefore, doses are reduced or may be held for elevated bilirubin.

Vinca alkaloids are vesicants and extravasation can cause skin and soft tissue damage; if this occurs, local heat, hyaluronidase, and topical steroids might be helpful.

CSF, cerebrospinal fluid.

Due to significant exacerbation of vincas' neurotoxicity, simultaneous administration of CYP3A4 inhibitors such as voriconazole, itraconazole, and posaconazole with vinca alkaloid is contraindicated.

TABLE 8.1 Vincristine Neurotoxicity

- Dose limiting; should cap the dose at 2 mg per injection and at least administer as a weekly schedule
- Preexisting neurologic disorders can potentiate neurotoxities to severe and debilitating forms. Duloxetine, gabapentin, and pregabalin may be useful in the management of neurotoxicity due to vinca alkaloids; although no randomized clinical trial has shown objective benefit, some patients feel improved symptoms.
- Neurotoxicity initially presents as symmetrical sensory impairment:
  - Paresthesia presents as "stocking and glove" tingling in distal extremities; increasing cumulative dose of vincristine exacerbates paresthesia, which can progress to disabling pain and loss of function (patient cannot pick up coins or fasten buttons).
  - Neuropathic pains, demyelination of nerve fibers; unmyelinated nerves most sensitive
  - May be reversible; however, some patients report persisting symptoms years after treatment.
- Irreversible or minimally reversible motor nerve impairment with continued use can occur and presents as
  - Loss of deep tendon reflexes
  - Ataxia
  - Foot and wrist drop as well as paralysis
- Central nervous system and cranial nerve toxicities may occur with continued use, and can present as
  - Hoarseness, diplopia, facial palsy, hearing loss
  - Jaw, parotid and pharyngeal pains
  - Confusion, agitation, hallucinations and seizures
- Autonomic neuropathy can present as
  - Gut hypomotility and constipation
  - Paralytic ileus; it is recommended that patients be on stool softener and have 1–2 bowel movements daily.
- Syndrome of inappropriate antidiuretic hormone (SIADH) secretion, causing hyponatremia
- Cardiac autonomic dysfunction, which can manifest as orthostatic hypotension
- Bladder atony resulting in urinary retention or urinary incontinence; simultaneous anticholinergic drugs should be avoided if clinically possible

TAXANES

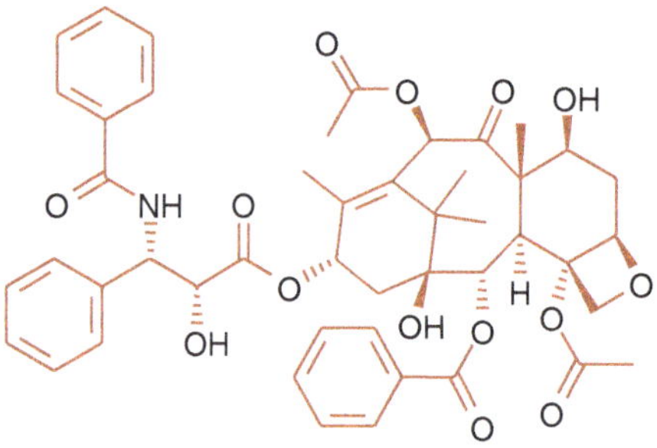

Paclitaxel (Taxol)

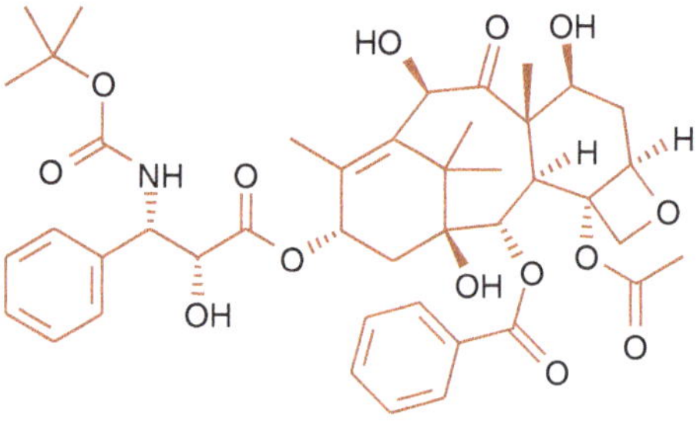

Docetaxel (Taxotere)

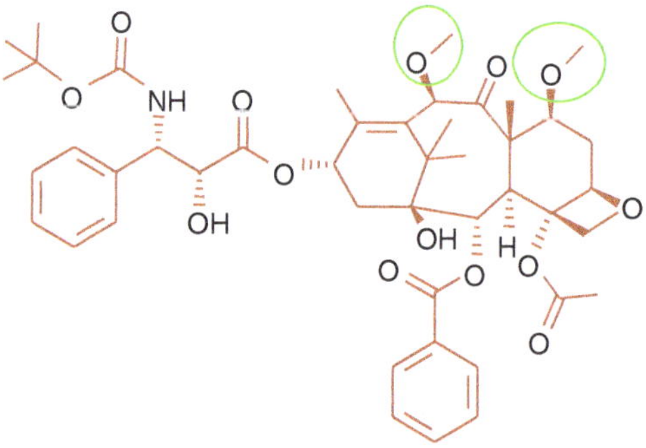

Cabazitaxel (Jevtana)

FIGURE 8.6 Complex chemical structures of taxanes.
The originally approved drug paclitaxel was first identified in the bark of the Pacific yew tree. Taxanes approved for use in clinical practice include paclitaxel, docetaxel, and cabazitaxel, an analogue of docetaxel.

Paclitaxel is approved for (a) adjuvant treatment of breast cancer sequentially after an anthracycline-containing regimen, (b) metastatic or relapsed breast cancer, (c) use in combination with cisplatin or carboplatin for NSCLC, (d) advanced ovarian cancer, and (e) second-line AIDS-related Kaposi sarcoma. The common and frequent off-label uses of paclitaxel include (but are not limited to) the treatment of advanced head and neck cancers, preoperative chemoradiation for esophageal or gastric cancers, relapsed/refractory small cell lung cancer, advanced thymoma/thymic carcinoma, neoadjuvant/advanced or metastatic bladder cancer, metastatic penile cancer, relapsed/refractory testicular germ cell tumors, advanced cervical cancer, and adenocarcinoma of unknown primary.

Docetaxel is approved for (a) squamous cell carcinoma of the head and neck with cisplatin and 5-FU; (b) use as a single agent for locally advanced or metastatic breast cancer after chemotherapy failure; (c) use with doxorubicin and cyclophosphamide as adjuvant therapy for breast cancer; (d) use as a single agent for locally advanced or metastatic NSCLC after platinum therapy failure; (e) use with cisplatin for unresectable, locally advanced, or metastatic

(continued)

FIGURE 8.6 Complex chemical structures of taxanes. (*continued*)
untreated NSCLC; (f) use with cisplatin and fluorouracil for untreated, advanced gastric adenocarcinoma including the gastroesophageal junction; and (h) use with prednisone in hormone refractory metastatic prostate cancer.

Cabazitaxel is approved for hormone-refractory metastatic prostate cancer previously treated with a docetaxel-containing regimen.

5-FU, 5-fluorouracil; NSCLC, non-small cell lung cancer.

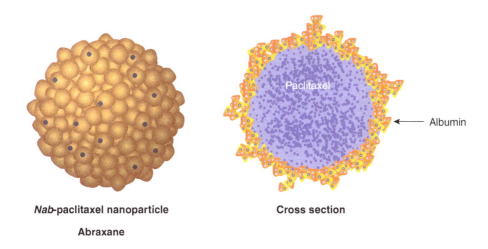

Nab-paclitaxel nanoparticle

Abraxane

Cross section

Albumin

FIGURE 8.7 Abraxane, paclitaxel albumin-bound nanoparticles for injectable suspension.
Nab-paclitaxel nanoparticle albumin-bound (abraxane) is approved for treatment of (a) metastatic breast cancer, and breast cancer relapses within 6 months of adjuvant chemotherapy; (b) locally advanced or metastatic NSCLC, as first-line treatment in combination with carboplatin; and (c) metastatic adenocarcinoma of the pancreas as first-line treatment in combination with gemcitabine. For pancreatic adenocarcinoma, nab-paclitaxel is not recommended if bilirubin is greater than1.5 times the upper limit of normal.

NSCLC, non-small cell lung cancer.

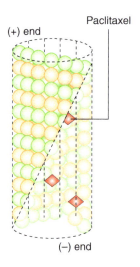

FIGURE 8.8 Taxanes as microtubule polymer stabilizers.
Taxanes bind to a site on β-tubulin distinct from that of the vincas and promote abnormal assembly of short, stubby, abnormally functioning microtubule-like structures that cannot participate in normal mitosis. Abnormal tubulin structures promote apoptosis.

    Taxanes bind to subunits inside of microtubules. The biophysical properties of the cell (e.g., intracellular viscosity, microtubule stiffness, cell deformation) can affect stabilization of microtubules in the formation and progression of the bundles.

TABLE 8.2 Taxane-Related Clinical and Pharmacologic Points

- *Hepatic impairment:* Taxanes are cleared by hepatic metabolism; adverse events can be triggered by coadministration with other cytochrome P450 substrates; concomitant medications and consultation with an oncology pharmacy specialist might be considered. Patients with elevations of bilirubin or abnormal AST/ALT concurrent elevation of alkaline phosphatase are at increased risk for the development of severe neutropenia, febrile neutropenia, infections, severe thrombocytopenia, severe stomatitis, and severe skin toxicity. It is strongly recommended to avoid treatment with taxanes in patients with bilirubin greater than upper limit of normal (ULN), or patients with AST and/or ALT >1.5 × ULN.
- *Renal impairment:* Dose adjustment of taxanes with abnormal creatinine is not necessary.
- *Severe hypersensitivity:*
  - Paclitaxel injection contains polyoxyethylated castor oil (Cremophor EL), which is associated with hypersensitivity reactions.
  - Docetaxel contains polysorbate 80, which is associated with hypersensitivity reactions.
  - Severe hypersensitivity reactions are characterized by generalized rash or erythema, hypotension, and/or bronchospasm, which can progress to a fatal condition if not aggressively treated. Patients should not be rechallenged if they have a history of severe hypersensitivity reactions. Patients who have previously experienced a hypersensitivity reaction to paclitaxel/docetaxel may develop a hypersensitivity reaction to docetaxel/paclitaxel, which may include anaphylaxis. All patients should be premedicated with an oral corticosteroid, antihistamines, and H2 blockers prior to the initiation of the infusion of paclitaxel/docetaxel.

(continued)

TABLE 8.2 Taxane-Related Clinical and Pharmacologic Points (*continued*)

- *Fluid retention:* Severe fluid retention as a sign of vascular leak syndrome owing to damage to endothelial cell tight junctions can occur following taxane therapy. Peripheral edema usually begins in the lower extremities and may become generalized with a median weight gain of 2 kg. Patients should be premedicated with oral corticosteroids before each taxane administration to reduce the incidence and severity of fluid retention. Fluid retention can be managed by salt restriction, with diuretics and compression stockings, and slowly resolves with a median of 16 weeks from the last infusion of a taxanes.
- *Neurotoxicity:* Severe neurosensory symptoms including paresthesia, dysesthesia, pain, and distal extremity weakness can occur after administration of different taxane products. The incidence of ileus is less than what is observed with vinca alkaloids. Severe asthenia can occur in ~15% of patients receiving taxanes.
- *Eye disorders:* Lacrimal duct stenosis causing constant and severe tearing, which may require stent placement in the lacrimal ducts, and cystoid macular edema may develop with administration of taxanes.
- *Alcohol content:* The alcohol content in a dose of docetaxel injection may affect the CNS and cause impairment of ability to drive or use machines immediately after infusion. Each docetaxel injection at 100 mg/m^2 delivers 2.0 g/m^2 of ethanol; patients with BSA of 2–2.2 will receive ~4–4.5 g ethanol.
- *Cutaneous reactions:* Erythema of the extremities with edema followed by desquamation may occur. Stevens-Johnson syndrome (SJS), toxic epidermal necrolysis (TEN), and acute generalized exanthematous pustulosis (AGEP) may rarely occur after administration of taxanes.
- Taxanes are multidrug resistant P-glycoprotein substrates.
- *Hematologic effects:* Myelosuppression including severe neutropenia occurs after administration of taxanes. Neutropenia (<2,000 neutrophils/µL) occurs in all patients given 60–100 mg/m^2 docetaxel. Grade 4 neutropenia (<500 neutrophils/µL) occurs in 85% and 75% of patients given 100 mg/m^2 and 60 mg/m^2 docetaxel, respectively. Docetaxel should not be administered to patients with neutrophils <1,500/µL. A 25% reduction in the dose of docetaxel is recommended during subsequent cycles following severe neutropenia (<500 neutrophils/µL) lasting 7 days or more, or febrile neutropenia. Second primary malignancies, including treatment-related myeloid neoplasms (t-MNs) can occur several months to years after administration of taxanes.
- *Neutropenic colitis (typhlitis) and enterocolitis:* These types of colitis may occur with a taxane monotherapy or in combination with other chemotherapeutic agents, despite the coadministration of G-CSF.
- *Cardiac electrophysiology effects:* Taxanes can cause dysrhythmias including sinus bradycardia.

ALT, alanine transaminase; AST, aspartate transaminase; BSA, body surface area; CNS, central nervous system; G-CSF, granulocyte colony-stimulating factor.

NEWER MICROTUBULE-DIRECTED AGENTS

Ixabepilone

Ixabepilone, as a nontaxane microtubule-targeting agent, as a single agent or in combination with capecitabine is approved for use in advanced breast cancer resistant to anthracyclines and other taxanes. It binds directly to β-tubulin subunits near the taxane site in a distinct manner compared to that of taxanes, and causes aberrant tubulin depolymerization. Ixabepilone is a less prominent multidrug resistance P-glycoprotein substrate, concordant with its clinical activity in taxane-resistant tumors. It has an adverse-event profile similar to that of taxanes, including hepatotoxicity, myelosuppression and peripheral neuropathy, hypersensitivity reactions, and cognitive impairment from dehydrated alcohol.

Eribulin

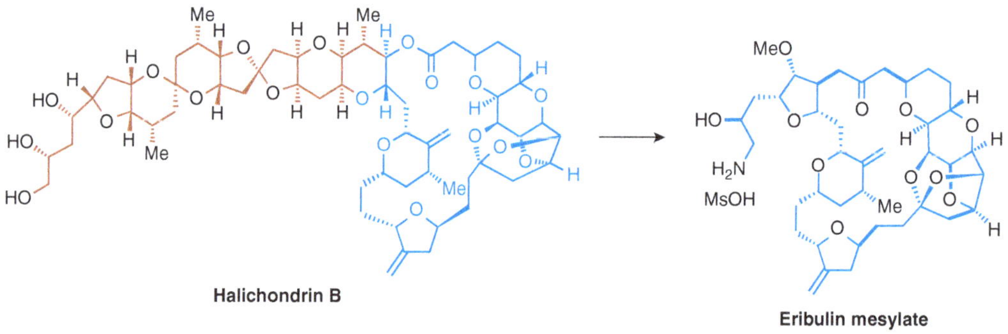

Halichondrin B

Eribulin mesylate

FIGURE 8.9 **Eribulin as a halichondrin B analog.**
Halichondrin B is a polyether macrolide, which was originally isolated from the marine sponge *Halichondria okadai* and was listed for development as a tubulin-targeted mitotic inhibitor anticancer by the NCI in the 1990s. Eribulin is a structurally simplified and pharmaceutically optimized analogue of halichondrin B.

Eribulin is approved for the treatment of (a) patients with metastatic breast cancer who have previously received at least two prior chemotherapy regimens including an anthracycline and a taxane in either the adjuvant or metastatic setting, and (b) patients with unresectable or metastatic liposarcoma who have received a prior anthracycline-containing regimen. A statistically significant improvement in overall survival was observed in patients with liposarcoma randomized to receive eribulin compared with dacarbazine.

Eribulin has an adverse event profile similar to that of vinca alkaloids and taxanes. Eribulin can prolong the QT interval. QT prolongation usually occurs in the second week posttreatment and is independent of eribulin concentration. In patients with congestive heart failure, bradyarrhythmias, or those who receive drugs known to prolong the QT interval, ECG monitoring is recommended. Hypokalemia and hypomagnesemia should be corrected prior to initiating eribulin, and potassium and magnesium should be monitored periodically during therapy.

NCI, National Cancer Institute.

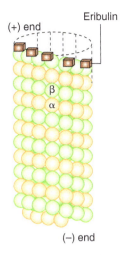

FIGURE 8.10 Eribulin as an altering microtubule growth dynamics agent.
Eribulin binds to β-subunits of microtubules that are partially overlapping the vinca site and distinct from taxanes, resulting in inhibition of microtubule assembly and elongation. Eribulin does not affect microtubule shortening but does generate nonproductive tubulin aggregates.

Eribulin is administered 1.4 mg/m² IV over 2–5 minutes on days 1 and 8 of a 21-day cycle. Eribulin dose should be reduced in patients with hepatic impairment or with moderate or severe renal impairment.

For injection, eribulin should not be mixed with other drugs or be administered with dextrose-containing solutions.

IV, intravenous.

CHAPTER SUMMARY

Anti-microtubule–directed drugs can either affect the assembly of microtubules or induce the formation of abnormal, functionally useless microtubule-related structures. In either case, these can lead to blockade of cell cycle progression and induction of apoptosis, leading to cell death. Common side effects include cytopenias and the occurrence of neuropathy as well as hypersensitivity reactions, which can limit the drug dosage or frequency of treatment.

CLINICAL PEARLS

- Treatment-related mortality risk with taxanes increases with abnormal liver function. Taxanes should not be given or significant dose reduction should occur if bilirubin exceeds the upper limit of normal (ULN), or if aspartate aminotransferase (AST) and/or alanine aminotransferase (ALT) >1.5 × ULN concomitant with alkaline phosphatase >2.5 × ULN. No dose adjustment in taxanes is necessary for renal failure.

- The alcohol content in a dose of docetaxel injection may affect the central nervous system or cause impairment of ability to drive or use machines immediately after infusion.
- The growing preclinical and clinical evidence suggests to combine a taxane with a checkpoint inhibitor targeting the PD-1/PD-L (programmed cell death) pathway due to the complementary effects of the role of tubulin/microtubule inhibitors in the expression and function of immune checkpoints. For example, a randomized multicenter Phase 3 clinical trial of ~700 patients showed a significant and clinically meaningful improvement in overall survival (OS) and a significant improvement in progression-free survival (PFS) with atezolizumab (1,200 mg intravenously every 3 weeks) plus chemotherapy (carboplatin [AUC 6 mg/mL/min IV every 3 weeks] plus nab-paclitaxel [100 mg/m^2 IV every week]) versus chemotherapy as first-line treatment of patients with stage IV nonsquamous non-small cell lung cancer and no ALK or EGFR mutations.

MULTIPLE-CHOICE QUESTIONS

1. Ado-trastuzumab emtansine is approved for the treatment of patients with HER2$^+$, stage IV breast cancer who previously received a taxane and trastuzumab. Which one of the following does NOT describe this agent accurately?

   A. In the EMILIA study, it improved PFS and OS compared with lapatinib plus capecitabine in patients with HER2$^+$ advanced breast cancer, who had previously been treated with trastuzumab and a taxane.
   B. DM1, the cytotoxic component of ado-trastuzumab emtansine, is a DNA minor groove inhibitor.
   C. Hepatotoxicity, liver failure, and death have occurred in patients treated with ado-trastuzumab emtansine.
   D. Thrombocytopenia is the most common hematologic adverse event of ado-trastuzumab emtansin.
   E. Neurotoxicity, predominantly sensory, can occur in approximately 20% of patients receiving ado-trastuzumab emtansine.

2. A 16-year-old man presents with relapsed acute lymphoblastic leukemia. He complains of progressive ptosis and exotropia along with vertical misalignment of the eye, vertical diplopia characterized by ipsilateral hypertropia that increases in contralateral gaze and ipsilateral head tilt, and binocular horizontal double vision. The diagnosis of third, fourth, and sixth cranial nerve palsy was made on examination. The patient requires lumbar puncture with administration of intrathecal (IT) chemotherapy. Which of the IT chemotherapy combination should be used in an attempt to alleviate his symptoms?

   A. Vincristine and methylprednisolone
   B. Methotrexate and vincristine
   C. Cytarabine, methotrexate, and hydrocortisone
   D. Vincristine and cytarabine
   E. Vincristine followed by cranial nerve radiation

3. Abraxane (paclitaxel albumin-bound nano particles for injectable suspension) is approved for which of the following neoplasms?

   A. Metastatic penile cancer
   B. Glioblastoma multiforme relapsed after radiation and temozolomide
   C. Gastric adenocarcinoma combined with cisplatin and fluorouracil
   D. AIDS-related Kaposi sarcoma
   E. Metastatic adenocarcinoma of the pancreas as first-line treatment, in combination with gemcitabine

4. A 49-year-old Caucasian woman was diagnosed with left-sided breast cancer and underwent lumpectomy followed by radiation. Pathology revealed a grade 2, 3-cm tumor (T2) with two sentinel lymph nodes positive with cancer (N1). The cancer is ER = 90%, PR = 35%, and HER2⁻. She is started on chemotherapy with cyclophosphamide and docetaxel. Three days after the first cycle of chemotherapy, she experiences shortness of breath. She has +2 pitting edema. Chest x-ray shows moderate pleural effusion; echo reveals mild pericardial effusion. Pretreatment with which one of the medications may help prevent these issues during future cycles?

   A. Dexamethasone
   B. Mesna
   C. Albumin infusion
   D. Ranitidine and acetaminophen
   E. Albuterol inhaler

5. A 36-year-old woman with metastatic breast cancer is referred to you for a second opinion on the use of U.S. Food and Drug Administration (FDA)-approved antimitotic inhibitors. She has had triple-negative breast cancer, which has failed to respond to two prior lines of treatment including an anthracycline and a taxane. She gives you a list of statements that she has found on social media and asks your opinion about their accuracy. Her performance status is 0, and she has mild renal insufficiency. Which one of the following statements is NOT accurate?

   A. Ixabepilone is an epothilone that is approved as monotherapy or in combination with capecitabine for metastatic or locally advanced breast cancer in patients in her condition.
   B. Myelosuppression (primarily neutropenia) and peripheral neuropathy (primarily sensory) may occur with 30% to 60% probability in patients treated with ixabepilone.
   C. The dose of ixabepilone should be reduced by 50% due to renal insufficiency.
   D. Eribulin is approved for treatment of patients with metastatic breast cancer in her condition.
   E. QT interval prolongation may occur in the second week of treatment with eribulin.

6. A 27-year-old woman with progressive headache, nausea and vomiting, and difficulty in word finding presents for further evaluation. Imaging of her brain shows a 4 × 6 cm mass involving the subcortical white matter, with low attenuation on CT, hypointense compared to gray matter on T1-weighted and hyperintense compared to gray matter on T2-weighted MRI scans. Brain biopsy shows histologic features

compatible with grade 2 oligodendroglioma, IDH1-R132H mutation positive on immunohistochemistry. Next-generation sequencing and 1p19q co-deletion status were not available. What is the best management step for this patient?

A. Subtotal resection of the tumor followed by radiation therapy
B. High-dose methotrexate
C. Subtotal resection of the tumor followed by radiation therapy concomitant with high-dose methotrexate as a radiation sensitizer
D. Palliative dexamethasone combined with palliative radiation
E. Procarbazine, lomustine (CCNU), and vincristine (PCV regimen) after radiation therapy

7. Patients who are treated with paclitaxel, docetaxel, nab-paclitaxel, or oxaliplatin, cisplatin can develop painful chemotherapy-induced peripheral neuropathy (CIPN), which may persist from weeks to years beyond chemotherapy completion, significantly affecting quality of life. Which of the following agents has some evidence of clinical benefit to decrease pain after chemotherapy?

A. Duloxetine (Cymbalta)
B. Olanzapine
C. Acetyl-L-carnitine
D. Gabapentin/pregabalin
E. Oral cannabinoids

8. A 37-year-old woman was diagnosed with T2/N1/M0, ER⁻, PR⁻, HER2⁺ immunohistochemistry findings for breast cancer while she is 24 weeks pregnant with a male fetus. After mastectomy, what do you recommend to this woman for adjuvant therapy?

A. Start paclitaxel, carboplatin, and trastuzumab now during pregnancy.
B. Start paclitaxel, carboplatin now during the pregnancy and doxorubicin, cyclophosphamide and trastuzumab after delivery.
C. Doxorubicin, cyclophosphamide now during the pregnancy and trastuzumab plus pertuzumab plus paclitaxel after delivery.
D. Start trastuzumab plus pertuzumab immunotherapy now during pregnancy and chemotherapy after delivery.
E. Do not start any treatment until after delivery.

9. A 44-year-old Iranian-American man with 20 pack–year smoking history and family history of brain tumor in his brother presented to the ED with gross hematuria. The patient underwent CT of the abdomen, which showed an 8-cm fungating mass at the left posterior wall of the bladder extending to the left ureteral orifice. No lymphadenopathy was identified. Cystoscopy showed a muscle invasive bladder cancer. The plan is to treat him with neoadjuvant MVAC (methotrexate 30 mg/m² IV day 1, 15, 22; vinblastine 3 mg/m² IV day 2, 15, 22; doxorubicin (Adriamycin) 30 mg/m² IV day 2; cisplatin 70 mg/m² IV day 2). The patient insist that if he were to develop significant nausea/vomiting, he would stop chemotherapy immediately. Which medication do you recommend to be added to ondansetron, aprepitant, and dexamethasone to optimally prevent/diminish nausea/vomiting for him?

A. Lorazepam (Ativan)

B. Rhizomes of *Zingiber officinale* (ginger)

C. Olanzapine (Zyprexa)

D. Prochlorperazine (Compazine)

E. Tofacitinib (Xeljanz)

10. A 55-year-old man with history of metastatic prostate cancer and otherwise no past medical history presents to the ED with severe bone pain and inability to urinate. He was recently told that his cancer stopped responding to hormone therapy. MRI scan shows several lytic lesions in ribs, vertebrae, and femur, without evidence of spinal cord compression, but with a significantly enlarged prostate. Prostate-specific antigen is 340 ng/mL. What is the best next step for his treatment?

A. Radium-223 or strontium-89 or Samarium-153

B. Docetaxel + prednisone

C. Radical prostatectomy followed by radiation

D. Degarelix

E. Bicalutamide for 1 week and then leuprolide depot injection

ANSWERS TO MULTIPLE-CHOICE QUESTIONS

1. **B.** Mertansine, or DM1, the cytotoxic component of ado-trastuzumab emtansine, is not a DNA minor groove inhibitor; it is a tubulin inhibitor, inhibiting the assembly of microtubules by binding to tubulin (see also Chapter 17). Ado-trastuzumab emtansine (Kadcyla) is a HER2-targeted antibody and microtubule inhibitor (DM1) conjugate that is indicated, as monotherapy, for the treatment of patients with HER2+, metastatic breast cancer who previously received trastuzumab and a taxane, for metastatic disease or developed disease recurrence during or within 6 months of completing adjuvant therapy. The efficacy of the agent was evaluated in a randomized, multicenter, open-label trial (EMILIA) of 991 patients with HER2+, unresectable, locally advanced, or metastatic breast cancer who were randomly allocated (1:1) to receive lapatinib plus capecitabine or ado-trastuzumab emtansine. In the EMILIA study, ado-trastuzumab emtansine statistically significantly improved progression-free survival (PFS) and overall survival (OS) compared with lapatinib plus capecitabine in patients with HER2+ advanced breast cancer who had previously been treated with trastuzumab and a taxane. It is also approved for the adjuvant treatment of patients with HER2+ early breast cancer who have residual invasive disease after neoadjuvant taxane and trastuzumab-based treatment. Hepatotoxicity, liver failure, and death have occurred in patients treated with ado-trastuzumab emtansine. Thrombocytopenia is the most common hematologic adverse event of ado-trastuzumab emtansine. Neurotoxicity, predominantly sensory, can occur in approximately 20% of patients receiving ado-trastuzumab emtansine.

2. **C.** The commonly used chemotherapeutic agents for intrathecal administration include methotrexate and cytarabine with or without a steroid (e.g., hydrocortisone). If given intrathecally by accident, vincristine can cause ascending radiculomyeloencephalopathy, which is always fatal.

3. **E.** Abraxane is a microtubule inhibitor indicated for the treatment of (1) metastatic adenocarcinoma of the pancreas as first-line treatment, in combination with gemcitabine; (2) metastatic breast cancer, after failure of combination chemotherapy for metastatic disease or relapse within 6 months of adjuvant chemotherapy (prior therapy should have included an anthracycline); and (3) locally advanced or metastatic non-small cell lung cancer, as first-line treatment in combination with carboplatin, in patients who are not candidates for curative surgery or radiation therapy.

4. **A.** All patients receiving docetaxel should be premedicated with oral corticosteroids (e.g., dexamethasone 16 mg daily or 8 mg twice daily) for 3 days starting 1 day prior to docetaxel administration in order to reduce the incidence and severity of fluid retention as well as the severity of hypersensitivity reactions. Severe fluid retention occurred in 6.5% of patients despite use of a 3-day dexamethasone premedication regimen. The fluid retention was characterized by one or more of the following signs/symptoms: generalized edema, peripheral edema, pleural effusion requiring urgent drainage, dyspnea at rest, cardiac tamponade, or pronounced abdominal distention due to ascites.

5. **C.** Ixabepilone (Ixempra) is a microtubule inhibitor that is indicated, as single agent, for the treatment of metastatic or locally advanced breast cancer in patients after failure of an anthracycline, a taxane, and capecitabine. It is also indicated in combination with capecitabine for the treatment of metastatic or locally advanced breast cancer in patients after failure of an anthracycline and a taxane. Ixabepilone is minimally excreted via kidney and as monotherapy; there was no meaningful effect of renal insufficiency (CrCL >30 mL/min) on the pharmacokinetics of ixabepilone. Hence, unless in rare circumstances, the dose of ixabepilone does not need to be reduced due to renal insufficiency.

    Eribulin mesylate (Halaven) is a microtubule inhibitor that is indicated for the treatment of patients with (1) unresectable or metastatic liposarcoma who have received a prior anthracycline-containing regimen, and (2) metastatic breast cancer who have previously received at least two chemotherapeutic regimens (including an anthracycline and a taxane) for the treatment of metastatic disease. Patients receiving eribulin should be monitored for prolonged QT intervals particularly with history of congestive heart failure, bradyarrhythmias, and electrolyte abnormalities.

6. **E.** A study by Buckner et al. (2016) enrolled of 251 eligible patients with grade 2 astrocytoma, oligoastrocytoma, or oligodendroglioma who were <40 years of age and had gone through subtotal resection or biopsy or who were ≥40 years of age and had biopsy or resection of any of the tumor. Patients who received radiation therapy plus PCV chemotherapy had longer median OS than did those who received radiation therapy alone (13.3 vs. 7.8 years; hazard ratio for death, 0.59; p = .003). The rate of PFS at 10 years was 51% in the group that received radiation therapy+PCV versus 21% in the group that received radiation therapy alone; the corresponding rates of OS at 10 years were 60% and 40%.

7. **A.** There is no agent that is recommended for the prevention of CIPN. Duloxetine is the only agent that has adequate evidence to support its use for patients with established painful CIPN. In a multicenter randomized clinical trial (Lavoie Smith et al., 2013) that enrolled 231 adult patients with ≥grade 1 sensory CIPN to receive either duloxetine followed by placebo or placebo followed by duloxetine (duloxetine/placebo 30 mg/one capsule daily for the first week, then 60 mg/two capsules for 4 additional weeks), patients receiving duloxetine as initial treatment (weeks 1–5) reported a larger mean decrease in average pain (1.06; 95% CI: 0.72, 1.40) compared to placebo-treated patients (0.34; 95% CI: 0.01, 0.66, p = .003, effect size = 0.513). Also approximately 60% of duloxetine-treated patients compared to approximately 40% of placebo-treated patients reported decreased pain of any amount.

    According to the American Society of Clinical Oncology (ASCO) Guideline for Prevention and Management of Chemotherapy-Induced Peripheral Neuropathy in Survivors of Adult Cancers, outside the context of a clinical trial, the use of the following interventions for the treatment of CIPN cannot be recommended: exercise therapy, acupuncture, scrambler therapy, gabapentin/pregabalin, topical gel treatment containing baclofen, amitriptyline +/− ketamine, tricyclic antidepressants, or oral cannabinoids.

    The use of acetyl-L-carnitine for the prevention of CIPN in patients with cancer should not be recommended as harms outweigh benefits (Campone et al., 2013).

8. **C.** Taxanes and anti-HER2 antibodies can cause harm to fetus when administered to a pregnant woman. In animal reproduction studies, administration of taxanes to pregnant rats and rabbits during the period of organogenesis caused embryo-fetal toxicities, including intrauterine death even at very small dosages. Use of trastuzumab during pregnancy can cause oligohydramnios and oligohydramnios sequence manifesting as pulmonary hypoplasia, skeletal abnormalities, and neonatal death. Exposure to trastuzumab during pregnancy or within 7 months prior to conception can result in fetal harm. Cyclophosphamide and doxorubicin are pregnancy category D agents; however, potential benefits may justify treatment with these agents during pregnancy during the second and third trimesters (Ring et al., 2005).

9. **C.** Olanzapine has appropriate evidence for prevention and treatment of chemotherapy-induced nausea and vomiting (CINV). The addition of 5 mg daily of oral olanzapine to standard therapy has been shown to reduce the frequency of CINV and improve quality of life of patients receiving moderately or highly emetogenic chemotherapy (Mizukami et al., 2014). A randomized, double-blind, Phase 3 clinical trial (Navari et al., 2016), compared olanzapine (10 mg orally or matching placebo daily on days 1 through 4) with placebo, in combination with dexamethasone, aprepitant or fosaprepitant, and a 5-HT receptor antagonist, in patients with no previous chemotherapy who were receiving cisplatin or cyclophosphamide–doxorubicin. The doses of the three concomitant drugs administered before and after chemotherapy were similar in the two groups. Among 380 enrolled patients, the proportion of patients with no CINV was significantly greater with olanzapine than with placebo in the first 24 hours after chemotherapy, day 2 to day 5, and the overall 120-hour period.

10. **B.** In a randomized clinical trial (Tannock et al., 2004) approximately 1,000 men with metastatic hormone-refractory prostate cancer received 5 mg of prednisone twice daily and were randomly assigned to receive 12 mg/m^2 of mitoxantrone every 3 weeks, 75 mg/m^2 of docetaxel every 3 weeks, or 30 mg/m^2 of docetaxel weekly for 5 of every 6 weeks. The primary endpoint of the trial was overall survival. As compared with the men in the mitoxantrone group, men in the group given docetaxel every 3 weeks had a hazard ratio for death of 0.76 (95% CI, 0.62 to 0.94; p = .009 by the stratified log-rank test) and those given weekly docetaxel had a hazard ratio for death of 0.91 (95% CI, 0.75 to 1.11; p = .36). The median survival was 16.5 months in the mitoxantrone group, 18.9 months in the group given docetaxel every 3 weeks, and 17.4 months in the group given weekly docetaxel.

SELECTED REFERENCES

Banach M, Juranek JK, Zygulska AL. Chemotherapy-induced neuropathies—A growing problem for patients and health care providers. Brain Behav. 2017;7(1):e00558. https://doi.org/10.1002/brb3.558

Brunton LL, Knollman BC. Goodman & Gilman's: The Pharmacological Basis of Therapeutics, 14th ed. New York: McGraw-Hill Education; 2022.

Buckner JC, Shaw EG, Pugh SL, et al. Radiation plus procarbazine, CCNU, and vincristine in low-grade glioma. N Engl J Med. 2016;374(14):1344–55. https://doi.org/10.1056/NEJMoa1500925

Campone M, Berton-Rigaud D, Joly-Lobbedez F, et al. A double-blind, randomized phase II study to evaluate the safety and efficacy of acetyl-L-carnitine in the prevention of sagopilone-induced peripheral neuropathy. Oncologist. 2013;18(11):1190–1. https://doi.org/10.1634/theoncologist.2013-0061

Eli S, Castagna R, Mapelli M, Parisini E. Recent approaches to the identification of novel microtubule-targeting agents. Front Mol Biosci. 2022;9:841777. https://doi.org/10.3389/fmolb.2022.841777

Hou S, Huh B, Kim HK, et al. Treatment of chemotherapy-induced peripheral neuropathy: Systematic review and recommendations. Pain Phys. 2018 Nov;21(6):571–92. https://doi.org/10.36076/ppj.2018.6.571

Lavoie Smith EM, Pang H, Cirrincione C, et al. Effect of duloxetine on pain, function, and quality of life among patients with chemotherapy-induced painful peripheral neuropathy: A randomized clinical trial. JAMA. 2013;309(13):1359–67. https://doi.org/10.1001/jama.2013.2813

Lee JJ, Swain SM. Peripheral neuropathy induced by microtubule-stabilizing agents. J Clin Oncol. 2006;24(10):1633–42. https://doi.org/10.1200/JCO.2005.04.0543

Mizukami N, Yamauchi M, Koike K, et al. Olanzapine for the prevention of chemotherapy-induced nausea and vomiting in patients receiving highly or moderately emetogenic chemotherapy: A randomized, double-blind, placebo-controlled study. J Pain Symptom Manage. 2014;47(3):542–50. https://doi.org/10.1016/j.jpainsymman.2013.05.003

Moriyama B, Henning SA, Leung J, et al. Adverse interactions between antifungal azoles and vincristine: Review and analysis of cases. Mycoses. 2012;55(4):290–7. https://doi.org/10.1111/j.1439-0507.2011.02158.x

Navari RM, Qin R, Ruddy KJ, et al. Olanzapine for the prevention of chemotherapy-induced nausea and vomiting. N Engl J Med. 2016;375(2):134–42. https://doi.org/10.1056/NEJMoa1515725

Ring AE, Smith IE, Jones A, et al. Chemotherapy for breast cancer during pregnancy: An 18-year experience from five London teaching hospitals. J Clin Oncol. 2005;23(18):4192–7. https://doi.org/10.1200/JCO.2005.03.038

Schiff PB, Fant J, Horwitz SB. Promotion of microtubule assembly in vitro by Taxol. Nature. 1979;277(5698):665–7. https://doi.org/10.1038/277665a0

Smith EM, Pang H, Cirrincione C, et al. Effect of duloxetine on pain, function, and quality of life among patients with chemotherapy-induced painful peripheral neuropathy: A randomized clinical trial. JAMA. 2013;309(13):1359–67. https://doi.org/10.1001/jama.2013.2813

Tannock IF, de Wit R, Berry WR, et al. Docetaxel plus prednisone or mitoxantrone plus prednisone for advanced prostate cancer. N Engl J Med. 2004;351(15):1502–12. https://doi.org/10.1056/NEJMoa040720

West H, McCleod M, Hussein M, et al. Atezolizumab in combination with carboplatin plus nab-paclitaxel chemotherapy compared with chemotherapy alone as first-line treatment for metastatic non-squamous non-small-cell lung cancer (IMpower130): A multicentre, randomised, open-label, phase 3 trial. Lancet Oncol. 2019;20(7):924–37. https://doi.org/10.1016/S1470-2045(19)30167-6

Wiernik PH, Schwartz EL, Einzig A, et al. Phase I trial of Taxol given as a 24-hour infusion every 21 days: Responses observed in metastatic melanoma. J Clin Oncol. 1987;5(8):1232–9. https://doi.org/10.1200/JCO.1987.5.8.1232

Exploiting Cellular and Extracellular Pathways

CHAPTER 9

Drugs Targeting DNA Repair, Cell Cycle, and Apoptosis

MIRA A. KOHORST • SCOTT H. KAUFMANN

INTRODUCTION

A wide variety of established and investigational anticancer drugs target topoisomerases, enzymes that adjust the torsional strain in DNA during normal physiologic processes, or components of the DNA damage response, a series of biochemical reactions that recognize DNA alterations and help cells respond to them. If not properly repaired, damage induced by topoisomerases or perpetuated by inhibitors of DNA repair can lead to apoptosis. Thus, the processes of DNA metabolism, DNA repair, and apoptosis play critical roles in current anticancer therapies.

When targeting processes as fundamental as these, one might think that there would be no therapeutic window for successful anticancer treatment. However, many neoplasms have underlying DNA repair defects, as evidenced by their genomic instability. As a result of these defects, the cancer cells are often dependent on alternative DNA repair pathways for their survival, and targeting these alternative pathways can be quite beneficial. A now classical example of this so-called synthetic lethality is the extreme sensitivity of homologous recombination-deficient cancers to inhibitors of the repair enzyme poly(ADP-ribose) polymerase 1 (PARP1), an ADP (adenosine diphosphate) ribosyl transferase. Likewise, many oncogenic kinases lead to enhanced activation of antiapoptotic pathways. Because of their exposure to a variety of stresses, including elevated reactive oxygen species, proteotoxic stress, and nutrient deficiencies, neoplastic cells are often dependent on these hyperactivated antiapoptotic pathways for their survival. In this context, small molecule inhibitors called BH3 mimetics that inactivate antiapoptotic proteins may sometimes be effective antineoplastic agents, either alone or in combination with cytotoxic chemotherapeutic agents.

In this chapter we briefly review the cellular physiology and pharmacology of agents that target topoisomerases, the DNA damage response, antiapoptotic proteins, and cyclin-dependent kinases.

TOPOISOMERASES: ENDOGENOUS ENZYMES THAT BECOME AGENTS OF DNA DAMAGE

DNA in somatic cells is constantly undergoing extensive structural changes. During transcription, the two strands of DNA are pried apart to allow RNA polymerases to synthesize messenger, ribosomal, and transfer RNAs. During replication, the parental strands are separated to serve as templates for the daughter strands. Both transcription and replication generate torsional strain in the DNA, and both processes quickly grind to a halt if this torsional strain is not relieved. Accordingly, enzymes that relieve this torsional strain play very important roles in DNA metabolism.

Mammalian cells contain a variety of enzymes called DNA topoisomerases that have evolved to resolve torsional strain (Figure 9.1). Topoisomerase I (TOP1) and topoisomerase III (TOP3) nick the DNA backbone, allow rotation of one strand of the DNA with respect to the other, and reseal the DNA. In contrast, topoisomerase II (TOP2) isoenzymes introduce a double-strand break in the DNA, pass an intact piece of double-stranded DNA through the break, and reseal the DNA. These various enzymes play critical but distinct roles during various aspects of DNA metabolism. In particular, nuclear TOP1 relieves torsional strain in the vicinity of transcription complexes. TOP2α, which is expressed in a cell cycle–dependent manner, appears to facilitate decatenation of intertwined daughter strands during and after DNA replication. TOP2β adjusts torsional strain in promoters to allow gene activation.

These enzymes are critical targets for a variety of anticancer drugs. For example, camptothecins and indinoisoquinolines stabilize TOP1-DNA covalent complexes that ordinarily form as transient intermediates in the TOP1 catalytic cycle. These covalent complexes stall advancing replication forks, triggering part of the DNA damage response described later in this chapter. If the TOP1-DNA covalent complexes cannot be reversed, either by restarting the enzyme or by proteolytically cleaving it and hydrolyzing the peptide-DNA adduct, DNA double-strand breaks result and lead to further damage. Agents in clinical practice that target TOP1 include topotecan, SN-38 (the active metabolite of irinotecan), and exatecan (Tables 9.1 and 9.2). Building on the activity of these agents, topotecan, SN-38, and exatecan have been coupled to targeting antibodies as exemplified by fam-trastuzumab-deruxtecan (Enhertu), which consists of exatecan conjugated to the anti-HER2 antibody trastuzumab. In addition, irinotecan is U.S. Food and Drug Administration (FDA) approved as a nanoliposomal formulation (Onivyde); and additional formulations of SN-38 and exatecan continue to undergo preclinical and clinical testing.

A growing body of preclinical evidence indicates that TOP1 inhibitors also sensitize neoplastic cells to immunotherapy. Accordingly, several studies of TOP1 inhibitors in combination with immune checkpoint blockers are currently ongoing.

Agents that target TOP2 likewise stabilize covalent complexes between TOP2 isoenzymes and DNA that transiently form during the normal TOP2 catalytic cycle. Helicases that pry the DNA apart for replication or transcription can then convert these trapped complexes into DNA double-strand breaks, with dire consequences for the cell. Agents with this mechanism of action include anthracyclines such as doxorubicin, epipodophyllotoxins such as etoposide, and anthracenediones such as mitoxantrone (Tables 9.1 and 9.2). Interestingly, the secondary leukemias associated with these agents have been traced, in part, to effects of these drugs on TOP2β. Likewise, the MLL (mixed lineage leukemia)-rearranged infant leukemias have been traced to dietary flavonoids acting on topoisomerase II in utero.

In addition to these anticancer drugs, a number of endogenous DNA lesions cause trapping of TOP1- or TOP2-containing DNA–protein crosslinks. For example, incorporation of ribonucleotides into DNA during replication results in trapping of TOP1 covalently bound to DNA. Likewise, abasic sites and other base excision repair intermediates cause trapping of TOP2-DNA covalent complexes. Accordingly, cells have evolved a number of enzymatic strategies for dealing with endogenous DNA lesions, including trapped topoisomerases.

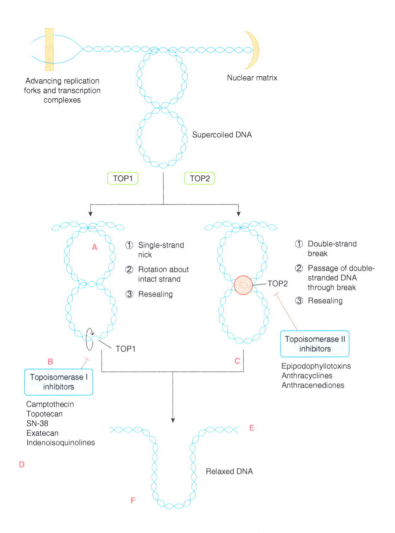

FIGURE 9.1 **Function and therapeutic targeting of DNA topoisomerase I and II.**
(A) Advancing replication forks and transcription complexes create DNA supercoiling.
This torsional strain is relieved by both topoisomerase I (TOP1) and topoisomerase II
(TOP2) by different mechanisms. **(B)** TOP1 acts by nicking one of the strands of DNA
and allowing controlled rotation about the intact strand, resulting in DNA relaxation.
TOP1, which is covalently bound to the DNA, then enables religation of the DNA
backbone and is released from the DNA. **(C)** TOP2 is active at areas of double-
stranded DNA overlap (i.e., supercoiled or catenated DNA). The enzyme creates a
double-strand break in one of the DNA segments, allowing passage of the other
double-stranded DNA segment through the break. It then reseals the gating strand
and is released. **(D)** TOP1 inhibitors (e.g., camptothecin, topotecan, exatecan, and
SN-38 [7-ethyl-10-hydroxycamptothecin]) intercalate into the DNA at the TOP1 active
site and prevent the religation step. This results in increased TOP1-DNA covalent
complexes, which impede advancing replication forks and transcription machinery,
ultimately leading to DNA damage and cell death by apoptosis. **(E)** TOP2 inhibitors
(e.g., epipodophyllotoxins, anthracyclines, and anthracenediones) stabilize TOP2-
DNA covalent complexes, which similarly results in significant DNA damage and cell
death. **(F)** Torsional strain relieved by TOP1 and TOP2 results in relaxed DNA.
Source: Adapted from Nitiss JL., Nat Rev Cancer, 2009.

TABLE 9.1 Topoisomerase Inhibitors: Clinical Considerations

AGENTS	DISEASES	TOXICITIES	DOSE MODIFICATIONS
Topoisomerase I inhibitors		BM, oral, and GI mucosa	
Topotecan	Ovarian, small cell lung cancer, endometrial		Renal
Irinotecan (prodrug of SN-38)	GI malignancies, lung cancer		Hepatic, UGTIA1 deficiency
Nanoliposomal irinotecan	Pancreatic cancer (with fluoropyrimidines)	Interstitial lung disease	UGT1A1 deficiency
Trastuzumab deruxtecan (exatecan conjugated to anti-HER2 antibody)	Recurrent breast and gastric cancers	Interstitial lung disease	
Sacituzumab govitecan (SN-38 conjugated to anti-TROP2 antibody)	Triple negative breast cancer and advanced uroepithelial cancer	Hypersensitivity reactions	UGT1A1 deficiency
Topoisomerase II inhibitors		BM, oral, GI mucosa, and t-AML	
Anthracyclines		Cardiac	Hepatic
Daunorubicin	Acute leukemias		
Idarubicin	Acute leukemias		
Doxorubicin	Breast, lymphomas		
Mitoxantrone	Acute leukemias, lymphomas, prostate		
Epirubicin	Breast, upper GI		
Podophyllins		Hepatic, infusional	Renal, hepatic
Etoposide	AML, testicular, lung, neuroblastoma		
Teniposide	ALL, lung, bladder, neuroblastoma		

ALL, acute lymphocytic leukemia; AML, acute myeloid leukemia; BM, bone marrow; GI, gastrointestinal; HER2, human epidermal growth factor receptor 2; t-AML, treatment-related AML; TROP-2, trophoblast cell surface antigen-2; UGT1A1, uridine diphosphate glucuronosyl transferase.

TABLE 9.2 Topoisomerase Inhibitors: Pharmacologic Considerations

AGENT	ADMINISTRATION/ ELIMINATION	MECHANISMS OF RESISTANCE*
Topoisomerase I inhibitors		Decreased TOP I Increased PARP DNA repair pathways ATR/CHK I DNA repair pathway Decreased cell proliferation
Topotecan	IV, oral/renal	Increased ABCB1, ABCC4, ABCC1, ABCG2
Irinotecan	IV, renal, hepatic	Increased ABCC1, ABCG2
Topoisomerase II inhibitors		Decreased TOP2 Decreased cell proliferation Increased ABCB1, ABCC1, ABCG2 and other ABC transporters
Anthracyclines		
Daunorubicin	IV, hepatic	
Idarubicin	IV, oral/hepatic	
Doxorubicin	IV, hepatic	
Mitoxantrone	IV, hepatic	
Epirubicin	IV, oral/hepatic	
Epipodophyllotoxins		
Etoposide	IV, oral/hepatic	
Teniposide	IV, hepatic	

*ABCB1 (MDR1), ABCC1 (MRP), ABCC4 and ABCG2 (BCRP) are multidrug transporters that act as efflux pumps in many types of cancer cells when overexpressed.

ATR, ataxia-telangiectasia and Rad3-related; BCRP, breast cancer resistance protein; CHK1, checkpoint kinase 1; IV, intravenous; MDR, multidrug resistance; MRP, multidrug resistance protein; PARP, poly(ADP-ribose) polymerase; TOP1, topoisomerase I.

Elevated expression of these components of the DNA damage response are among the mechanisms implicated in resistance to topoisomerase poisons.

TARGETING THE DNA DAMAGE RESPONSE

During normal DNA metabolism and as a consequence of environmental exposure, DNA in each cell sustains tens of thousands of damaging lesions each day. Types of DNA damage include covalent modifications of DNA bases, single- and double-strand breaks in the DNA backbone, covalent adducts between the DNA backbone and proteins, and nucleotide

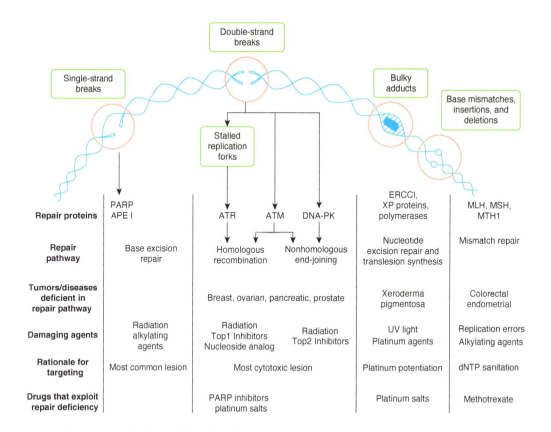

FIGURE 9.2 Targeting the DNA damage response pathway.

DNA damage response (DRR) proteins are summarized in this figure, along with descriptions of their associated repair pathways, examples of tumors that exemplify deficiencies in these pathways, agents that induce specific types of dama, the rationale for targeting, and drugs that exploit the specific repair deficiencies.

ADP, adenosine diphosphate; AP, apurinic/apyrimidinic; APE1, AP endonuclease 1; ATM, ataxia-telangiectasia mutated; ATR, ataxia-telangiectasia and Rad3-related; DNA-PK, DNA-dependent protein kinase; dNTP, deoxyribonucleoside triphosphate; ERCC1, excision repair, complementing deficient, in Chinese hamster, 1; MLH, MutL homolog; MSH, MutS homolog; MTH1, MutT homolog 1; PARP, poly(ADP-ribose) polymerase; XP, xeroderma pigmentosa.

Source: Adapted from Lord CJ, Ashworth A., Nature, 2012; O'Connor MJ., Mol Cell, 2015.

insertions, deletions, or substitutions. To deal with this wide variety of lesions, cells have developed a series of biochemical reactions that are able to reverse or repair these various types of DNA damage (**Figure 9.2**).

As understanding of various components of the DNA damage response has developed, efforts have been made to target these various pathways. Current understanding suggests that these inhibitors are most effective in neoplasms that have underlying defects in parallel or complementary pathways, as illustrated in the following text and **Figure 9.3**.

Targeting the ATR–CHK1–WEE1 Pathway to Inhibit the Replication Checkpoint

DNA polymerases stall when they encounter a variety of lesions, including bulky adducts (e.g., TOP1-DNA covalent complexes), nucleoside analogs incorporated into DNA (e.g., after

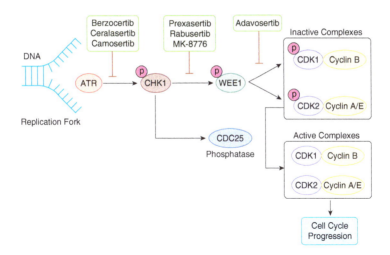

FIGURE 9.3 **Targeting the ATR–CHK1–WEE1 pathway to inhibit the replication checkpoint.**
Replication fork stalling or DNA damage activates the protein kinase ATR, which activates CHK1 and WEE1. Activated WEE1 then phosphorylates and inactivates CDK2–cyclin A/E and CDK1–cyclin B complexes. CHK1 also inhibits CDC25 phosphatases, which otherwise would dephosphorylate the CDK2–cyclin A/E and CDK1–cyclin B complexes, resulting in activation of the complexes and cell cycle progression. Because many malignancies have a deficient G1 checkpoint, they are often more dependent on the S and G2/M checkpoints to prevent cells with excessive DNA damage from entering mitosis, resulting in mitotic collapse and ultimately apoptosis. Therapeutic targeting of the ATR–CHK1–WEE1 pathway may therefore be particularly advantageous in malignancies with G1 checkpoint deficiencies or those under significant replication stress.

ATR, ataxia-telangiectasia and Rad3-related; CDC25, cell division cycle 25; CDK, cyclin-dependent kinase; CHK1, checkpoint kinase 1; WEE1, Wee1 homolog.
Source: Adapted from Karnitz LM, Zou L., Clin Cancer Res, 2015.

treatment with gemcitabine or cytarabine), or certain DNA crosslinks such as those introduced by cisplatin or melphalan. This replication fork stalling leads directly to activation of the protein kinases ATR (ataxia telangiectasia and Rad3-related protein), checkpoint kinase 1 (CHK1), and WEE1 that initiate a series of biochemical processes that stop firing of additional replication origins, stabilize replication forks, and attempt to restart the DNA polymerases (**Figure 9.3**).

Importantly, inhibition of ATR has been shown to enhance the cytotoxicity of TOP1 poisons, nucleoside analogs, and platinum agents in preclinical studies, with CHK1 inhibitors having somewhat more limited sensitizing effects. Accordingly, early-phase clinical trials of ATR inhibitors (berzosertib, ceralasertib camonsertib, BAY1895344, IMP9064) and CHK1 inhibitors (prexasertib) as modulators of the replication checkpoint are ongoing. For example, in a recently reported Phase 2 trial in patients with recurrent, platinum-resistant high-grade serous ovarian cancer, the ATR inhibitor berzosertib combined with the nucleoside analog gemcitabine was more effective than gemcitabine alone. Subsequent laboratory studies have suggested that the increased response reflects the ability of berzosertib to increase replication stress, thus sensitizing cancers to gemcitabine.

WEE1 kinase plays a critical role in S and G2/M checkpoint integrity and is highly expressed in many malignancies, including leukemia, breast cancers, melanoma, and both adult and pediatric brain tumors. WEE1 inhibition is thought to potentiate DNA-damaging therapy and has been targeted with the potent inhibitor adavosertib, which is currently being tested in clinical trials in combination with gemcitabine, platinum compounds, and other DNA damaging agents.

Targeting DNA-Dependent Protein Kinase

DNA double-strand breaks arise in cells as a consequence of exposure to ionizing radiation and when replication forks collapse. Accordingly, cells have evolved several pathways for dealing with these very toxic lesions. During S and G2 phases of the cell cycle, DNA double-strand breaks are repaired by homologous recombination, a process in which a second DNA double strand with identical sequence serves as a template for repair of the damaged DNA double strand. In G0 and G1 phases of the cell cycle, however, the sister chromatid that can serve as a template for homologous recombination is not present and multiple components of the homologous recombination pathway are missing from cells. Under these conditions, DNA double-strand breaks are repaired by a process known as nonhomologous end-joining (NHEJ). This repair process involves initial binding of KU70/KU80 heterodimers to the broken DNA ends and recruitment of the kinase DNA-PKcs (DNA-dependent protein kinase, catalytic subunit) phosphorylation and recruitment of downstream components such as the nuclease artemis, the scaffolding protein XRCC4, and DNA ligase IV; and processing and ligation of the broken ends. Because of its critical role in this process, DNA-PKcs has emerged as a potential drug target. Inhibitors of DNA-PKcs have been shown to enhance sensitivity to ionizing radiation. Whether these will have any impact on the treatment of hematologic malignancies remains to be determined.

PARP Inhibitors

Poly(ADP-ribose) polymerase (PARP1) is the most abundant member of a family of enzymes that transfer ADP-ribose monomer or polymer to a series of protein substrates. PARP1 synthesizes long-branched chains of ADP-ribose polymer attached to proteins after stimulation by either DNA single- or double-strand breaks. The resulting polymer modifies the action of a series of nuclear proteins and also serves as a docking scaffold for additional DNA repair components. PARP1 has been reported to modulate a number of different DNA repair processes, including homologous recombination, classical NHEJ, alternative NHEJ, and base excision repair.

Early studies showed that inhibition of PARP1 activity not only results in failure to synthesize polymer but also in trapping of PARP1 at sites of DNA damage. This reflects the fact that attachment of poly(ADP-ribose) polymer to PARP1 diminishes the affinity of this protein for damaged DNA. More recent studies have demonstrated that inhibition of PARP1 is particularly toxic to cells with certain types of DNA repair deficiencies, specifically loss of BRCA1, BRCA2, and other components of the homologous recombination pathway (Figure 9.4). Various explanations have been put forward for this so-called synthetic lethality, including (a) excess conversion of DNA single-strand breaks into double-strand breaks in the presence of PARP inhibitor, (b) excess error-prone nonhomologous end-joining in the absence of homologous recombination, (c) a requirement for PARP1 in order for alternative NHEJ to occur, (d) excess incorporation of ribonucleotides into DNA, leading to enhanced trapping of TOP1-DNA covalent complexes in the absence of PARP activity, (e) failure to stabilize and restart stalled replication forks, and (f) failure to properly join nascent DNA fragments during replication.

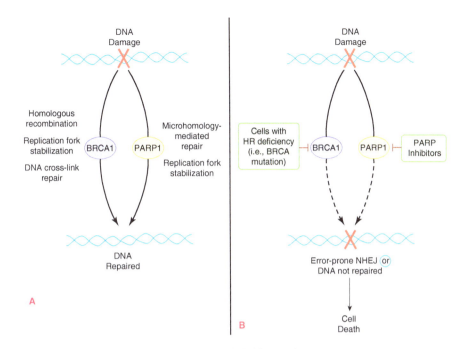

FIGURE 9.4 **PARP inhibitors exemplify synthetic lethality.**
(A) Under normal conditions, DNA damage is repaired by multiple, often redundant, mechanisms. BRCA1 is an important protein in homologous recombination, replication fork stabilization, and DNA cross-link repair. PARP1 contributes to microhomology-mediated DNA repair and replication fork stabilization. If BRCA1 (or another protein involved in homologous recombination) is lost, DNA can still be repaired through the PARP1-mediated pathways. Similarly, if PARP1 inhibitors are administered, DNA can still be repaired through the BRCA1 pathways. **(B)** However, when cells with a deficiency in homologous recombination (HR) are treated with a PARP1 inhibitor, both repair pathways are disabled, resulting in error-prone nonhomologous end-joining (NHEJ) or unrepaired DNA damage and ultimately cell death in a process termed synthetic lethality.

BRCA1, breast cancer susceptibility gene 1; PARP 1, poly(ADP-ribose) polymerase 1.

Source: Adapted from Scott CL, Swisher EM, Kaufmann SH., J Clin Oncol, 2015.

Whatever the explanation, PARP inhibitors have demonstrated promising activity in a variety of clinical settings. In platinum-sensitive *BRCA1*- and *BRCA2*-mutant ovarian cancer, PARP inhibitors as single agents exhibited response rates of 40% to 80%. After their initial approval as monotherapy or maintenance where homologous recombination deficiencies were known or suspected, they have been widely tested as single agents and in combinations. A summary of current FDA approvals is shown in Table 9.3. While the approvals in ovarian cancer are broad and do not require a *BRCA1* or *BRCA2* mutation, efforts to better define the settings in which these agents produce the most benefit are currently ongoing.

The FDA-approved PARP inhibitors universally inhibit two PARP family members, PARP1 and PARP2, which are both involved in DNA repair. Their impact on other PARP family members, which share extensive homology in their ADP-ribosyl transferase domains, varies from agent to agent. Common side effects of PARP inhibitors include fatigue, nausea, and myelosuppression, with one of them (talazoparib) also causing alopecia. A more selective PARP1 inhibitor is currently undergoing clinical testing.

TABLE 9.3 FDA Approvals for PARP Inhibitors

PARP INHIBITOR	DISEASE	SETTING	SPECIAL CONSIDERATIONS
Niraparib	Ovarian cancer (OC)	First-line maintenance of OC if in PR or CR after surgery and adjuvant/neoadjuvant chemotherapy	FDA approved regardless of HR status, but shows largest median survival benefit in *BRCA1/BRCA2*-mutant OC
Olaparib	Ovarian cancer (OC)	First-line maintenance of *BRCA1/2*-mutated ovarian cancer if in PR or CR after surgery and adjuvant/neoadjuvant chemotherapy	Approved for both germline and somatic *BRCA1/2* mutations.
	Prostate cancer (PC)	Metastatic castration-resistant PC with *BRCA1/2* mutations	
	Breast cancer (BC)	First-line maintenance for germline *BRCA1/2* mutated HER2⁻ early high risk BC in older patients	Maintenance after adjuvant or neoadjuvant chemohormonal therapy
Rucaparib	Ovarian cancer (OC)	Second-line maintenance of platinum-sensitive OC	Efficacy greatest in monotherapy trials if OC harbors *BRCA1/BRCA2* mutation
	Prostate cancer (PC)	Metastatic castration-resistant PC with *BRCA1/2* mutations	
Talazoparib	Breast cancer (BC)	Germline *BRCA1/2* mutated HER2⁻ locally advanced or metastatic BC	

CR, complete response; FDA, U.S. Food and Drug Administration; HER2, human epidermal growth factor receptor 2; HR, homologous recombination: PARP, poly(ADP-ribose) polymerase; PR, partial response.

Importantly, PARP inhibitor treatment has also been associated the development of therapy-related myelodysplastic syndrome and acute myeloid leukemia (AML). All reported cases have occurred in ovarian cancer patients who had received prior carboplatin therapy, a treatment that has previously been associated with development of secondary myeloid neoplasms. Comparison across arms in randomized trials comparing chemotherapy plus PARP inhibitor to chemotherapy alone suggests that PARP inhibitors increase the risk of these myeloid neoplasms ~2.6-fold. Because these myeloid neoplasms have generally lost both copies of the *TP53* tumor suppressor gene, they tend to be resistant to chemotherapy. Accordingly, there is a growing sentiment to use PARP inhibitor maintenance only in those patients who have been shown to benefit the most.

ACTIVATING APOPTOSIS: BH3 MIMETICS AND BEYOND

As indicated in the introduction, all of the drugs described previously induce apoptosis in susceptible cells when they are active. Apoptosis is a form of cell suicide in which individual cells undergo an increasingly well-defined series of biochemical changes that result in loss of viability and packaging of cell fragments for disposal. These biochemical changes reflect, at least in part, the action of a series of intracellular proteases called caspases, which are activated through two distinct pathways.

Activation of the mitochondrial or intrinsic pathway results in mitochondrial release of cytochrome c, which is a cofactor for the activation of caspase 9 (Figure 9.5). Release of cytochrome c from mitochondria is in turn regulated by a series of protein–protein interactions involving

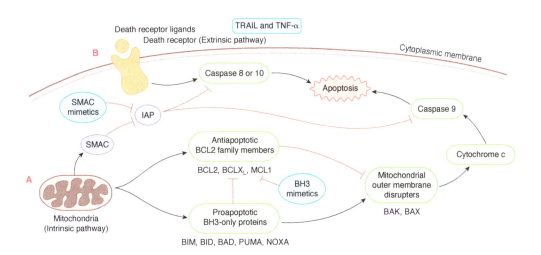

FIGURE 9.5 Therapeutic activation of apoptosis.
(A) The mitochondrial or intrinsic pathway results in mitochondrial release of cytochrome c, which activates an intracellular protease, caspase 9, leading to an intracellular protease cascade and digestion of cellular substrates to yield the process recognized as apoptosis. The process of cytochrome c release is tightly regulated by antiapoptotic proteins (i.e., BCL2 family members, including BCL2, $BCLX_L$, and MCL1) and proapoptotic proteins (i.e., BH3-only proteins, including BIM, PUMA, NOXA, and a fragment of BID) that ultimately control BAK and BAX, the mitochondrial outer membrane disruptors that lead to the release of cytochrome c. BH3 mimetics, which act like BH3-only proteins, promote apoptosis by this pathway. Aside from cytochrome c, other mitochondrial intermembrane proteins are released, including second mitochondrial activator of caspases (SMAC), which neutralizes caspase inhibitors termed IAP (inhibitor of apoptosis) proteins. Thus, SMAC has also been mimicked therapeutically (i.e., SMAC mimetics) as an anticancer drug. **(B)** The death receptor or extrinsic pathway is activated by death receptor ligands (e.g., TRAIL and TNF-α), which then activate caspase 8 or 10 to trigger apoptosis.

TNF-α, tumor necrosis factor alpha; TRAIL, TNF-related apoptosis-inducing ligand.

Sources: Adapted from Dai H, Meng XW, Kaufmann SH., F1000Res, 2016; Taylor RC, Cullen SP, Martin SJ., Nat Rev Mol Cell Biol, 2008.

BCL2 family members. Through a process that remains poorly understood, two of these family members, BAX and BAK, are able to permeabilize the outer mitochondrial membranes to allow cytochrome c release. BAX and BAK are present in a variety of normal and neoplastic cells but are prevented from acting unless other events occur. BAX and BAK can be activated by binding to a series of small proteins (e.g., Bim, PUMA, NOXA, BAD, and a fragment of BID), termed BH3-only proteins, that serve as sensors of various types of cellular stress, including DNA damage, loss of adhesion-mediated signaling, interruption of microtubule function, and intracellular protease activation. Through a series of competing interactions, both BAX/BAK and the BH3-only proteins are held in check by antiapoptotic BCL2 family members, including $BCLX_L$, MCL1, and the eponymous BCL2 itself. In neoplasms in which these antiapoptotic proteins are overexpressed as a consequence of gene rearrangements or amplification, there is enhanced ability to neutralize the proapoptotic proteins and resist apoptotic stimuli.

To counteract the antiapoptotic effects of overexpressed BCL2, $BCLX_L$, and MCL1, a series of small molecules termed BH3 mimetics (because they mimic BH3-only proteins) have been developed. Venetoclax is a potent and highly selective BCL2 antagonist that is FDA approved, alone or in combination with the anti-CD20 antibody rituximab, for the treatment of chronic lymphocytic leukemia, a disease in which BCL2 is overexpressed as a consequence of loss of two BCL2-suppressive microRNAs. In addition, venetoclax is approved for treatment of newly diagnosed AML in adults who are age 75 years or older, or who have comorbidities that preclude use of intensive induction chemotherapy, in combination with azacitidine or decitabine or low-dose cytarabine. Based on these results, venetoclax is currently being tested in combination with intensive induction and consolidation therapy in younger patients with a goal of increasing the depth and durability of complete remissions. Venetoclax as monotherapy has less promising activity for newly diagnosed AML. Moreover, venetoclax as monotherapy or in combination has shown limited activity in treatment of patients with relapsed or refractory AML, most likely because the antiapoptotic protein MCL1 is prominently upregulated at the time of AML relapse.

Targeting of other antiapoptotic BCL2 family members has lagged behind targeting of BCL2. The potent and selective MCL1 inhibitors MIK665 (S64315), tapotoclax (AMG176), AMG397, and AZD5991 have shown promising single-agent activity against multiple myeloma, acute leukemia, and solid tumor preclinical models. These agents have entered clinical testing in lymphoma, multiple myeloma, and/or AML. Clinical testing, however, has been halted on three of these four agents due to concerns of cardiotoxicity. The BCL2/$BCLX_L$ dual inhibitor navitoclax and selective $BCLX_L$-directed BH3 mimetics such as A1331852 underwent late preclinical and early clinical testing, but their development was halted due to thrombocytopenia, which reflects the important role of $BCLX_L$ in platelet survival in the circulation.

Current efforts to target MCL1 and $BCLX_L$ are focusing on two alternative approaches. One involves coupling an MCL1 or $BCLX_L$ inhibitor to an antibody to achieve greater selectivity in delivery of the BH3 mimetic. The other involves creating a proteolysis targeting chimera (ProTaC), a small molecule that contains both a BH3 mimetic group and a protease targeting moiety, typically a ligand for a ubiquitin E3 ligase that is present in tumor cells but not normal cells. For example, the ProTaC DT2216 contains the BCL2/$BCLX_L$ binding motif from navitoclax hooked to a ligand that binds the VHL E3 ligase, leading to proteasome-mediated degradation of $BCLX_L$ in cells expressing von Hippel-Lindau (VHL; many neoplastic cells) but not in cells such as platelets that lack VHL. DT2216 is currently undergoing extensive clinical testing; and there is an active effort to target MCL1 in a similar fashion.

Additional approaches to directly targeting the apoptotic machinery have been less successful. In addition to cytochrome c, another mitochondrial intermembrane protein that is released when BAX or BAK breaches the outer mitochondrial membrane is the second mitochondrial activator of caspases (SMAC), which facilitates caspase activation and apoptosis by neutralizing cell-intrinsic caspase inhibitors called IAP (inhibitor of apoptosis) proteins. Recognition of this apoptotic regulatory pathway led to the development of SMAC mimetics, small molecules like birinapant, LCL161, and AZD5582, that enhance apoptosis by inhibiting IAP proteins. Despite extensive clinical testing as single agents and in combination with chemotherapy, none of these agents displayed enough activity to gain regulatory approval.

A second pathway for triggering apoptosis involves ligation of cell surface death receptors, which are members of the tumor necrosis factor alpha (TNF-α) receptor superfamily (Figure 9.5). Ligation of these receptors causes assembly of several intracellular signaling complexes, one of which results in activation of caspase 8 and subsequent cleavage of the BH3-only protein BID as well as direct activation of downstream caspases. Because this pathway can be selectively activated in neoplastic cells by treatment with TNF-α-related apoptosis-inducing ligand (TRAIL), there was substantial interest in developing TRAIL as an antineoplastic biologic. Unfortunately, the short half-life of TRAIL in the circulation (20 minutes) limited its clinical activity. At the present time, ongoing clinical studies are testing an IgM antibody (IGM-8444) that binds and activates the TRAIL receptor DR5 (TNFRSF10B), which is expressed almost exclusively on neoplastic cells. Additional studies have shown that the death receptor pathway can also be activated in AML cells by low concentrations of ATR, CHK1, and WEE1 inhibitors through the induction of TNF-α and subsequent binding of this protein to its receptor. Whether this leukemia-specific TNF-α-mediated killing can be parlayed into a selective AML therapy remains to be established.

CDK INHIBITORS: TARGETING THE CELL CYCLE, ANTIAPOPTOTIC PROTEINS, AND MORE

As indicated in the section on DNA damage repair inhibitors, transition through the phases of the cell cycle is driven by the activity of cyclin-dependent kinases (CDKs), a group of kinases that are activated by CDK-binding proteins called cyclins, which are expressed during specific phases of the cell cycle. As indicated in Figure 9.6, CDKs 4 and 6 are activated during G1, CDK2 is most active during S phase, and CDK1 is active at the G2/M transition. Among the substrates of CDK4/6 is the protein RB (retinoblastoma), which ordinarily binds and sequesters E2F transcription factors. Upon phosphorylation by activated CDK4/6, RB releases E2F1, which then activates genes encoding for several enzymes that contribute to synthesis of nucleotides required for DNA synthesis, including thymidine kinase, dihydrofolate reductase, and DNA polymerase alpha. The importance of CDK4/6-mediated phosphorylation is underscored by the fact that RB is a tumor suppressor that is lost in retinoblastoma, sarcomas, glioblastomas, and ovarian cancer, among others. Conversely, CCND1 (the gene-encoding cyclin D1) is activated by chromosomal translocation in mantle cell lymphoma and CCNE is amplified in a number of solid tumors, including breast and ovarian cancers. Given the frequent alteration in these cell cycle regulatory pathways, substantial effort has gone into the design and testing of CDK inhibitors.

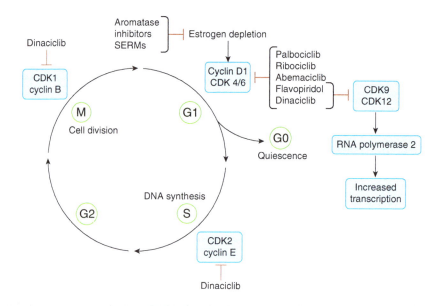

FIGURE 9.6 Inhibition of the cell cycle and transcription through CDK inhibition.
This schematic depicts the classical mammalian cell cycle model with G1 (gap 1),
G0 (quiescence), S (DNA synthesis/replication), G2 (gap 2), and M (mitosis) phases.
The progression through these phases is driven by the activity of cyclin-dependent
kinases (CDKs), which are activated when they bind their respective cyclins.
Specific cyclins are only present at certain phases of the cell cycle. CDKs 4 and 6
are active during G1 and are regulated by cyclin D isoforms. CDK2 is most active
during DNA replication in S phase and is associated with cyclins A and E. CDK1/
cyclin B is active at the G2/M transition. Inhibitors have been developed to target
CDK4/6, including palbociclib, ribociclib, abemaciclib, and flavopiridol. Interestingly,
flavopiridol as well as dinaciclib also inhibit CDK9 and CDK12, which are not
involved in the cell cycle but are involved in transcription through activation of RNA
polymerase 2. Estrogen enhances synthesis of the cyclin D1 protein, providing an
explanation for the synergistic effects of antiestrogens and CDK4/6 inhibitors.

SERMs, selective estrogen receptor modulators.

Sources: Adapted from Blazek D, Kohoutek J, Bartholomeeusen K, et al., Genes Dev, 2011; Johnson SF, Cruz
C, Greifenberg AK, et al., Cell Rep. 2016.

At the present time, the CDK4/6 inhibitors palbociclib, ribociclib, and abemaciclib are
FDA-approved for hormone receptor-positive HER2⁻ breast cancer in a number of settings,
including adjuvant therapy in high-risk cases, in the first-line metastatic setting in combination with endocrine therapy, and in combination with fulvestrant in cases that fail endocrine
thearpy (Table 9.4). The known ability of the estrogen receptor to activate transcription of
CCND1 gene in breast cancer, along with the role of cyclin D1 in activating CDKs 4 and 6,
provides an explanation for the beneficial effects of combining hormonal manipulations with
CDK4/6 inhibitors. These CDK4/6 inhibitors have also shown single-agent activity in mantle
cell lymphoma, liposarcoma, and teratoma. As a class, these agents induce neutropenia as
their main toxicity, although diarrhea and fatigue have also been noteworthy.

In contrast to these highly selective CDK4/6 inhibitors, earlier CDK inhibitors modulated the activity of the additional CDKs and exhibited broader effects on tumor cell biology (Table 9.4). For example, alvocidib and dinaciclib also inhibit CDK9, a cyclin T–dependent kinase that catalyzes activating phosphorylation of RNA polymerase II, leading to broad inhibition of RNA synthesis and rapid loss of proteins with short half-lives such as MYC or MCL1. In addition, dinaciclib inhibits CDK12, an atypical kinase that plays a role in the

TABLE 9.4 FDA Approvals for CDK Inhibitors

DRUG	CDK TARGETS	DISEASE TARGETS	FDA APPROVAL	SPECIAL CONSIDERATIONS
Palbociclib	CDKs 4 and 6	HR⁺ HER2⁻ advanced or metatastic breast cancer	Yes	1) With an aromatase inhibitor as initial endocrine therapy for women or men 2) With fulvestrant in patients who have progressed following endocrine therapy
Ribociclib	CDKs 4 and 6	HR⁺ HER2⁻ advanced or metatastic breast cancer	Yes	1) With an aromatase inhibitor as initial endocrine therapy for women or men 2) With fulvestrant as initial endocrine therapy or in patients who have progressed following endocrine therapy
Abemaciclib	CDKs 4 and 6	HR⁺ HER2⁻ breast cancer	Yes	1) In early breast cancer: as adjuvant therapy along with endocrine therapy in cases with positive lymph nodes, Ki67 >20%, and a high risk of recurrence 2) In advanced or metatstatic breast cancer: with aromatase inhibitor for initial endocrine therapy
Alvocidib	CDKs 1, 2, 4 6, 7, and 9	CLL and AML	No	Tested in AML with cytarabine + mitoxantrone, with venetoclax and in other combinations
Dinaciclib	CDKs 1, 2, 5, 9 and 12	CLL, ovarian and breast cancers	No	Tested as single agent and in combination with PARP inhibitors due to CDK 12 inhibition

AML, acute myeloid leukemia; CDK, cyclin-dependent kinase; CLL, chronic lymphocytic leukemia; FDA, U.S. Food and Drug Administration; HER, human epidermal growth factor receptor; HR, (steroid) hormone receptor; Ki67, a nuclear protein that is present in cells that are actively progressing through the cell cycle; PARP, poly(ADP-ribose) polymerase.

synthesis and stabilization of several DNA repair proteins, including BRCA1, ATR, and Fanconi anemia pathway proteins. Although alvocidib showed promise in AML in combination with cytarabine and mitoxantrone, possibly because of high dependency of many AMLs on MCL1, and dinaciclib showed promise in combination with PARP inhibitors in preclinical models, possibly because of BRCA1 downregulation, these agents did not achieve FDA approval. Nonetheless, there remains interest in selectively targeting atypical CDKs such as CDK9 and CDK12 to assess whether the resulting effects on apoptotic and DNA repair pathways can be effectively harnessed for cancer therapy.

CHAPTER SUMMARY

In this chapter, we have highlighted the physiologic roles of topoisomerases, components of the DNA damage response, antiapoptotic proteins, and cyclin-dependent kinases. Agents that target these proteins impact critical cellular processes and induce cytotoxic effects either by themselves (as with the topoisomerase inhibitors and cyclin-dependent kinase inhibitors) or by overcoming cellular mechanisms of resistance (inhibitors of DNA damage response/ repair and inhibitors of antiapoptotic molecules). Importantly, differences between normal and neoplastic cells, some of which are still poorly understood, provide a therapeutic window for clinical use of some of these agents.

CLINICAL PEARLS

- Drugs that target TOP1 are effective as small molecules and when delivered as the cargo of antibody-drug conjugates.
- Drugs that target topoisomerase II cause significant oropharyngeal mucositis that is dose- and schedule-dependent and is enhanced by prior or concomitant radiation therapy or concomitant administration of PARP inhibitors.
- PARP inhibitors exhibit single-agent activity and are most active in ovarian, breast, pancreatic, and prostate cancers that harbor inactivating mutations in *BRCA* genes and exhibit a resultant defect in homologous recombination repair.
- PARP inhibitors, which can cause dose-limiting fatigue and myelosuppression, might contribute to secondary myeloid neoplasms as well.
- BCL2 inhibitors are associated with induction of tumor lysis syndrome (TLS) in chronic lymphocytic leukemia (CLL) and acute leukemias. To decrease the risk and intensity of TLS, venetoclax is given initially in gradually increasing doses ("ramp up").

MULTIPLE-CHOICE QUESTIONS

1. A 50-year-old woman with a history of stage IIA breast cancer presents with a white blood cell count of 35,000/μL, gingival hypertrophy, and multiple skin chloromata. One year previously, she completed adjuvant chemotherapy with an

anthracycline-containing regimen. Bone marrow shows M4 (myelomonocytic) AML. Which of the following genes is likely to be involved in a translocation, rearrangement, and development of a leukemia-related fusion gene?

A. *IDH1*
B. *FLT3-ITD*
C. *MLL (KMT2A)*
D. *NPM1*
E. *TP53*

2. A 39-year-old woman with a family history of hereditary breast and ovarian cancer (HBOC) was diagnosed with stage IIIB ovarian cancer and received initial cytoreductive surgery followed by platinum-based adjuvant therapy with carboplatin and paclitaxel. She relapsed within 6 months of completing platinum-based therapy and was deemed to be platinum-refractory. Salvage therapy with the anti-vascular endothelial growth factor (VEGF) monoclonal antibody bevacizumab yielded no response. What would be the next therapy?

A. Cytarabine plus daunorubicin
B. High-dose methotrexate
C. Temozolomide
D. Cisplatin plus etoposide
E. Single-agent PARP inhibitor

3. A 43-year-old woman with relapsed colon cancer was started on FOLFIRI (an irinotecan-containing regimen). She asks you about the potential adverse events of irinotecan. Which of the following is NOT true about irinotecan?

A. Patients homozygous/heterozygous for the UGT1A1*28 allele are at increased risk of neutropenia. A test is available for genotyping of UGT1A1; however, use of the test is not widely accepted and a dose reduction is already recommended in patients who have experienced toxicity.
B. Early diarrhea occurs within 24 hours of receiving drug, accompanied by symptoms such as runny nose, increased salivation, watery eyes, sweating, flushing, and abdominal cramping, which may be prevented or ameliorated by atropine.
C. Late-onset diarrhea can be life-threatening and should be treated promptly with loperamide.
D. It has primarily hepatic metabolism to SN-38 (active metabolite) by carboxylesterase enzymes. SN-38 undergoes conjugation by UDP-glucuronosyl transferase 1A1 (UGT1A1) to form a glucuronide metabolite. SN-38 is increased by UGT1A1*28 polymorphism.
E. If she tolerates the first dose well, liposomal irinotecan can be substituted with conventional irinotecan to improve bioavailability and clinical outcome.

4. Mitomycin C is a benzoquinone-based antitumor antibiotic. In vitro studies have shown significant antineoplastic activity of this agent mainly by increasing intracellular reactive oxygen species generated by reductive-oxidative (redox) activity

of quinone. In which of the following conditions has mitomycin C shown clinical efficacy (and is approved by regulatory agencies)?

A. Intravesical therapy after transurethral resection of bladder tumor (TURBT) for noninvasive (stage 0) or minimally invasive (stage I) bladder cancers
B. Intracervical therapy for HPV (human papillomavirus)-negative in situ cervical cancer
C. Intratonsilar therapy for HPV-negative early-stage head and neck cancer
D. Intracardiac malignant right atrial myxoma
E. Intraocular B-RAF wild-type malignant melanoma

5. A 49-year-old man is receiving dose-adjusted R-EPOCH (rituximab, etoposide, prednisone, vincristine, cyclophosphamide, and doxorubicin) for his *BCL2/MYC* gene–rearranged, stage IV, diffuse, large B cell lymphoma (DLBCL). On the second day, the nurse reports marked erythema, swelling, and pain of his left arm. Over the next 6 hours, his left antecubital area has become more indurated. He also complains of left-hand paresthesia. What is the best next step in the management of this patient?

A. Duplex ultrasound of left upper extremity
B. Consult soft tissue or plastic surgery
C. Heating pad for 4 hours followed by cooling pad for 8 hours
D. Dexrazoxane
E. Administration of anti-vincristine (Oncovin) antibody

6. A 62-year-old woman with a history of breast cancer 20 years ago and a recently resected stage IIIC *BRCA2*-mutant ovarian cancer is about to complete her sixth cycle of carboplatin/paclitaxel adjuvant chemotherapy. You are asked to discuss the pros and cons of PARP inhibitor maintenance therapy. Which of the following are among the reported toxicities of PARP inhibitor?

A. Nausea
B. Fatigue
C. Myelosuppression
D. Therapy-related myeloid neoplasms, including myelodysplastic syndrome and acute myeloid leukemia
E. All of the above

7. A 72-year-old woman with newly diagnosed acute myeloid leukemia is about to begin azacytidine and venetoclax induction therapy. Her white blood cell (WBC) count is 25,000 and her marrow aspirate has 90% blasts. Which of the following considerations need to be factored into the initial venetoclax dose and schedule?

A. The patient's age
B. The patient's risk of tumor lysis syndrome
C. Your decision to administer posaconazole prophylactically as antifungal prophylaxis.
D. A and B
E. B and C

8. A 79-year-old man with metastatic breast cancer is about to start therapy with the CDK4/6 inhibitor ribociclib. Which agent should be prescribed along with ribociclib?

    A. Gemcitabine
    B. Letrozole
    C. Capecitabine
    D. Trastuzumab deruxtecan
    E. Oxaliplatin

ANSWERS TO MULTIPLE-CHOICE QUESTIONS

1. **C.** World Health Organization classification of myeloid malignancies recognizes two types of therapy-related myeloid neoplasms including t-MDS (therapy-related myelodysplastic syndrome) and t-AML: (1) an alkylating agent/radiation–related type, and (2) a topoisomerase II inhibitor–related type. AML developing post-topoisomerase II inhibitors (etoposide, anthracyclines, etc.) often presents 1 to 3 years after treatment with these agents, with a prominent monocytic component, and is associated with balanced translocations involving chromosome bands 11q23 and the *KMT2A* gene encoding a lysine (K)–specific histone methyltransferase 2A, which functions as an epigenetic regulator of transcription. The other name for *KMT2A* is MLL (mixed lineage or myeloid/lymphoid leukemia).

2. **E.** PARP inhibitors (e.g., olaparib, rucaparib, niraparib, and talazoparib) are approved for treatment of patients with germline *BRCA* mutated advanced ovarian cancer.

3. **E.** Irinotecan liposome injection (Onivyde) is a topoisomerase I inhibitor that is indicated, in combination with 5-fluorouracil (5-FU) and leucovorin, for the treatment of patients with metastatic adenocarcinoma of the pancreas after disease progression following gemcitabine-based therapy. Liposomal irinotecan SHOULD NOT substitute irinotecan in other regimens. IrinotecanH+s metabolized by carboxylesterases to its active form SN-38 (see the following figure), which is inactivated via glucuronidation by uridine diphosphate glucuronosyltransferases (UGTs). Hepatic UGT1A1 and UGT1A9 have a major role in the detoxification of SN-38. Patients who are homozygous, and to a lesser extent heterozygous carriers, for the UGT1A1*28 allele are at increased risk of neutropenia.

Patients treated with irinotecan may develop severe, and potentially fatal, diarrhea. Early-onset diarrhea occurs during or within 24 hours of receiving irinotecan and is characterized by cholinergic symptoms; it may be prevented or treated with atropine. Late-onset diarrhea should be promptly treated with loperamide. Irinotecan should be interrupted and dose reduced for the subsequent doses if severe diarrhea occurs.

Mitomycin C

4. **A.** Mitomycin C is a benzoquinone antineoplastic agent that is clinically used for (1) intravesical therapy after transurethral resection of bladder tumor (TURBT) for noninvasive (stage 0) or minimally invasive (stage I) bladder cancers, and (2) chemoradiation (XRT/mitomycin C/5-FU) for stage I to III anal cancer. It can cause hemolytic uremic syndrome (HUS).

5. **D.** Dexrazoxane is a cytoprotective agent indicated for reducing the incidence and severity of cardiomyopathy associated with doxorubicin administration in women with metastatic breast cancer who have received a cumulative doxorubicin dose of 300 mg/m^2 and who will continue to receive doxorubicin therapy to maintain tumor control (Muthuramalingam et al., 2013).

6. **E.** Although PARP inhibitor-related fatalities are rare, as many as 74% of patients on PARP inhibitor monotherapy experience a grade <u>3 or greater</u> treatment-related adverse event at some time during their maintenance therapy (González-Martín et al., 2022). As a class, PARP inhibitors cause nausea, emesis, and fatigue, which can cause discontinuation in some patients. PARP inhibitors are also myelosuppressive, causing grade 3 or greater anemia, thrombocytopenia, and neutropenia in a substantial fraction of patients (op cit.). Emerging data indicate an increased risk of therapy-related myeloid neoplasms in women receiving PARP inhibitor treatment (Morice et al., 2021). While the risk appears to be lower in first-line maintenance than in the recurrent setting (approximately 1% vs. up to 8%), further studies are required to better define the risk factors and understand the pathogenesis of this life-threatening adverse event.

7. **E.** Recommended dosing for venetoclax would involve (1) escalating to the final dose over 3–4 days and (2) capping the dose at 70 or 100 mg rather than the FDA-approved dose of 400 mg in combination with azacytidine. As summarized by Waggoner et al. (2022), the daily dose of venetoclax needs to be decreased by 75% to 80% in the presence of a strong cytochrome P450 3A4 inhibitor such as posaconazole and by 50% in the presence of a weaker 3A4 inhibitor such as fluconazole. Moreover, to diminish the risk of tumor lysis syndrome, venetoclax is slowly ramped up to the final dose in CLL over a 5-week period. While the risk of tumor lysis syndrome is somewhat lower in AML, the present patient has a high tumor burden (high

percentage of blasts in the marrow and elevated WBC count), which puts her at elevated risk when venetoclax is started. In AML, where treatment initiation is felt to be more urgent, the venetoclax dose is also started low but is ramped up over 3–4 days; and tumor lysis studies (including potassium, phosphate, creatinine and uric acid) are monitored multiple times per day for the first several days in the inpatient setting to allow early detection and treatment of tumor lysis syndrome when it occurs.

8. **B.** As a class, CDK4/6 inhibitors are administered in conjunction with endocrine therapy. The mechanistic rationale is that estrogen deprivation inhibits the production of cyclin D1 in estrogen receptor–positive cells and CDK4/6 inhibitors inhibit activity of the cyclin D1–dependent kinases, thereby resulting in two impediments to cell cycle progression. In this case, administration of letrozole, a competitive inhibitor of aromatase, would constitute an FDA-approved initial endocrine therapy to partner with ribociclib, although some studies also add leuprolide or goserelin as part of the endocrine therapy of male breast cancer (Campone et al., 2022).

SELECTED REFERENCES

Abraham J, Coleman R, Elias A, et al. Use of cyclin-dependent kinase (CDK) 4/6 inhibitors for hormone receptor-positive, human epidermal growth factor receptor 2-negative, metastatic breast cancer: A roundtable discussion by the Breast Cancer Therapy Expert Group (BCTEG). Breast Cancer Res Treat. 2018;171(1):11–20. https://doi.org/10.1007/s10549-018-4783-1

Arora S, Narayan P, Osgood CL, et al. U.S. FDA drug approvals for breast cancer: A decade in review. Clin Cancer Res. 2022;28(6):1072–86. https://doi.org/10.1158/1078-0432.CCR-21-2600

Ashkenazi A, Fairbrother WJ, Leverson JD, Souers AJ. From basic apoptosis discoveries to advanced selective BCL-2 family inhibitors. Nat Rev Drug Discov. 2017;16(4):273–84. https://doi.org/10.1038/nrd.2016.253

Ashworth A. A synthetic lethal therapeutic approach: Poly(ADP) ribose polymerase inhibitors for the treatment of cancers deficient in DNA double-strand break repair. J Clin Oncol. 2008;26(22):3785–90. https://doi.org/10.1200/JCO.2008.16.0812

Bjornsti MA, Kaufmann SH. Topoisomerases and cancer chemotherapy: Recent advances and unanswered questions. F1000Res. 2019 Sep 30;8:F1000 Faculty Rev-1704. https://doi.org/10.12688/f1000research.20201.1

Blazek D, Kohoutek J, Bartholomeeusen K, et al. The cyclin K/Cdk12 complex maintains genomic stability via regulation of expression of DNA damage response genes. Genes Dev. 2011;25(20):2158–72. https://doi.org/10.1101/gad.16962311

Campone M, De Laurentiis M, Zamagni C, et al. Ribociclib plus letrozole in male patients with hormone receptor-positive, human epidermal growth factor receptor 2-negative advanced breast cancer: Subgroup analysis of the phase IIIb CompLEEment-1 trial. Breast Cancer Res Treat. 2022;193(1):95–103. https://doi.org/10.1007/s10549-022-06543-1

Dai H, Meng XW, Kaufmann SH. Mitochondrial apoptosis and BH3 mimetics. F1000Res. 2016;5:2804. https://doi.org/10.12688/f1000research.9629.1; Taylor RC, Cullen SP, Martin SJ. Apoptosis: Controlled demolition at the cellular level. Nat Rev Mol Cell Biol. 2008;9:231–41. https://doi.org/10.1038/nrm2312

Diepstraten ST, Anderson MA, Czabotar PE, et al. The manipulation of apoptosis for cancer therapy using BH3-mimetic drugs. Nat Rev Cancer. 2022;22(1):45–64. https://doi.org/10.1038/s41568-021-00407-4

Forment JV, O'Connor MJ. Targeting the replication stress response in cancer. Pharmacol Ther. 2018;188:155–67. https://doi.org/10.1016/j.pharmthera.2018.03.005

Gonzalez-Martin A, Matulonis UA, Korach J, et al. Niraparib treatment for patients with *BRCA*-mutated ovarian cancer: Review of clinical data and therapeutic context. Future Oncol. 2022;18(23):2505–36. https://doi.org/10.2217/fon-2022-0206

Hanahan D, Weinberg RA. Hallmarks of cancer: The next generation. Cell. 2011;144(5):646–74. https://doi.org/10.1016/j.cell.2011.02.013

Johnson SF, Cruz C, Greifenberg AK, et al. CDK12 inhibition reverses de novo and acquired PARP inhibitor resistance in BRCA wild-type and mutated models of triple-negative breast cancer. Cell Rep. 2016;17(9):2367–81. https://doi.org/10.1016/j.celrep.2016.10.077

Karnitz LM, Zou L. Molecular pathways: Targeting ATR in cancer therapy. Clin Cancer Res. 2015;21(21):4780–5. https://doi.org/10.1158/1078-0432.CCR-15-0479

Kaufmann SH, Karp JE, Svingen PA, et al. Elevated expression of the apoptotic regulator Mcl-1 at the time of leukemic relapse. Blood. 1998;91(3):991–1000. https://doi.org/10.1182/blood.V91.3.991.991_991_1000

Konstantinopoulos PA, Cheng SC, Wahner Hendrickson AE, et al. Berzosertib plus gemcitabine versus gemcitabine alone in platinum-resistant high-grade serous ovarian cancer: A multicentre, open-label, randomised, phase 2 trial. Lancet Oncol. 2020;21(7):957–68. https://doi.org/10.1016/S1470-2045(20)30180-7

Konstantinopoulos PA, da Costa AABA, Gulhan D, et al. A Replication stress biomarker is associated with response to gemcitabine versus combined gemcitabine and ATR inhibitor therapy in ovarian cancer. Nat Commun. 2021;12(1):5574. https://doi.org/10.1038/s41467-021-25904-w

Konstantinopoulos PA, Matulonis UA. PARP inhibitors in ovarian cancer: A trailblazing and transformative journey. Clin Cancer Res. 2018;24(17):4062–5. https://doi.org/10.1158/1078-0432.CCR-18-1314

Kwan TT, Oza AM, Tinker AV, et al. Preexisting TP53-variant clonal hematopoiesis and risk of secondary myeloid neoplasms in patients with high-grade ovarian cancer treated with rucaparib. JAMA Oncol. 2021;7(12):1772–81. https://doi.org/10.1001/jamaoncol.2021.4664

Lachowiez CA, Atluri H, DiNardo CD. Advancing the standard: Venetoclax combined with intensive induction and consolidation therapy for acute myeloid leukemia. Ther Adv Hematol. 2022;13:20406207221093964. https://doi.org/10.1177/20406207221093964

Lachowiez C, DiNardo CD, Konopleva M. Venetoclax in acute myeloid leukemia—Current and future directions. Leuk Lymphoma. 2020;61(6):1313–22. https://doi.org/10.1080/10428194.2020.1719098

Lheureux S, Cristea MC, Bruce JP, et al. Adavosertib plus gemcitabine for platinum-resistant or platinum-refractory recurrent ovarian cancer: A double-blind, randomised, placebo-controlled, phase 2 trial. Lancet. 2021;397(10271):281–92. https://doi.org/10.1016/S0140-6736(20)32554-X

Lord CJ, Ashworth A. The DNA damage response and cancer therapy. Nature. 2012;481(7381):287–94. https://doi.org/10.1038/nature10760

Malumbres M, Barbacid M. Cell cycle, CDKs and cancer: A changing paradigm. Nat Rev Cancer. 2009;9(3):153–66. https://doi.org/10.1038/nrc2602

Minchom A, Aversa C, Lopez J. Dancing with the DNA damage response: Next-generation anti-cancer therapeutic strategies. Ther Adv Med Oncol. 2018;10:1758835918786658. https://doi.org/10.1177/1758835918786658

Moore KN, Pothuri B. Poly(ADP-ribose) polymerase inhibitor inhibition in ovarian cancer: A comprehensive review. Cancer J. 2021;27(6):432–40. https://doi.org/10.1097/PPO.0000000000000558

Morice PM, Leary A, Dolladille C, et al. Myelodysplastic syndrome and acute myeloid leukaemia in patients treated with PARP inhibitors: A safety meta-analysis of randomised controlled trials and a retrospective study of the WHO pharmacovigilance database. Lancet Haematol. 2021;8(2):e122–34. https://doi.org/10.1016/S2352-3026(20)30360-4

Muthuramalingam S, Gale J, Bradbury J. Dexrazoxane efficacy for anthracycline extravasation: Use in UK clinical practice. Int J Clin Pract. 2013;67(3):244–9. https://doi.org/10.1111/ijcp.12103

Nitiss JL. DNA topoisomerase II and its growing repertoire of biological functions. Nat Rev Cancer. 2009;9:327–37. https://doi.org/10.1038/nrc2608

O'Connor MJ. Targeting the DNA damage response in cancer. Mol Cell. 2015;60(4):547–60. https://doi.org/10.1016/j.molcel.2015.10.040

Pommier Y, Nussenzweig A, Takeda S, Austin C. Human topoisomerases and their roles in genome stability and organization. Nat Rev Mol Cell Biol. 2022;23(6):407–27. https://doi.org/10.1038/s41580-022-00452-3

Scott CL, Swisher EM, Kaufmann SH. Poly (ADP-Ribose) polymerase inhibitors: Recent advances and future development. J Clin Oncol. 2015;33:1397–406. https://doi.org/10.1200/JCO.2014.58.8848

Taylor RC, Cullen SP, Martin SJ. Apoptosis: Controlled demolition at the cellular level. Nat Rev Mol Cell Biol. 2008;9(3):231–41. https://doi.org/10.1038/nrm2312

Waggoner M, Katsetos J, Thomas E, et al. Practical management of the venetoclax-treated patient in chronic lymphocytic leukemia and acute myeloid leukemia. J Adv Pract Oncol. 2022;13(4):400–15. https://doi.org/10.6004/jadpro.2022.13.4.4

Wethington SL, Wahner-Hendrickson AE, Swisher EM, et al. PARP inhibitor maintenance for primary ovarian cancer—A missed opportunity for precision medicine. Gynecol Oncol. 2021;163(1):11–3. https://doi.org/10.1016/j.ygyno.2021.08.002

CHAPTER 10

Epigenetic Modulators

SERGIU PASCA • LUKASZ P. GONDEK

INTRODUCTION

All cells in a single organism share identical genetic information encoded in DNA, yet they differ tremendously in function. These variations in cellular fate are mainly dictated by the distinct transcriptional programs. Gene expression is orchestrated by epigenetic information that interconnects genome sequence and environmental/extracellular factors. This fine-tuning of cellular fate and function can happen at multiple levels: DNA modifications, post-translational modifications of histones, and changes at the level of higher-order chromatin structures.

DNA methylation is a process of covalent modification of cytosine at the DNA level that is usually associated with gene silencing. This process is catalyzed by one of three DNA methyltransferases: DNMT1, DNMT3A, and DNMT3B. These repressive marks can be erased either by cell division in the absence of DNMT1 activity or by ten-eleven translocation (TET) dioxygenases. Thus, DNMT and TET confer opposing effects on DNA methylation status. Somatic mutations in DNMT3A and TET2 are among the most frequently mutated genes in hematologic malignancies and premalignant clonal hematopoiesis.

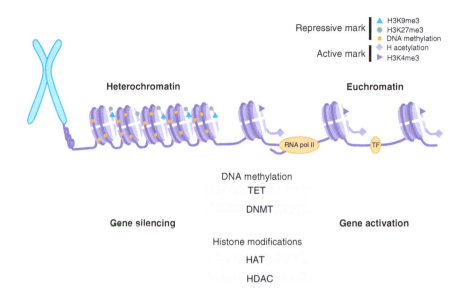

FIGURE 10.1 Chromatin structure and epigenetic marks.
Chromatin remodeling and bidirectional transition from transcriptionally active euchromatin to compacted heterochromatin are orchestrated by multiple epigenetic modifications at DNA and nucleosome levels.

CpG sites (or islands) are repeated cytosine and guanine nucleotides with the "p" representing the phosphate linker. CpG sites are usually in the vicinity of the promoters of actively expressed genes. DNA methylation of cytosines in CpG sites is generally associated with gene silencing, and the methylation pattern is heritable during cell division. This process is catalyzed by one of the three DNA methyltransferases identified in mammals. DNMT1 is considered the main maintenance methyltransferase and is responsible for preserving the methylation pattern after cell division. DNMT3A and DNMT3B are so-called de novo methyltransferases that establish a DNA methylation pattern during development. DNA methylation is a physiologically reversible process. Ten-eleven translocation (TET) genes are members of enzymes called dioxygenases. TET1 and TET2 catalyze the conversion of 5-methylcytosine to 5-hydroxymethylcytosine, which constitutes the initial step of DNA demethylation.

Histone modifications represent the second level of epigenetic control of the overall transcriptional program. Over 200 histone modifications have been described. The most common and best understood are histone methylation and acetylation. The latter process is usually associated with the relaxation of chromatin that facilitates access of transcription factors (TFs) and RNA polymerase complex to DNA. Histone acetylation is catalyzed by histone acetyltransferases (HATs). Conversely, histone deacetylation catalyzed by histone deacetylases (HDACs) marks chromatin compaction (heterochromatin) and subsequent inhibition of transcription. Activation and inhibition of gene expression are also dependent on the methylation of histone tails either on lysine (K) or on arginine (R) residues. The methylation pattern commonly associated with active transcription includes H3K4, H3K48, and H3K79. Transcription repression is achieved by methylation of H3K9 and H3K27.

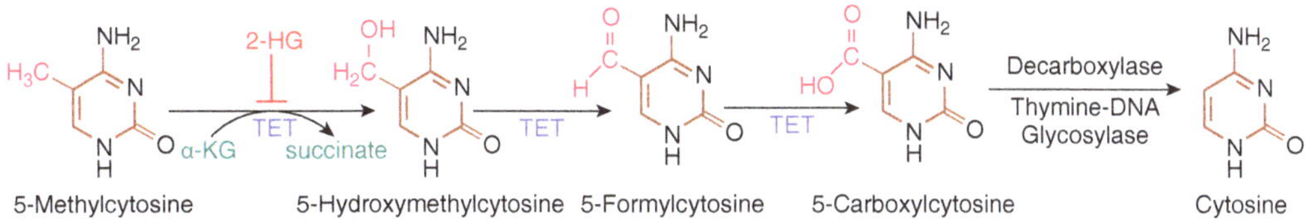

FIGURE 10.2 DNA demethylation steps.
DNA demethylation reactions are mediated by the effect of TET (ten-eleven translocation) enzymes. 5-Methylcytosine in DNA is partially converted to 5-hydroxymethylcytosine by the TET dioxygenases. In DNA, 5-hydroxy-methylcytosines are subsequently oxidized to an aldehyde (5-formylcytosine) and further oxidized to an acid (5-carboxylcytosine) by TET enzymes. TET enzymes use alpha-ketoglutarate (α-KG) as coenzyme. 2-Hydroxyglutarate (2-HG) produced by IDH (isocitrate dehydrogenase) mutant enzymes inhibits these reactions mediated by TET enzymes and the ultimate outcome of IDH mutations and presence of 2-HG is aberrant hypermethylation of DNA.

Source: Courtesy of Professor Ashkan Emadi.

Post-translational histone modifications include methylation, acetylation, phosphorylation, ubiquitination, and sumoylation of histones at different residues. The functional consequences of such modifications rely not only on the type of modification but also on the modified residues. Thus, the same chemical modification may have distinct effects on gene expression. The most common histone marks and their transcriptional effects are depicted in Figure 10.2.

Both DNA methylation and histone modifications participate in the third layer of epigenetic modification, that is, chromatin remodeling. Certain histone marks, particularly acetylation, result in chromatin relaxation (euchromatin) and active transcription. Conversely, deacetylation of histones is associated with chromatin compaction (heterochromatin) that blocks transcriptional machinery from binding to DNA and results in the repression of gene expression (Figure 10.3).

Lysine-specific histone demethylase (LSD1) is a monoamine oxidase involved in the demethylation of lysine 4 and 9 on histone H3 (H3K4/H3K9). LSD1 is a component of several multiprotein complexes and can act as both a transcriptional repressor and activator. High expression of LSD1 has been found in acute myeloid leukemia (AML) stem cells. Preclinical studies suggested that AML (formerly known as mixed lineage leukemia, or MLL) with lysine methyltransferase 2A (*KMT2A*) and *RUNX1* rearrangements as well as erythroleukemia may be particularly sensitive to LSD1 inhibition. *KMT2A* rearrangements (*KMT2Ar*) are present in 5% to 10% of acute leukemia patients and indicate a very poor prognosis. They result in an in-frame fusion of the N-terminal region of KMT2A to one of over 60 fusion partners that interact directly with the disruptor of telomeric silencing 1-like (DOT1L). DOT1L is a histone methyltransferase enzyme that catalyzes mono-, di-, or trimethylation of H3K79 at KMT2A-target genes that results in the activation of leukemogenic genes including *HOXA9* and *MEIS1*. DOT1L inhibitor, pinometostat, has been tested in Phase 1 clinical trials and showed modest activity in relapsed/refractory AML.

Menin is a ubiquitously expressed nuclear protein that facilitates the binding of KMT2A/KMT2A-fusion partner (KMT2A-FP) to target genes such as *HOXA* genes. Menin inhibitors are a novel class of agents disrupting protein-protein interaction between menin and KMT2A/KMT2A-FP. The competitive inhibition of either KMT2A-FP in *KMT2Ar* or native

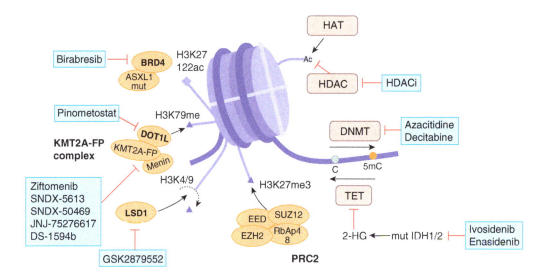

FIGURE 10.3 Epigenetic modifying agents and their mechanism of action.
DNMT inhibitors: **Azacitidine** (5-azacytidine) and its analog **decitabine** (5-aza-2-deoxycytidine) are clinically available DNMT (DNA methyltransferase) inhibitors. Both drugs are metabolized intracellularly and incorporated into DNA during replication and exert DNMT inhibition through the covalent binding of DNMT to azacytosine (see Figure 10.4).

TET (ten-eleven translocation) dioxygenases require α-KG (alpha-ketoglutarate) for enzymatic conversion of methylcytosine to 5-hydroxymethylcytosine (see Figure 10.1). α-KG is a product of the enzymatic oxidative decarboxylation of isocitrate by isocitrate dehydrogenase (IDH1 and IDH2) localized in cytoplasm and mitochondria, respectively. Point mutations in *IDH1* R132 and *IDH2* R140 and R172 result in the loss of normal enzymatic activity and accumulation of 2-hydroxyglutarate (2-HG). 2-HG is a competitive inhibitor of α-KG-dependent dioxygenases such as TET and results in DNA hypermethylation. **Ivosidenib** and **enasidenib** are selective inhibitors of mutant IDH1 and IDH2, respectively. Both are currently approved for the treatment of acute myeloid leukemia (AML).

Histone acetylation: Acetylation and deacetylation of histone tails is an important mechanism of gene expression control. These modifications are catalyzed by histone acetylases (HATs) and deacetylases (HDACs), respectively. Although several HDAC inhibitors have been approved for the treatment of lymphoid malignancies, some of these agents, like panobinostat, have been withdrawn given the fact that postapproval clinical trials did not confirm the favorable risk-benefit (Table 10.1). The efficacy of these agents in myeloid malignancies is not yet well defined.

Histone methylation: EZH2 is a histone-lysine *N*-methyltransferase that catalyzes the addition of a methyl (CH_3) group to H3K27. H3K27-CH_3 is associated with transcriptional repression and heterochromatin formation. EZH2 is a catalytic component of the polycomb repressive complex 2 (PRC2). *EZH2* mutations, both gain, and loss of function have been identified in numerous hematologic malignancies and solid tumors. Of note, increased EZH2/PRC2 activity has been found in stem and progenitor cells. Thus, inhibition of EZH2 could potentially shut off the stem cell programs and promote differentiation. Phase 1/2 clinical trials suggested that EZH2 inhibition was well tolerated and produced antitumor activity in patients with refractory B-cell non-Hodgkin lymphoma and advanced solid tumors.

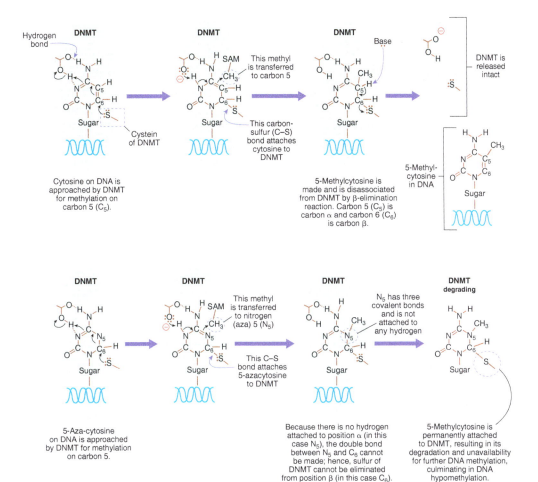

FIGURE 10.4 DNA methylation reaction by DNMT (top) and DNMT inhibition by 5-azacytosine analogs (bottom).
The chemical reactions result in the formation of 5-methylcytosine and its release from DNA methyltransferase (DNMT) mediated by a β-elimination reaction (top panel). The incorporation of 5-azanucleoside alters the interaction between DNA and DNMTs through the presence of nitrogen instead of carbon in the 5-position of the pyrimidine ring. DNMT remains covalently bound to 5-methylcytosine and its function is blocked, thus resulting in the passive loss of cytosine methylation in the daughter cells after replication. The DNA demethylating effect is usually seen at a lower drug concentration while higher doses may also induce direct cytotoxicity.

Source: Courtesy of Professor Ashkan Emadi.

KMT2A in *NPM1* mutated AML prevents downstream activation of key mediators of leukemogenesis, proliferation, and self-renewal such as *HOXA9, MEIS1,* and *CDK9.* Preclinical studies using *KMT2A*r and *NPM1* mutant patient-derived xenograft models demonstrated very strong activity in these well-defined subsets of AML. Several clinical studies are currently ongoing to test this class of agents in humans.

BROMODOMAIN INHIBITORS

Bromodomain and extraterminal (BET) proteins, including BRD4, are "reader" proteins that bind to acetylated histones and recruit several chromatin modifiers and mediators of transcription. BRD4 after binding to acetylated histone recruits P-TEFb and CDK9, enabling transcript elongation by RNA polymerase II. Thus, BRD4 links histone acetylation with active transcription especially at the enhancers and promoters of such oncogenes as *MYC* and *BCL2*. *ASXL1* frameshift mutations are relatively frequent in myeloid neoplasm and the aberrant interaction of truncated ASXL1 and BRD4 enhances the expression of genes involved in stem cell maintenance and differentiation. In preclinical models, *ASXL1* mutated cells were explicitly sensitive to BET bromodomain inhibitors.

TABLE 10.1 Epigenetic Modifying Agents Approved for Clinical Use (as of September 2022)

Drug	Class	Indication	Response	Approval Year
Azacitidine	DNMT inhibitor	MDS	14%–19% CR + PR	2004
Decitabine	DNMT inhibitor	MDS	17%–26% ORR	2006
Vorinostat	HDAC inhibitor	r/r CTCL	31% ORR	2006
Romidepsin	HDAC inhibitor	TCL	35% ORR	2009
Belinostat	HDAC inhibitor	r/r PTCL	26% ORR	2015
Enasidenib	IDH2 inhibitor	r/r AML	23% CR/CRh	2017
Ivosidenib	IDH1 inhibitor	r/r AML Cholangiocarcinoma[*]	32% CR/CRh improvement in PFS[†]	2018 2022
Decitabine and cedazuridine	DNMT inhibitor	MDS	18–21% CR	2020
Azacitidine and cedazuridine	DNMT inhibitor	AML	Remission maintenance 24.7 months OS vs. 14.8 months placebo	2020

[*]Locally advanced or metastatic.
[†]A statistically significant improvement in PFS, hazard ratio 0.37 (0.25, 0.54), $p < .0001$.
AML, acute myeloid leukemia; CR, complete response; CRh, complete remission with partial blood cells recovery; CTCL, cutaneous T-cell lymphoma; DMNT, DNA methyltransferase; HDAC, histone deacetylase; IDH, isocitrate dehydrogenase; MDS, myelodysplastic syndromes; ORR, overall response rate; OS, overall survival; PFS, progression free survival; PR, partial response; PTCL, peripheral T-cell lymphoma; r/r, relapsed refractory; TCL, T-cell lymphoma.

COMBINATION THERAPIES

As hypomethylating agents remain an important therapeutic modality for patients with hematologic malignancies, it is of no surprise that they constitute a backbone for less intensive combination therapies. Hypomethylating agents combined with B-cell lymphoma 2 (BCL-2) inhibitor, venetoclax, demonstrated an impressive response in older patients with AML ineligible for intensive chemotherapy. BCL-2 is an antiapoptotic protein that is crucial in the survival and therapeutic resistance of AML cells, including the leukemia stem cell (LSC) population. Hypomethylating agents also demonstrated a synergistic effect in combination with ivosidenib and enasidenib, small molecules approved for the treatment of AML with *IDH1* and *IDH2* mutations, respectively. The therapeutic effect is achieved mostly through increased differentiation of AML blasts.

TABLE 10.2 Combinations of Epigenetic Modifying Agents Most Frequently Used

Drug	Class	Indication	Response	Approval Year
Azacitidine + venetoclax	DNMT inhibitor + BCL-2 inhibitors	AML	66% CR	2020
Decitabine + venetoclax	DNMT inhibitor + BCL-2 inhibitors	AML	74% ORR	2020
Azacitidine + enasidenib	DNMT inhibitor + IDH2 inhibitor	AML	74% ORR; 63% CR	2017
Azacitidine + ivosidenib	DNMT inhibitor + IDH1 inhibitor	AML	55% ORR; 42% CR	2022

AML, acute myeloid leukemia; BCL-2, B-cell lymphoma 2; CR, complete response; DNMT, DNA methyltransferase; IDH1, isocitrate dehydrogenase; ORR, overall response rate.

CHAPTER SUMMARY

Somatic mutations, amplifications, and translocations involving genes that encode proteins responsible for epigenetic modifications of DNA have been found in myeloid malignancies. This includes genes involved in DNA methylation (TET2, DNMT3A, IDH1/IDH2) and post-translational histone modifications (EZH2, ASXL1, KMT2A, DOT1L). In this chapter, we focused on the function of these proteins as well as available targeted therapies. The recent efforts to develop more selective and less toxic therapies focused on direct inhibition of mutated proteins or disruption of downstream pathways may result in the restoration of normal epigenetic patterns and improvement in hematopoietic differentiation rather than the direct cytotoxic effect on leukemic cells.

CLINICAL PEARLS

- A significant and dose-limiting toxicity of all epigenetic modifiers (DNA methyltransferase inhibitors, histone deacetylase inhibitors, lysine demethylase-1 inhibitors) is fatigue.
- Azacitidine and decitabine as monotherapy or combined with several targeted therapies are used in clinical practice for the treatment of patients with myelodysplastic syndrome and AML.
- Clinical responses to epigenetic modifiers, as single agents, occur gradually over a protracted period, with responses often not evinced until 4 to 6 months after beginning treatment. This aligns with the mechanism of action of these agents.
- Histone deacetylase inhibitors (HDACi) have shown clinical activity and have been approved for use in treating relapsed or refractory T-cell lymphoma.

MULTIPLE-CHOICE QUESTIONS

1. A 74-year-old woman was treated with azacitidine (5-azacytidine) for her intermediate-risk myelodysplastic syndrome. She was treated at 75 mg/m^2 daily for 7 days via subcutaneous injection. You see her 1 week after the completion of her last dose. She is surprised that her anemia is not improved. What do you tell the patient?

   A. Switching to decitabine is indicated.
   B. Evaluation of the myeloid mutation panel is warranted to investigate resistance mutations.
   C. Subcutaneous infection is inferior to intravenous injection.
   D. Patients should be treated for a minimum of four to six cycles. A complete or partial response may require additional treatment cycles.

2. What are the maximum cycles of treatment in patients who are treated with DNA methyltransferase inhibitors (DNMTI), decitabine, and azacitidine, and have responded?

    A. Four
    B. Six
    C. 12 (once monthly)
    D. There is no maximum.

3. Romidepsin is a histone deacetylase (HDAC) inhibitor that has shown responses in relapsed or refractory cutaneous T-cell lymphoma (CTCL) and peripheral T-cell lymphoma (PTCL) in Phase 2 trials. Patients receiving romidepsin should be monitored for EKG changes. Which one of the following treatment-emergent morphologic changes in EKGs have been observed several times in clinical studies?

    A. QT-interval prolongation
    B. T-wave and ST-segment changes
    C. Second-degree heart block
    D. Frequent premature atrial contractions (PACs)

4. Which of the following indications related to epigenetic modulators has NOT been approved by the FDA?

    A. Panobinostat as monotherapy for the treatment of refractory multiple myeloma (MM)
    B. Belinostat as monotherapy for the treatment of relapsed or refractory PTCL
    C. Ivosidenib as monotherapy for the treatment of patients with newly diagnosed or relapsed/refractory AML with isocitrate dehydrogenase 1 (IDH1) mutation
    D. Ivosidenib in combination with azacitidine for the treatment of patients with newly diagnosed or relapsed/refractory AML with IDH1 mutation

5. A 42-year-old female with relapse refractory AML and *IDH1* and *TET2* mutations presented to your office 3 weeks ago with a white blood cell (WBC) count of 7,000/μL and 25% circulating blasts. You decided to start ivosidenib 500 mg daily. The patient presents to the ED with new-onset dyspnea now requiring 4 L supplemental oxygen via nasal cannula. Chest CT showed diffuse pulmonary infiltrates. Her WBC count is now 25,000/μL, predominantly neutrophils, and 2% circulating blasts. What is the most likely diagnosis?

    A. Multifocal pneumonia
    B. Differentiation syndrome
    C. Progressive disease with leukostasis
    D. Pulmonary edema

6. What is the most appropriate therapy for the patient in Question 5?

    A. Emergent cytotoxic chemotherapy
    B. Antibiotics alone
    C. Systemic corticosteroids and hydroxyurea
    D. Discontinuation of ivosidenib permanently

7. A 76-year-old man with newly diagnosed AML with normal karyotype and *DNMT3A* and *TET2* mutations and pancytopenia is started on azacitidine 75 mg/m^2 daily for 7 days and venetoclax 400 mg daily after the initial ramp-up. He is also on prophylactic levofloxacin, valacyclovir, and posaconazole. After 28 days of therapy, the patient remained profoundly aplastic, transfusion-dependent of red blood cells and platelets with no neutrophils. Bone marrow aspirate and biopsy showed aplastic bone marrow with no residual disease. Venetoclax was stopped but 2 weeks later the patient remains pancytopenic. What could have been done differently to minimize the risk of prolonged aplasia?

    A. Azacitidine 5-day course
    B. Discontinuation of venetoclax at day 21
    C. Discontinuation of posaconazole prior to initiation of venetoclax
    D. 25% dose reduction of venetoclax

8. Oral azacitidine is FDA approved for which of the following conditions?

    A. MDS
    B. Newly diagnosed and relapsed AML patient >65 years of age
    C. AML patients in first complete remission or complete remission with incomplete blood count recovery who are not candidates for curative therapies
    D. After hematopoietic stem cell transplant maintenance in patients with AML

9. In preclinical studies, menin inhibitors demonstrated therapeutic activity in which of the following conditions:

    A. Chronic lymphocytic leukemia with 17p deletion
    B. AML with *NPM1* mutation or *KMT2A* rearrangement
    C. MDS with *TP53* mutation
    D. T-cell lymphomas

ANSWERS TO MULTIPLE-CHOICE QUESTIONS

1. **D.** When 5-cytidine analogs are used, they are incorporated into the DNA methyltransferase enzymes instead of the cytosine. The process of methylation of N_5 is very similar to the methylation of C_5. However, due to the lack of hydrogen (proton) attached to the N_5, the critical beta-elimination reaction cannot proceed. The lack of beta-elimination results in the permanent attachment of 5-azacytosine to DNA methyltransferase via the covalent bond between sulfide and C_6. The net outcome is the "entrapment" of the DNA methyltransferase enzyme by 5-azacytosine analogs and its eventual degradation, leading to hypomethylation and achievement of the desired antineoplastic effects. This chemical process requires time.

2. **D.** DNMTI should be continued as long as the patient continues to benefit.

3. **B.** Several treatment-emergent morphologic changes in EKGs (including T-wave and ST-segment changes) have been reported in clinical studies. The clinical significance of these changes is unknown.

4. **A.** Panobinostat is not approved to be used as a single agent. Furthermore, its approval was withdrawn.

5. **B.** Differentiation syndrome due to IDH1 and IDH2 inhibitors may affect up to 20% of patients. Dyspnea, leukocytosis, and pulmonary infiltrates are the most common symptoms that can occur within days of starting the therapy and up to 3 months. Baseline bone marrow blasts >50% and peripheral blasts >25% are associated with an increased risk of differentiation syndrome

6. **C.** Systemic steroids (dexamethasone 10 mg given intravenously every 12 hours) are recommended as soon as differentiation syndrome is suspected. Cytoreduction with hydroxyurea should be initiated in a patient with concomitant leukocytosis. Temporary discontinuation of IDH1 or IDH2 inhibitors may be necessary.

7. **C.** Strong CYP3A inhibitors such as posaconazole should be avoided in a patient treated with venetoclax. Alternatively, if azole antifungal agents are clinically necessary, venetoclax dose should be adjusted (dose reduction to 70–100 mg) to avoid myelosuppression.

8. **C.** Oral azacitidine is approved in AML patients in first complete remission or complete remission with incomplete blood count recovery after intensive induction chemotherapy who are not candidates for curative therapies.

9. **B.** Menin inhibitors disrupt protein-protein interaction between menin and KMT2A or KMT2A-fusion partner. They appear to have therapeutic activity in AML with *NPM1* mutation or *KMT2A* rearrangement and prevent activation of genes involved in leukemogenesis.

SELECTED REFERENCES

Ahuja N, Sharma AR, Baylin SB. Epigenetic therapeutics: A new weapon in the war against cancer. Annu Rev Med. 2016;67:73–89. https://doi.org/10.1146/annurev-med-111314-035900

DiNardo CD, Jonas BA, Pullarkat V, et al. Azacitidine and venetoclax in previously untreated acute myeloid leukemia. N Engl J Med. 2020;383(7):617–29. https://doi.org/10.1056/NEJMoa2012971

DiNardo CD, Maiti A, Rausch CR, et al. 10-day decitabine with venetoclax for newly diagnosed intensive chemotherapy ineligible, and relapsed or refractory acute myeloid leukaemia: A single-centre, phase 2 trial. Lancet Haematol. 2020;7(10):e724–36. https://doi.org/10.1016/S2352-3026(20)30210-6

DiNardo CD, Schuh AC, Stein EM, et al. Enasidenib plus azacitidine versus azacitidine alone in patients with newly diagnosed, mutant-IDH2 acute myeloid leukaemia (AG221-AML-005): A single-arm, phase 1b and randomised, phase 2 trial. Lancet Oncol. 2021;22(11):1597–608. https://doi.org/10.1016/S1470-2045(21)00494-0

DiNardo CD, Stein AS, Stein EM, et al. Mutant isocitrate dehydrogenase 1 inhibitor ivosidenib in combination with azacitidine for newly diagnosed acute myeloid leukemia. J Clin Oncol. 2021;39(1):57–65. https://doi.org/10.1200/JCO.20.01632 [published correction appears in J Clin Oncol. 2021 February 1;39(4):341]

Emadi A, Faramand R, Carter-Cooper B, et al. Presence of isocitrate dehydrogenase mutations may predict clinical response to hypomethylating agents in patients with acute myeloid leukemia. Am J Hematol. 2015;90(5):E77–9. https://doi.org/10.1002/ajh.23965

Fathi AT, Wander SA, Faramand R, Emadi A. Biochemical, epigenetic, and metabolic approaches to target IDH mutations in acute myeloid leukemia. Semin Hematol. 2015;52(3):165–71. https://doi.org/10.1053/j.seminhematol.2015.03.002

Feinberg AP. The key role of epigenetics in human disease prevention and mitigation. N Engl J Med. 2018;378(14):1323–34. https://doi.org/10.1056/NEJMra1402513

Garnock-Jones KP. Panobinostat: First global approval. Drugs. 2015;75(6):695–704. https://doi.org/10.1007/s40265-015-0388-8 [published correction appears in Drugs. 2015 May;75(8):929. https://doi.org/10.1007/s40265-015-0403-0]

Kaminskas E, Farrell A, Abraham S, et al. Approval summary: Azacitidine for treatment of myelodysplastic syndrome subtypes. Clin Cancer Res. 2005;11(10):3604–8. https://doi.org/10.1158/1078-0432.CCR-04-2135

Kantarjian H, Issa JP, Rosenfeld CS, et al. Decitabine improves patient outcomes in myelodysplastic syndromes: Results of a phase III randomized study. Cancer. 2006;106(8):1794–803. https://doi.org/10.1002/cncr.21792

Kim N, Norsworthy KJ, Subramaniam S, et al. FDA approval summary: Decitabine and cedazuridine tablets for myelodysplastic syndromes. Clin Cancer Res. 2022;28(16):3411–6. https://doi.org/10.1158/1078-0432.CCR-21-4498

Lee HZ, Kwitkowski VE, Del Valle PL, et al. FDA approval: Belinostat for the treatment of patients with relapsed or refractory peripheral T-cell lymphoma. Clin Cancer Res. 2015;21(12):2666–70. https://doi.org/10.1158/1078-0432.CCR-14-3119

Mann BS, Johnson JR, Cohen MH, et al. FDA approval summary: Vorinostat for treatment of advanced primary cutaneous T-cell lymphoma. Oncologist. 2007;12(10):1247–52. https://doi.org/10.1634/theoncologist.12-10-1247

Norsworthy KJ, Luo L, Hsu V, et al. FDA approval summary: Ivosidenib for relapsed or refractory acute myeloid leukemia with an isocitrate dehydrogenase-1 mutation. Clin Cancer Res. 2019;25(11):3205–9. https://doi.org/10.1158/1078-0432.CCR-18-3749

Piekarz RL, Frye R, Turner M, et al. Phase II multi-institutional trial of the histone deacetylase inhibitor romidepsin as monotherapy for patients with cutaneous T-cell lymphoma. J Clin Oncol. 2009;27(32):5410–7. https://doi.org/10.1200/JCO.2008.21.6150

Popovic R, Licht JD. Emerging epigenetic targets and therapies in cancer medicine. Cancer Discov. 2012;2(5):405–13. https://doi.org/10.1158/2159-8290.CD-12-0076

Stahl M, Kohrman N, Gore SD, et al. Epigenetics in cancer: A hematological perspective. PLOS Genet. 2016;12(10):e1006193. https://doi.org/10.1371/journal.pgen.1006193

Stein EM, DiNardo CD, Pollyea DA, et al. Enasidenib in mutant IDH2 relapsed or refractory acute myeloid leukemia. Blood. 2017;130(6):722–31. https://doi.org/10.1182/blood-2017-04-779405

Wouters BJ, Delwel R. Epigenetics and approaches to targeted epigenetic therapy in acute myeloid leukemia. Blood. 2016;127(1):42–52. https://doi.org/10.1182/blood-2015-07-604512

CHAPTER 11

Differentiating Agents and Microenvironment

YUYA NAGAI • GABRIEL GHIAUR

INTRODUCTION

The pharmacokinetic and pharmacodynamics properties of cancer therapies within the circulation have been extensively studied in order to balance the therapeutic efficacy of a drug with its toxicity; however, drug levels and their effects on cancer cells are profoundly altered by the local tumor microenvironment (TME). The TME is shaped by the presence or absence of essential nutrients, concentrations of signaling molecules, and nearby nonmalignant cells. This chapter focuses on the impact of the TME on the pharmacokinetics and pharmacodynamics of cancer therapeutics.

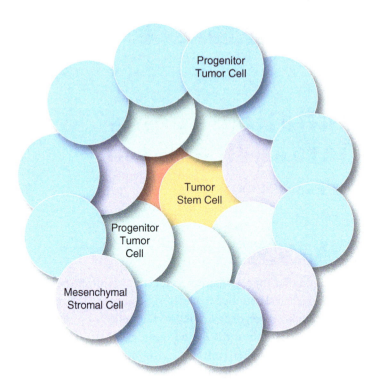

FIGURE 11.1 Tumor stem cells and their microenvironment.
One of the greatest challenges of cancer therapy is not the effective elimination
of the bulk of the tumor, but instead the elimination of the small population
of stem cells from which the tumor originated. These cells are hardy and
possess the capacity for quiescence and self-renewal. More so, these cells are
capable of producing the malignant progenitor cells that eventually recreate the
original disease. The tumor can recruit and manipulate nonmalignant stromal
and immune cells to create a protective niche where cancer stem cells can
survive initial therapy and persist as minimal residual disease. New therapeutic
approaches will have to overcome the microenvironmental factors that limit
the impact of chemotherapy on tumor stem cells in order to eliminate minimal
residual disease and provide cure in patients with cancer.

Depending on their specific chemical properties, each drug is expected to have a unique
volume of distribution and tissue penetration. In solid tumors, for instance, chemotherapy
may reach therapeutic concentrations within the organ of origin, and metastasis to another
organ, perhaps less permeable to chemotherapy, provides the tumor with a mechanism
of escape. Similarly, for liquid tumors, such as acute leukemia, circulating blasts may be
exposed to drug pharmacokinetics significantly different from malignant cells residing in
various bone marrow microenvironments (**Figures 11.2** and **11.3**).

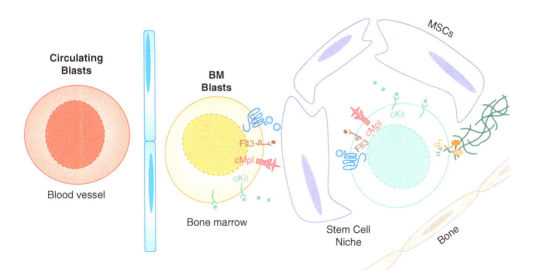

FIGURE 11.2 Leukemia cells reside in different compartments.
In liquid tumors, much as in solid tumors, malignant cells can be found in various compartments that have characteristically different soluble factors and cell-to-cell interactions. Thus, combined with divergent pharmacokinetics, the pharmacodynamics of various chemotherapeutics, including differentiation agents, may be profoundly different among these compartments. For instance, Flt3 inhibitors such as gilteritinib may induce apoptosis of circulating blasts. Growth factors present in the bone marrow rescue leukemia blasts from apoptosis and thus, gilteritinib may induce differentiation of these cells. Lastly, blasts found in specialized niches in which gilteritinib levels are insufficient may be completely resistant to treatment with this agent, and this can explain persistence of minimal residual disease.

BM, bone marrow; MSCs, mesenchymal stromal cells.

Mechanisms that have a profound impact on drug pharmacokinetics in the TME include:

A. Limited blood flow: Poor blood flow not only reduces delivery of drugs to the TME, but also produces a hypoxic and acidic environment, which may further impair drug delivery. An acidic environment favors protonation of basic drugs, resulting in low cellular uptake. Cancer cells preferentially reside within supportive niches and actively sculpt the local vasculature to achieve an even more favorable microenvironment. For example, the bone marrow has several distinct niches, including the vascular and endosteal niches, which differ in terms of blood flow, pH, and oxygen tension. Leukemic cells anchored within the endosteal niche may be less exposed to therapeutic agents and are responsible for residual disease upon initial treatment. Heterogeneity of microenvironments within the tumors themselves allows the cancer to diversify its portfolio—benefiting from high blood flow environments when nutrients are rich and from low blood flow environments when toxic drugs are in circulation. The presence of necrosis within a tumor exemplifies this trade-off; tumor cells in necrotic regions grow slowly or not at all, but are shielded from the high concentrations of toxic drugs that would otherwise lead to their demise.

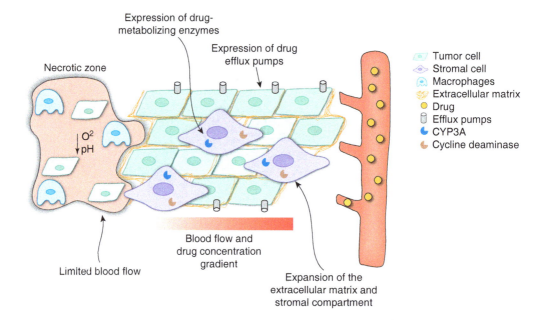

FIGURE 11.3 Effects of the tumor microenvironment on pharmacokinetics.
Pharmacokinetics describes the changes in drug concentrations over time and
are closely monitored for chemotherapeutics given their narrow therapeutic
index. Drugs are removed from the systemic circulation by the organs that
metabolize them, such as the liver or kidneys, and are subsequently excreted
through the urine, bile, or stool. The resulting plasma concentrations of a drug
may be significantly different from the concentrations of drug to which the
cancer cell is exposed. Factors that contribute to this disparity are illustrated
in the figure.

CYP, cytochrome P450.

B. Expansion of the extracellular matrix (ECM) and stromal compartment: Diverse
    ECM components, such as collagen, hyaluronan, fibronectin, and laminin, increase
    interstitial pressure and produce a physical barrier that reduces diffusion of drugs
    throughout the tumor.
C. TME expression of drug-metabolizing enzymes: Drug metabolism at the level of the
    TME creates unique local drug concentrations. Tumor cells and the surrounding
    stroma upregulate cytochrome P450 (CYP) enzymes in response to drug exposure,
    resulting in increased metabolism and locally reduced drug concentrations. CYP3A4,
    in particular, is responsible for the metabolism of a vast array of oncologic therapies,
    including topoisomerase inhibitors, vinca alkaloids and proteasome inhibitors, and
    also nearly all small-molecule inhibitors, most notably the large family of tyrosine
    kinase inhibitors. Similarly, mesenchymal stroma cells express high levels of cytidine
    deaminase (CDA) that can inactivate cytarabine and azacitidine, which are two active
    drugs in acute leukemia and myelodysplastic syndrome.

D. Expression of efflux pumps: Although expression of efflux pumps is not the focus of this chapter, it is worth noting that the drug concentrations in the TME may differ yet again from those in the tumor cells themselves. Although there are multiple mechanisms that can account for potential differences, perhaps the best characterized and most noteworthy is the overexpression of drug efflux pumps such as adenosine triphosphate (ATP)-binding cassette (ABC) transport proteins, which actively pump deleterious drugs out of the tumor cells.

Understanding TME-dependent mechanisms of impaired local pharmacokinetics may provide opportunities for novel therapeutic strategies. For instance, drugs that are repackaged within liposomes or nanoparticles have altered volumes of distribution and tissue penetration, favoring uptake within the TME. These larger drug particles preferentially extravasate into tumor sites that are supplied by fragile and relatively leaky vasculature. Liposomal doxorubicin as well as the liposomal combination of daunorubicin and cytarabine are two illustrative examples. The effectiveness of liposomal doxorubicin is dramatically improved in the treatment of patients with Kaposi sarcoma affecting the skin due to improved tumor penetration and retention. The liposomal formulation also reduces deposition in unaffected organs such as the heart, reducing adverse effects. The liposomal formulation of daunorubicin and cytarabine not only optimizes the delivery of both drugs into the tumor but may also ensure pharmacokinetic synchronization of the fixed 5:1 molar ratio to increase synergism and their uptake by leukemia cells. Another promising strategy is the coadministration of drugs that block drug-metabolizing enzymes such as CYP3A4. Clarithromycin is a potent CYP3A4 inhibitor and is used in combination with lenalidomide and dexamethasone (BiRD regimen) to optimize the pharmacokinetics and local effects of dexamethasone, resulting in improved responses compared to lenalidomide and dexamethasone alone. More so, a clinical trial of clarithromycin and cabazitaxel aims to test the efficacy of this same strategy in the treatment of metastatic, castration-resistant prostate cancer.

Some of the mechanisms by which TME changes the responsiveness of malignant cells to chemotherapy include:

A. Providing antiapoptotic survival and growth signals: Cancer cells are involved in a complex crosstalk with nonmalignant cells within the TME. Nonmalignant cells often elaborate prosurvival and growth signals that fortify malignant cells and attenuate the effects of the drug on the tumor, even at therapeutic concentrations. Leukemia cells, for example, overexpress a variety of receptors, including c-kit, Flt3, and AXL, which are typically expressed by hematopoietic stem cells. Activation of these receptors by signaling molecules produced by mesenchymal stromal cells leads to upregulation of antiapoptotic signaling programs that decrease the efficacy of chemotherapy.

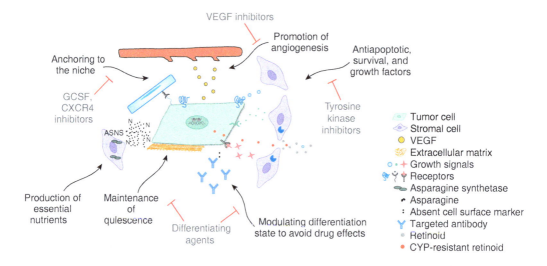

FIGURE 11.4 Effects of the tumor microenvironment on pharmacodynamics.
The tumor microenvironment promotes a unique phenotype in the malignant cells and, thus, modulates their response to otherwise adequate drug levels.

CXCR4, chemokine receptor type 4; CYP, cytochrome P450; GCSF, granulocyte colony-stimulating factor; VEGF, vascular endothelial growth factor.

B. Modulating differentiation state as a means of avoiding drug effect: Tumors contain a heterogeneous population of subclones, which differ in their state of differentiation. In the case of multiple myeloma, mesenchymal stroma cells promote an immature phenotype of malignant plasma cells characterized by decreased immunoglobulin production, low endoplasmic reticulum (ER) stress, and resistance to proteasome inhibitors. In fact, myeloma cells reinforce this protective mechanism by secreting hedgehog ligands that upregulate stromal CYP26 and create low retinoid niches where immature malignant cells can survive.

C. Maintenance of quiescence: The toxicities of many cancer therapies are dependent on active cell cycling. These include cytotoxic chemotherapies and CDK (cyclin-dependent kinase) inhibitors. Cancer cells escape toxicity by maintaining a quiescent state. The TME is a crucial mediator of quiescence. Hypoxic environments lead to upregulation of hypoxia inducible factor (HIF)-1α, which, in turn, maintains cells within a quiescent state. Adhesion of tumor cells to specific components of the ECM is necessary for proliferation. Laminin-rich ECM influences gene expression within mammary epithelial cells to produce a script that favors quiescence and suppression of apoptosis.

D. Production of essential nutrients: Upregulation of nutrient production occurs within the TME to overcome therapies aimed at depleting these same nutrients. Pegasparaginase is a pegylated enzyme that is used in the treatment of acute lymphoblastic leukemia and functions by depleting asparagine, a nonessential amino acid that is required for leukemic proliferation. Malignant cells are capable of inducing local mesenchymal stromal cells to overexpress asparagine synthetase in order to abrogate the effects of systemic asparagine depletion.

E. Vasculature: Cancer cells stimulate angiogenesis within the TME through the production of cytokines, such as vascular endothelial growth factor (VEGF), in order to increase delivery of nutrients necessary for proliferation. VEGF inhibitors, such as bevacizumab, and vascular endothelial growth factor receptor (VEGFR) inhibitors, such as sunitinib or sorafenib, block angiogenesis.

F. Anchoring: Tumor cells benefit from the TME in myriad ways, not least of which is the protection it provides cancer cells from existing therapies. Cancer cells anchor themselves to the TME via interactions with the ECM, the endothelium, and other inhabitants of the TME. For example, leukemic and prostate cancer cells express the chemokine receptor type 4 (CXCR4), which is responsible for homing and anchoring hematopoietic stem cells to the marrow.

In conclusion, interfering with these TME-dependent mechanisms holds promise to positively impact tumor stem cells and sensitize them to chemotherapy. To this end, tyrosine kinase inhibitors such as midostaurin and sorafenib inhibit activation of c-KIT and FLT3 to dampen survival and proliferation signals. A variety of new FLT3-specific and AXL inhibitors are being investigated as potential therapeutic options in clinical trials. As such, gilteritinib, a second-generation tyrosine kinase inhibitor, with dual inhibition of FLT3 and AXL is currently approved for treatment of relapsed/refractory FLT3 mutant acute myelogenous leukemia (AML).

Cellular differentiation blockade is a critical pathophysiologic feature of myeloid malignancies, and is commonly driven by epigenetic dysregulation. Drugs that induce differentiation, such as retinoids, DNA methyltransferase inhibitors such as azacitidine, and isocitrate dehydrogenase (IDH1/2) inhibitors, reduce tumor stem cells' inherent hardiness and resistance to apoptosis by differentiating them into more vulnerable progenitor cells. The prototypical differentiation therapy is the combination of all-trans retinoic acid (ATRA) and arsenic trioxide (ATO) for acute promyelocytic leukemia (APL), characterized by the fusion of promyelocytic leukemia (PML) gene with retinoic acid receptor-alpha (RARα). The PML-RARα fusion transcript extensively disturbs transcriptional regulation leading to myeloid differential block at promyelocytic stage. Pharmacologic doses of ATRA and ATO induce proteasome-mediated degradation of the fusion protein and resolve transcriptional disturbance, resulting in terminal differentiation of leukemic cells. Some cases develop differentiation syndrome (DS) characterized by acute onset of fever, weight gain, dyspnea, and renal failure during induction therapy. This syndrome is attributed to chemokines secretion and adhesion molecules expression of differentiating leukemic cells. Lately, oral arsenic has shown comparable clinical efficacy to that of intravenous formulations and better safety profile. Thus, the approach for APL is moving toward oral chemo-free treatment. ATRA and ATO combination for non-APL AML has been investigated. In vitro study shows the combination induces differentiation and apoptosis in AML cells with mutant NPM1 through proteasome-mediated degradation of mutant NPM1, although the utility of the combination therapy in clinical context remains to be elucidated.

Another successful differentiating agent is mutant IDH1/2 inhibitors such as ivosidenib and enasidenib. Approximately 20% of AML cases harbor mutation in IDH (IDH1 or IDH2). The IDH1/2 enzyme catalyzes isocitrate conversion to α-ketoglutarate (α-KG), whereas mutated IDH1/2 converts α-KG into oncometabolite 2-hydroxyglutarate (2-HG). Because TET2 and Jumonji C domain-containing histone demethylases are α-KG-dependent enzymes, the functions of them are interfered with by depletion of α-KG and also inhibited by elevated 2-HG itself. The resultant alteration in epigenetic machinery is partially responsible for the differential blockade of IDH1/2 mutated AML cells. IDH1/2 inhibitors suppress production of 2-HG and restore myeloid differentiation capacity.

Clinical DS has relatively commonly developed in some cases, although the median time to onset of DS is longer in AML cases treated with IDH1/2 inhibitors than that in APL cases treated with ATRA/ATO.

FLT3-internal tandem duplication (FLT3-ITD) represents one of the most frequently identified genetic alterations in AML, and has been classically thought of as a class I mutation conferring a proliferation and survival advantage to leukemic cells through activation of PI3K/AKT and RAS/ERK1/2 pathway. However, there is accumulating evidence that second-generation FLT3 inhibitors, such as quizartinib and gilteritinib, have a potential role of leukemic cell differentiation in the mechanism of clinical efficacy in sizable subset of AML patients with FLT3-ITD. Interestingly, these FLT3 inhibitors quickly induce apoptosis of leukemic cells in circulation, but not in the protective bone marrow microenvironment. Instead, these inhibitors induce terminal differentiation of leukemic blasts in bone marrow of AML patients over several weeks, accompanied with clinically modest DS in some cases (Figure 11.2). FLT3-ITD is demonstrated to induce aberrant signaling through strong activation of signal transducer and activator of transcription 5 (STAT5) leading to repression of myeloid transcription factors such as CCAAT/enhancer-binding protein α (C/EBPα) and PU.1. Thus, FLT3 inhibitors are thought to release the differentiation block through restoring expression of these transcription factors.

CHAPTER SUMMARY

The tumor microenvironment plays a critical role in modulating the impact of anticancer therapies on their targets. The TME contains multiple components that interact to influence net drug delivery to tumor cells and to modulate the net balance between tumor cell proliferation, differentiation, survival, and death. The TME is capable of reducing the cancer stem cells' exposure to anticancer agents and can attenuate their toxic effects through paracrine signaling and cell–cell interactions. Through better understanding of the interactions between tumors and their environments, we may be able to enhance the effectiveness of existing cancer treatments and to identify new targets for anticancer therapeutics. Successful differentiation therapy is perhaps best exemplified by the use of all-trans retinoic acid (ATRA) and arsenic trioxide (ATO) in acute promyelocytic leukemia (APL, M3-AML) and reflects the impact of tumor-directed therapies on both the TME and the malignant stem cell.

CLINICAL PEARLS

- Differentiation syndrome (DS) caused by both ATRA and ATO therapies for APL consists of hyperleukocytosis and cytokine release syndrome with pulmonary and renal dysfunctions. DS is successfully prevented and/or managed in high-risk APL patients with high-dose steroids and hydroxyurea.

- IDH1 and IDH2 inhibitors are also associated with a syndrome of differentiation that is clinically similar to that seen in APL. This syndrome can occur both early (e.g., days 3–7) and late (days 25–35) during therapy and is managed with high-dose steroids and hydroxyurea.

- Antiangiogenesis agents targeting VEGF isoforms and receptors are characteristically associated with hypertension and proteinuria. In addition, tumor necrosis at specific organ sites can lead to hemorrhage and/or perforations in the brain, lung, or gastrointestinal tract.

- Bevacizumab (Avastin), a VEGF-A–directed monoclonal antibody, is approved for use as a single agent or in combination with other antitumor modalities for melanoma, glioblastoma, and renal cell, ovarian, cervical, non-small cell lung, and colorectal carcinomas.

- ATRA can increase intracranial pressure, causing pseudotumor cerebri associated with headache, papilledema, and sensorineural hearing loss, and is managed with high-dose steroids and acetazolamide.

- To prevent cardiac complications of ATO, patients must have adequate plasma potassium levels (>4 mg/dL) and magnesium levels (>2 mg/dL), and QT interval <500 ms during each ATO administration. Agents that prolong QT interval should be avoided or used sparingly.

MULTIPLE-CHOICE QUESTIONS

1. TY is a 38-year-old obese woman who presents with right subconjunctival hemorrhage, multiple ecchymoses on the abdominal wall, and diplopia within 1 week of onset. Examination otherwise is unremarkable. Complete blood count showed hemoglobin 9.3 g/dL, leukocytes 1,250/μL, and platelets 35,000/μL; international normalized ratio 1.6, partial thromboplastin time normal, fibrinogen 95 mg/dL. Peripheral blood smear shows hypergranular cells with multiple Auer rods. CT scan of head suggests small intracranial hemorrhage in the thalamic area. Diagnosis of acute promyelocytic leukemia (APL) is highly suggested but it is not confirmed by bone marrow examination and cytogenetics. What is the best next step?

   A. Continue supporting care until the diagnosis is confirmed by bone marrow biopsy.
   B. Start all-trans retinoic acid (ATRA) without confirmed diagnosis.
   C. Hold transfusion of all blood products.
   D. Discuss end-of-life/hospice care with the patient and family.

2. TY tolerates the first 2 weeks of treatment with ATRA and arsenic trioxide (ATO) for her APL. She was doing well with normal mental status, diplopia resolving, and no bleeding. On day 15, the patient becomes hypoxic and develops fever. Chest CT scan demonstrates pulmonary infiltrates and a right-sided pleural effusion and mild pericardial effusion. She is transferred to the ICU. What is the most likely diagnosis?

    A. Pneumonia and associated parapneumonic effusion
    B. Extramedullary leukemia
    C. Transfusion-related acute lung injury (TRALI)
    D. Differentiation syndrome
    E. Pulmonary edema due to volume overload

3. TC, a 79-year-old man, was noted to have cytopenia during a routine follow-up. His blood test revealed a white blood cell (WBC) count of 2.5×10^9/L with 10% blasts, neutrophils 0.5×10^9/L, hemoglobin 8.0 g/dL, and platelets 110×10^9/L. Bone marrow examination confirmed AML with 40% myeloblasts and normal diploid karyotype on cytogenetic analysis. He received azacytidine as initial therapy, and achieved hematologic improvement after three cycles. Bone marrow test after six cycles confirmed complete remission. He was continued on treatment with azacitidine, but progressive cytopenia was noted after 10 cycles. Bone marrow showed relapse of AML with 32% blasts. An AML next-generation sequencing panel identified IDH1-R132C and RUNX1-G135D mutations. What therapy would be recommended next?

    A. Gemtuzumab ozogamicin
    B. Intensive chemotherapy
    C. Midostaurin
    D. Mutant IDH1 inhibitor (ivosidenib)

4. TC initiated ivosidenib 500 mg daily. Three weeks later, his blood test showed WBC count of 7.5×10^9/L with 50% neutrophils, 12% metamyelocytes, and 15% blasts. At 5 weeks, he presented with high-grade fever, shortness of breath (oxygen saturation 92%), and peripheral edema. His blood test showed increased WBC count of 25×10^9/L with similar differentials, and chest x-ray revealed bilateral infiltrates. What is the most likely diagnosis?

    A. Differentiation syndrome
    B. Pneumonia
    C. Pulmonary alveolar hemorrhage
    D. Progression of his disease

5. A 75-year-old man was diagnosed with AML. He was not considered fit for standard chemotherapy due to cardiac comorbidities. He was started on treatment with azacitidine, but had disease progression after five cycles. Bone marrow examination revealed hypercellularity with 72% myeloblasts. Mutational analysis identified IDH2-R140Q and DNMT3A-R882H mutations. What would be a reasonable next therapeutic strategy?

   A. ATRA
   B. Enasidenib
   C. Ivosidenib
   D. Quizartinib

6. A 48-year-old man is found to have pancytopenia while being investigated for recurrent infections over the last several weeks. His CBC shows WBCs of 5.0×10^9/L with 60% blasts, neutrophils 0.2×10^9/L, hemoglobin 7.0 g/dL, and platelets 50×10^9/L. Bone marrow examination confirmed AML with 80% blasts, and molecular analysis showed a FLT3-ITD (variant allelic frequency of 40%). Metaphase analysis shows 46,XY,t(15;17)(q24;q21) in 16/20 metaphases and normal 46,XY in 4/20. He has no comorbidities and good performance status. What initial therapy is recommended?

   A. Azacitidine + venetoclax
   B. Intensive chemotherapy + midostaurin
   C. All-trans retinoic acid (ATRA) and arsenic trioxide (ATO)
   D. Quizartinib monotherapy

7. A 48-year-old man visited a clinic due to fatigue and slight shortness of breath. His blood test revealed WBCs 35.0×10^9/L with 60% blasts, neutrophils 0.2×10^9/L, hemoglobin 7.0 g/dL, and platelets 50×10^9/L. Bone marrow examination confirmed AML with 80% blasts, and genomic analysis identified FLT3-ITD and NPM1 mutations. Cytogenetic analysis reveals a normal 46,XY karyotype in 20/20 metaphases. He has no comorbidities and good performance status. What initial therapy would be recommended?

   A. All-trans retinoic acid (ATRA) and arsenic trioxide (ATO)
   B. Azacitidine + venetoclax
   C. Intensive chemotherapy + midostaurin
   D. Quizartinib monotherapy

8. A 62-year-old man was diagnosed with AML with NPM1, DNMT3A R882H, and FLT3-ITD mutations. He initiated standard chemotherapy plus midostaurin but developed severe pneumonia during consolidation therapy, resulting in delayed subsequent therapy. He had progressive cytopenia and bone marrow examination confirmed relapse of AML with 30% blasts, and molecular profiling identified the same triple mutations at diagnosis. He eagerly desired allogeneic hematopoietic stem cell transplant as curative therapy. What therapy is recommended next?

   A. Azacitidine
   B. Gilteritinib
   C. Low-dose cytarabine
   D. Mitoxantrone, etoposide, and cytarabine (MEC)

9. A 66-year-old man with type 2 diabetes mellitus, hyperlipidemia, and stage III chronic renal disease (creatinine clearance 35m L/min) was found to have pulmonary aspergillosis while being evaluated for cough and fatigue. A 12-week course of posaconazole is recommended for him. After 2 weeks, the patient's clinical status has improved and a complete metabolic profile shows stable renal function and normal transaminases. Complete blood counts reveal worsening pancytopenia, WBC count of 1.0×10^9/L, neutrophils 0.2×10^9/L, hemoglobin 7.5 g/dL, and platelets 50×10^9/L. A bone marrow biopsy confirms a diagnosis of AML with 40% myoblasts. Molecular and cytogenetic studies are unremarkable. Which of the following interventions offer a balanced risk/benefit profile toward curative goal?

   A. Initiate azacitidine treatment.
   B. Initiate 7 + 3 therapy with idarubicin (12 mg) and cytarabine (200 mg).
   C. Switch posaconazole to micafungin and initiate therapy with azacitidine and venetoclax.
   D. Initiate therapy with azacitidine and 75% reduced dose of venetoclax.

10. A 32-year-old woman with no prior past medical history is diagnosed with AML. Initial analysis show normal karyotype and no targetable somatic mutations. She undergoes induction chemotherapy with idarubicin (12 mg) for 3 days and cytarabine (200 mg; 7 + 3 therapy) and she achieves a complete remission on day 35. She went on to receive consolidation with four cycles of high doses of cytarabine (3 g/m^2 every 12 hours every other day for 5 days). She tolerated the treatment well. Six months after completion of therapy, she is found to have relapsed disease on a routine bone marrow evaluation. Upon goals of care discussions, the decision for salvage therapy as a bridge to bone marrow transplantation is reached. She is enrolled in a clinical trial using mitoxantrone, cytarabine, and bevacizumab. During the salvage therapy, which of the following on-target side effects may require prophylaxis and close monitorization?

   A. Glucose intolerance induced by cytarabine
   B. Allergic reactions during bevacizumab infusion
   C. Neurotoxicity secondary to mitoxantrone
   D. Hypertension due to bevacizumab

ANSWERS TO MULTIPLE-CHOICE QUESTIONS

1. **B.** Any suspicion for APL, even without the confirmation of diagnosis with cytogenetics showing t(15:17), must prompt immediate initiation of ATRA (22.5 mg/m^2 twice daily).

2. **D.** In APL treated with ATRA and/or ATO or in AML with IDH mutation treated with enasidenib or ivosidenib, the presence of three or more events is sufficient for a confident clinical diagnosis of differentiation syndrome and should prompt the use of dexamethasone or other steroids. These symptoms/signs include fever ≥38°C, weight gain >5 kg, hypotension, dyspnea, radiographic opacities, pleural or pericardial effusion, and acute renal failure.

3. **D.** Ivosidenib is an oral IDH1 inhibitor that showed remarkable activity as single agent in patients with relapsed/refractory AML (DiNardo et al., 2018) and is currently approved by the FDA to be used in this group of patients. In addition, recent data suggest that ivosidenib + azacitidine is a reasonable initial treatment for patients with IDH1 mutant AML (Montesinos et al., 2022).

4. **A.** The use of IDH inhibitors may be associated with cellular differentiation and differentiation syndrome. Differentiation syndrome due to IDH inhibitors is a medical emergency and may lead to death if not treated. In addition, this "on target" side effect may have the appearance of disease progression due to increased number of blasts in peripheral blood and may require transient cytoreductive therapy with hydroxyurea.

5. **B.** Enasidenib is an oral IDH2 inhibitor that showed remarkable activity as single agent in patients with relapsed/refractory AML (Stein et al., 2017).

6. **C.** This patient suffers from acute promyelocytic leukemia (APL). The optimal initial treatment for patients with APL with t(15;17)(q24;q21) is a combination of ATRA and ATO (LoCoco et al., 2013), regardless of any additional molecular or cytogenetic abnormalities.

7. **C.** Patients with FLT3 mutant AML (FLT3ITD or FLT3TKD) and otherwise fit for intensive chemotherapy benefit from the addition of a FLT3 inhibitors to their initial therapy. Though the optimal FLT3 inhibitor to be added to induction therapy for these patients may change in the future, current studies support the use of midostaurin with intensive chemotherapy (Stone et al., 2017).

8. **B.** Relapsed FLT3ITD AML is a disease that is incredibly resistant to chemotherapy. Gilteritinib, an oral FLT3 inhibitor, has shown significant activity as single agent in this patient population (Perl et al., 2019) and is currently FDA approved for this indication.

9. **D.** This frail patient has two potentially fatal acute medical problems: invasive aspergillosis and AML. Azoles such as posaconazole and voriconazole are optimal initial therapy for invasive aspergillosis and alternative options (liposomal amphotericin) are limited given the patient has chronic kidney disease. Single-agent echinocandins is a suboptimal treatment strategy for invasive aspergillosis. Azacitidine plus venetoclax is a reasonable and perhaps most suited induction regimen to achieve complete remission for patients otherwise unfit for intensive chemotherapy (DiNardo et al., 2020). Venetoclax is predominantly metabolized by CYP3A and posaconazole (and voriconazole) is a strong CYP3A inhibitor. Thus, concomitant use of venetoclax and posaconazole requires a 75% dose reduction.

10. **D.** Hypertension may be seen in 20% to 40% of patients treated with bevacizumab. This is generally mild and easily managed with calcium channel blockers. The pathophysiology of bevacizumab-associated hypertension depends on inhibition of VEGF signaling and is expected to be reproduced by other VEGF inhibitors. Of note, allergic reactions to bevacizumab infusion are common and prophylaxis with H2 blockers are generally used prior to administration. These hypersensitivity reactions are not considered on-target.

SELECTED REFERENCES

Alonso S, Hernandez D, Chang YT, et al. Hedgehog and retinoid signaling alters multiple myeloma microenvironment and generates bortezomib resistance. J Clin Invest. 2016;126(12):4460–8. https://doi.org/10.1172/JCI88152

Alonso S, Su M, Jones JW, et al. Human bone marrow niche chemoprotection mediated by cytochrome P450 enzymes. Oncotarget. 2015;6(17):14905–12. https://doi.org/10.18632/oncotarget.3614

Boyerinas B, Zafrir M, Yesilkanal AE, et al. Adhesion to osteopontin in the bone marrow niche regulates lymphoblastic leukemia cell dormancy. Blood. 2013;121(24):4821–31. https://doi.org/10.1182/blood-2012-12-475483

Cortes JE, Goldberg SL, Feldman EJ, et al. Phase II, multicenter, randomized trial of CPX-351 (cytarabine:daunorubicin) liposome injection versus intensive salvage therapy in adults with first relapse AML. Cancer. 2015;121(2):234–42. https://doi.org/10.1002/cncr.28974

DiNardo CD, Jonas BA, Pullarkat V, et al. Azacitidine and venetoclax in previously untreated acute myeloid leukemia. N Engl J Med. 2020;383(7):617–29. https://doi.org/10.1056/NEJMoa2012971

DiNardo CD, Stein EM, de Botton S, et al. Durable remissions with ivosidenib in IDH1-mutated relapsed or refractory AML. N Engl J Med. 2018 Jun 21;378(25):2386–98. https://doi.org/10.1056/NEJMoa1716984

Lancet JE, Uy GL, Cortes JE, et al. CPX-351 (cytarabine and daunorubicin) liposome for injection versus conventional cytarabine plus daunorubicin in older patients with newly diagnosed secondary acute myeloid leukemia. J Clin Oncol. 2018;36(26):2684–92. https://doi.org/10.1200/JCO.2017.77.6112

Laranjeira AB, de Vasconcellos JF, Sodek L, et al. IGFBP7 participates in the reciprocal interaction between acute lymphoblastic leukemia and BM stromal cells and in leukemia resistance to asparaginase. Leukemia. 2012;26(5):1001–11. https://doi.org/10.1038/leu.2011.289

Lo-Coco F, Avvisati G, Vignetti M, et al. Retinoic acid and arsenic trioxide for acute promyelocytic leukemia. N Engl J Med. 2013 Jul 11;369(2):111–21. https://doi.org/10.1056/NEJMoa1300874

Montesinos P, Recher C, Vives S, et al. Ivosidenib and azacitidine in IDH1-mutated acute myeloid leukemia. N Engl J Med. 2022 Apr 21;386(16):1519–31. https://doi.org/10.1056/NEJMoa2117344

Perl AE, Martinelli G, Cortes JE, et al. Gilteritinib or chemotherapy for relapsed or refractory FLT3-mutated AML. N Engl J Med. 2019 Oct 31;381(18):1728–40. https://doi.org/10.1056/NEJMoa1902688

Stein EM, DiNardo CD, Pollyea DA, et al. Enasidenib in mutant IDH2 relapsed or refractory acute myeloid leukemia. Blood. 2017 Aug 10;130(6):722–31. https://doi.org/10.1182/blood-2017-04-779405

Stone RM, Mandrekar SJ, Sanford BL, et al. Midostaurin plus chemotherapy for acute myeloid leukemia with a FLT3 mutation. N Engl J Med. 2017 Aug 3;377(5):454–64. https://doi.org/10.1056/NEJMoa1614359

Whatcott CJ, Han H, Posner RG, et al. Targeting the tumor microenvironment in cancer: Why hyaluronidase deserves a second look. Cancer Discov. 2011;1(4):291–6. https://doi.org/10.1158/2159-8290.CD-11-0136

PART IV

Organ-Targeted Approaches

CHAPTER 12

Targeted Therapies (Small Molecules)

YUCHEN (JAKE) LIU • ASHKAN EMADI

INTRODUCTION

The unprecedented understanding of molecular alterations driving tumorigenesis in the genomic era has led to a paradigm shift away from the isolated use of cytotoxic chemotherapy designed to indiscriminately destroy rapidly dividing cells to a more precise approach of targeting cancer cells based on specific molecular alterations in tumor DNA. Targeted therapy preferentially damages malignant cells while sparing normal cells by blocking the action of mutated enzymes, proteins, or molecules that perpetuate or "drive" growth and survival of cancer cells. Several of these therapies directly target mutated kinases, most commonly tyrosine kinases. Enzyme-specific drugs target constitutively active mutated tyrosine kinases generated by somatic DNA alterations, while nonspecific "multikinase" inhibitors target several enzymes that are upregulated in cancer cells and are involved in cell survival, angiogenesis, and metastasis. Drugs that are designed to target different kinases are accounting for ~25% of all current drug discovery research and development efforts. The goal of this chapter is to describe frequently used targeted therapies, affected enzymatic pathways, and common clinical applications.

KINASE

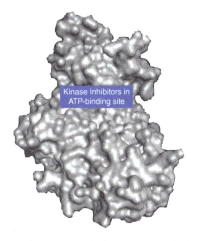

Kinase Inhibitors in ATP-binding site

FIGURE 12.1 Spatial structure of a kinase.

(continued)

FIGURE 12.1 Spatial structure of a kinase. (*continued*)
Kinases are enzymes that catalyze the transfer of a phosphate group (see the following) from adenosine triphosphate (ATP) to a protein within a cell, switching the cell from a state of inactivation to activation.

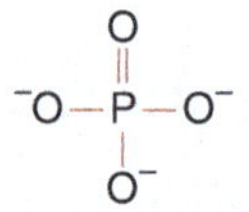

$$^-O-\overset{\overset{\displaystyle O}{\|}}{\underset{\underset{\displaystyle O^-}{|}}{P}}-O^-$$

Kinases share a secondary structure that folds into a twin-lobed catalytic core with ATP binding in a deep cleft located between the lobes. Kinases participate in signal transduction that regulate cytoskeletal rearrangement, differentiation, development, the immune response, nervous system function, DNA transcription, apoptosis, and cell cycle progression.

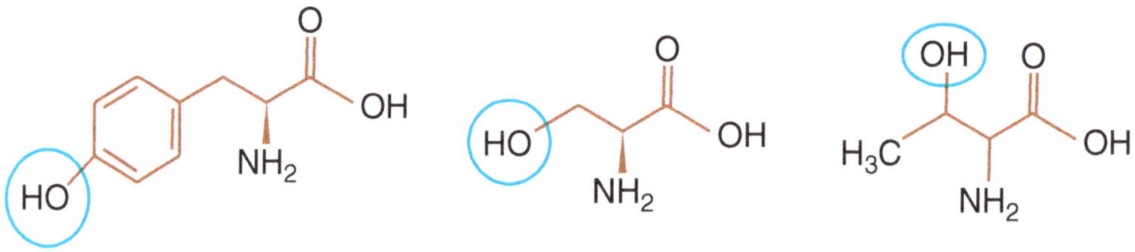

Tyrosine   **Serine**   **Threonine**

FIGURE 12.2 Structure of three hydroxyl (OH)-containing amino acids that can be phosphorylated in proteins by different types of kinases.
Kinases correspond to nearly 2% of all human genes. There are 518 human protein kinase genes, 478 typical and 40 atypical kinase

The protein kinase family includes:

- 385 serine/threonine kinases (e.g., CDK family, B-Raf, mTOR)
- 90 tyrosine kinases (e.g., ALK, EGFR family, platelet-derived growth factor receptor [PDGFR] α/β, vascular endothelial growth factor receptor [VEGFR] family, c-MET, RET, FLT3, BCR-ABL, Bruton tyrosine kinase [BTK] and JAK family, Scr family)
- 43 other proteinakinases (e.g., phosphatidylinositol 3-kinase [PI3K])

Of the 90 protein-tyrosine kinases:

- 58 are receptors with an extracellular, transmembrane, and intracellular domains (e.g., ALK, EGFR family, PDGFRα/β, VEGFR family, c-MET, RET; Figure 12.3).
- 32 are nonreceptor intracellular proteins (e.g., BCR-ABL, BTK, JAK [Figure 12.4], Src family); B-Raf and CDK family are examples of serine-threonine intracellular kinase.

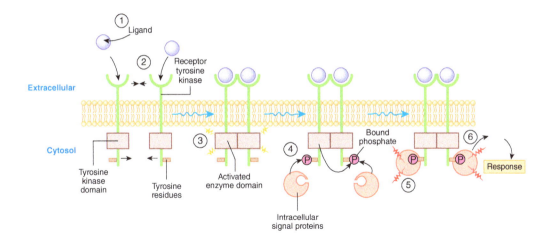

FIGURE 12.3 Receptor tyrosine kinase (e.g., FLT3).
(1) Ligands bind the receptor; (2) receptors dimerize; (3) receptor dimerization results in tyrosine kinase domain activation; (4) after activation, tyrosine kinase domain either autophosphorylates itself or the opposite tyrosine residue; (5) the phosphorylated tyrosine residues activate the intracellular signal proteins; (6) the activated intracellular signal proteins initiate an intracellular signaling pathway.

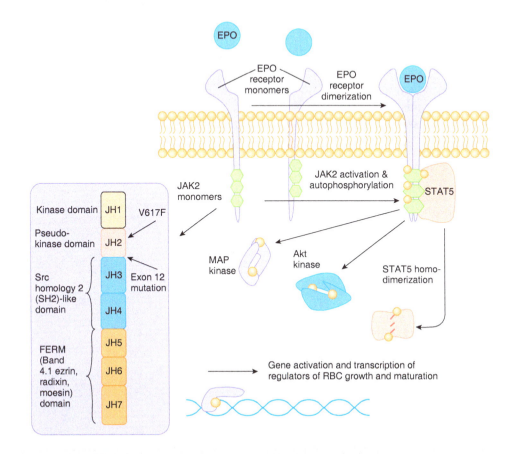

FIGURE 12.4 JAK, an example of non-receptor (intracellular) tyrosine kinase.

CLASSIFICATION OF PROTEIN KINASE INHIBITORS BASED UPON THE STRUCTURES OF THEIR DRUG-ENZYME COMPLEXES

1. Type I inhibitor: a small molecule that binds to the active conformation of a kinase in the ATP pocket (e.g., midostaurin, sunitinib, gilteritinib)
2. Type II inhibitor: a small molecule that binds to the inactive conformation of a kinase in the ATP pocket (e.g., ponatinib, sorafenib, quizartinib)
   a. Nearly all of the approved protein kinase type I and type II inhibitors occupy the adenine-binding pocket and form hydrogen bonds with the hinge region connecting the small and large lobes of the enzyme.
3. Type III: allosteric inhibitor bound next to the ATP site
4. Type IV: allosteric inhibitor not bound next to the ATP site (e.g., asciminib)
5. Type V: bivalent inhibitor spanning two regions
6. Type VI: covalent (irreversible) inhibitor (e.g., BTK inhibitors [ibrutinib, acalabrutinib, zanubrutinib], afatinib, neratinib)

BCR-ABL and BCR-ABL Inhibitors

The Philadelphia chromosome (Ph) was first discovered in 1959 by Dr. David Hungerford and Dr. Peter Nowell in Philadelphia. This was later found to lead to a gene fusion between the Abelson murine leukemia viral oncogene homolog (ABL) on chromosome 9 and the breakpoint cluster region (BCR) gene on chromosome 22 leading to constitutive activation of the tyrosine kinase (ABL), t(9;22)(q34;q11) (Figure 12.5). Different breakpoints were later identified and the two most commonly found breakpoints resulted in two different oncoproteins with different molecular weights (p190 and p210). The p190 product is more common in acute lymphoblastic leukemia (ALL) and the p210 product is more common in chronic myeloid leukemia (CML).

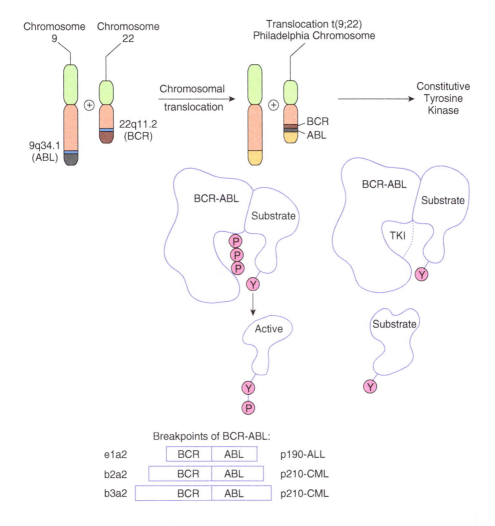

FIGURE 12.5 BCR-ABL translocation and the Philadelphia chromosome.
In this figure, the substrate with phosphorylated tyrosine (Y) is activated by BCR-ABL. Tyrosine kinase inhibitor (TKI) prevents phosphorylation, hence activation, of the substrates. The breakpoint in the *BCR* gene can occur in the 5.8 kb major breakpoint cluster region (M-bcr). This *BCR-ABL* gene is transcribed into a 8.5 kb mRNA with a b3a2 and/or b2a2 junction. The mRNA is translated into a 210-kD fusion protein. The breakpoint can also occur in the first intron of the *BCR* gene known as the minor breakpoint cluster region (m-bcr). This results in the fusion of *BCR* exon 1 to *ABL* exon 2 (e1a2) leading to a 7.0-kb mRNA transcript that is translated into the 190-kD protein.

ALL, acute lymphoblastic leukemia; CML, chronic myeloid leukemia; mRNA, messenger RNA.

The first generation BCR-ABL inhibitor imatinib was the first U.S. Food and Drug Administration (FDA)-approved targeted therapy in oncology, which has led to a revolution in the treatment of CML and Ph⁺ ALL. Imatinib is also FDA approved for the treatment of PDGFR rearranged myelodysplastic syndromes/myeloproliferative neoplasms (MDS/MPNs), hypereosinophilic syndrome, or chronic eosinophilic leukemia, aggressive systematic mastocytosis (SM) without a D816V c-kit mutation, and in c-Kit+ (CD117) unresectable or metastatic gastrointestinal stromal tumor.

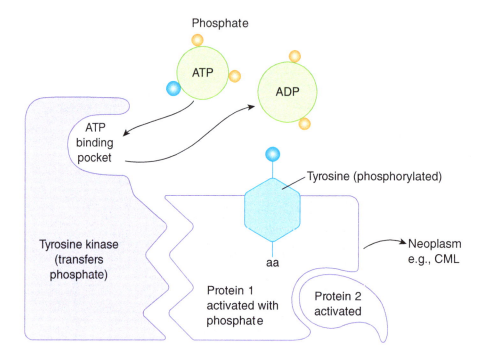

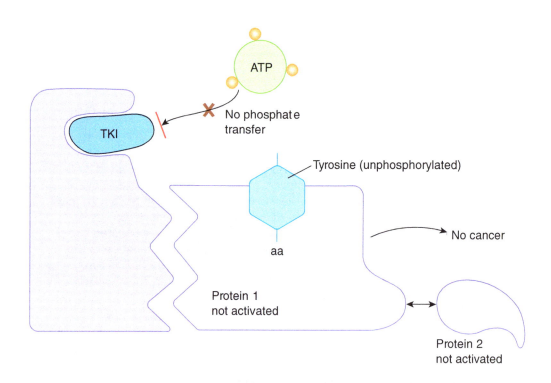

FIGURE 12.6 **Tyrosine kinase inhibitors (TKIs).**

aa, amino acid; ADP, adenosine diphosphate; ATP, adenosine triphosphate; CML, chronic myeloid leukemia.

Second-generation BCR-ABL inhibitors include dasatinib, nilotinib, and bosutinib, which are more potent than imatinib. Dasatinib and nilotinib have been shown to induce a more rapid decrease in BCR-ABL transcript levels.

- Dasatinib is approved for treatment of newly diagnosed adults with Ph$^+$ chronic phase (CP) CML; adults with CP, accelerated phase (AP), or myeloid or lymphoid blast phase (BP) Ph$^+$ CML with resistance or intolerance to prior therapy including imatinib; adults with Ph$^+$ ALL with resistance or intolerance to prior therapy; pediatric patients ≥ 1 year of age CP-CML; pediatric patients ≥ 1 year of age with newly diagnosed Ph$^+$ ALL in combination with chemotherapy. Dasatinib is associated with increased rates of bleeding, QT prolongation, and the development of fluid retention (e.g., pleural effusions, ascites) and pulmonary arterial hypertension (PAH).
- Nilotinib is the only BCR-ABL inhibitor that is taken twice daily and it is approved for treatment of adult and pediatric patients ≥ 1 year of age with newly diagnosed Ph$^+$ CML, adult patients with chronic and accelerated phase Ph$^+$ CML resistant to or intolerant to prior therapy that included imatinib, and pediatric patients ≥ 1 year of age with Ph$^+$ CP/AP-CML resistant or intolerant to prior tyrosine kinase inhibitor (TKI) therapy. Food should be avoided 2 hours before and 1 hour after taking a dose of nilotinib. Nilotinib has a black box warning for the risk of QT prolongation and the development of sudden death.
- Bosutinib is approved for the treatment of adult patients with newly diagnosed CP-CML and CP/AP/BP Ph$^+$ CML with resistance or intolerance to prior therapy. Bosutinib is commonly associated with gastrointestinal (GI) toxicity particularly diarrhea. The median time to onset for diarrhea is 2 days and the median duration per event is 2 days. Diarrhea is often self-limiting; however, its management may require withholding or dose reduction of bosutinib. Mild to moderate persistent diarrhea in majority of the cases can be managed by coadministration of loperamide (also known as Imodium).

Third-generation BCR-ABL inhibitor ponatinib was developed to overcome resistance that occurs due to the gatekeeper T315I mutation, which leads to resistance against all the earlier generation BCR-ABL inhibitors. Ponatinib is approved for treatment of (a) CP-CML with resistance or intolerance to at least two prior kinase inhibitors, (b) AP/BP CML or Ph$^+$ ALL when no other kinase inhibitors are indicated, (c) T315I-positive CML (CP, AP, BP) or T315I-positive Ph$^+$ ALL. Ponatinib has a black box warning for (a) arterial occlusive events including fatal myocardial infarction, stroke, stenosis of large arterial vessels of the brain, severe peripheral vascular disease, and the need for urgent revascularization procedures and patients with and without cardiovascular risk factors, including patients age 50 years or younger, who experienced these events; (b) venous thromboembolic events (VTEs); (c) heart failure; (d) hepatotoxicity, liver failure, and death. Ponatinib can also cause pancreatitis, and serum lipase should be monitored during treatment.

Asciminib is a newly developed BCR-ABL inhibitor that binds to the myristol pocket of the ABL protein, in contrast with previous BCR-ABL inhibitors that bind to the ATP binding site, and shows activity against the presence of the T315I mutation and is currently approved for CML with a T315I mutation and patients who had been previously treated with two prior BCR-ABL inhibitors. Asciminib is associated with pancreatitis, hypertension, and cardiovascular toxicity.

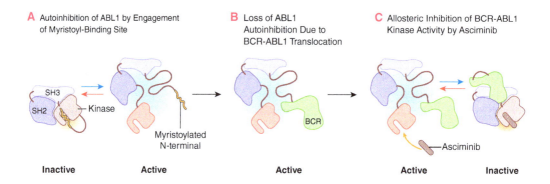

A Autoinhibition of ABL1 by Engagement of Myristoyl-Binding Site

B Loss of ABL1 Autoinhibition Due to BCR-ABL1 Translocation

C Allosteric Inhibition of BCR-ABL1 Kinase Activity by Asciminib

SH3

SH2 ——Kinase

Myristoylated N-terminal

BCR

——Asciminib

Inactive   Active   Active   Active   Inactive

FIGURE 12.7 Allosteric inhibitor not bound next to the adenosine triphosphate (ATP) site asciminib).

The fusion BCR-ABL1 protein leads to a loss of the autoinhibitory myristoyl-binding site present on ABL1. Asciminib mimics the native myristylated N-terminal of ABL1 to induce inhibition of the fusion of BCR-ABL1.

FMS-Like Tyrosine Kinase 3 (FLT3) and FLT3 Inhibitors

The FLT3 is a tyrosine kinase receptor that is expressed on early hematopoietic progenitor cells and dendritic cells. Binding of two FLT3 ligands forms a bridge that brings the FLT3 receptors in close proximity to one another and activates phosphorylation.

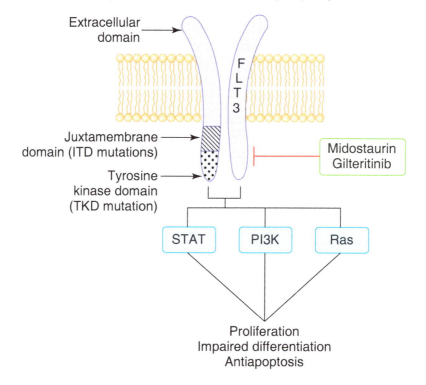

Extracellular domain

F L T 3

Juxtamembrane domain (ITD mutations)

Tyrosine kinase domain (TKD mutation)

Midostaurin Gilteritinib

STAT   PI3K   Ras

Proliferation
Impaired differentiation
Antiapoptosis

FIGURE 12.8 FLT3 receptor.

FLT3, FMS-like tyrosine kinase 3; ITD, internal tandem duplication; PI3K, phosphatidylinositol 3-kinase; STAT, signal transducer and activator of transcription; TKD, tyrosine kinase domain.

Mutations in either the juxtamembrane domain (internal tandem duplication [ITD]) or the tyrosine kinase domain (TKD) of FLT3 leads to its constitutive activity resulting in massive cell proliferation and cell survival. Approximately 30% of cases of acute myeloid leukemia (AML) harbor a FLT3 mutation, which has been proved to be a poor prognostic marker in AML and as such FLT3 has been an attractive therapeutic target. FLT3 inhibitors can be separated into two types: type 1 and type 2.

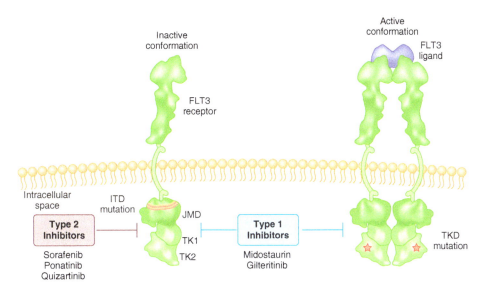

FIGURE 12.9 Different FLT3 inhibitors.
Type 1 FLT3 inhibitor binds to both the active and inactive conformations of FLT3 protein, and type 2 FLT3 inhibitors bind only to the inactive conformation.

The first FDA-approved FLT3 inhibitor is the multikinase (including FLT3, type 1) inhibitor midostaurin, which is used in combination with induction chemotherapy (daunorubicin and cytarabine) for patients who harbor either FLT3-ITD or FLT3-TKD mutation. Midostaurin is also approved as a single agent for the treatment of aggressive systemic mastocytosis and mast cell leukemia. Development of interstitial lung disease and pneumonitis have been associated with midostaurin.

Gilteritinib is also a type 1 FLT3 inhibitor that is approved as a single agent for relapsed or refractory AML with FLT3 mutations. Gilteritinib was found to be superior compared to investigator's choice of chemotherapy. There is a black box warning for gilteritinib for the development of differentiation syndrome, which is manifested by the development of fevers, volume overload, rash, and kidney damage, which can be managed with corticosteroids and hydroxyurea

Type 2 FLT3 inhibitor quizartinib is currently approved in Japan for the treatment of adult patients with relapsed/refractory FLT3-ITD AML. The FDA has granted priority review to quizartinib in combination with standard cytarabine and anthracycline induction followed by consolidation cytarabine and continuation of quizartinib monotherapy after consolidation in patients with newly diagnosed FLT3-ITD AML.

AML, acute myeloid leukemia; FDA, U.S. Food and Drug Administration; FLT3, FMS-like tyrosine kinase 3; ITD, internal tandem duplication; JMD, juxtamembrane domain; TK, tyrosine kinase;TKD, tyrosine kinase domain.

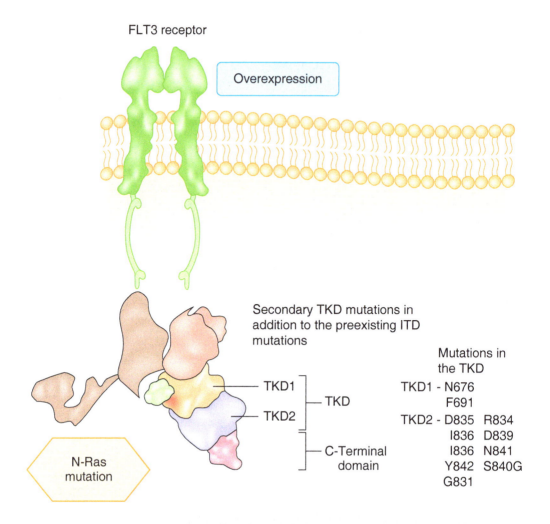

FIGURE 12.10 Common mechanisms of resistance to FLT3 inhibitors.
Resistance to the FLT3 inhibitors can occur via several mechanisms including
(a) treatment-emergent mutations that activate RAS/MAPK pathway signaling,
most commonly in NRAS or KRAS, (b) decreased drug-binding affinity by
secondary FLT3-F691L gatekeeper mutations, (c) BCR–ABL1 fusions identified at
progression, (d) FLT3 gene amplification or protein overexpression, (e) deletion or
insertion in TKD domain, (f) increased drug efflux pumps, and (g) overexpression
of anti-apoptotic Bcl-xL, survivin, and DNA repair molecule RAD51.

FLT3, FMS-like tyrosine kinase 3; ITD, internal tandem duplication; KRAS, Kirsten rat-sarcoma virus; MAPK,
mitogen-activated protein kinase; NRAS, neuroblastoma rat-sarcoma virus; TKD, tyrosine kinase domain.

ISOCITRATE DEHYDROGENASE AND IDH INHIBITORS AND TEN-ELEVEN TRANSLOCATION

Isocitrate dehydrogenase 1 and 2 (IDH1 and IDH2) are essential enzymes for oxidative decarboxylation (as well as reductive carboxylation) involved in oxidative phosphorylation that
are a part of the Krebs cycle.

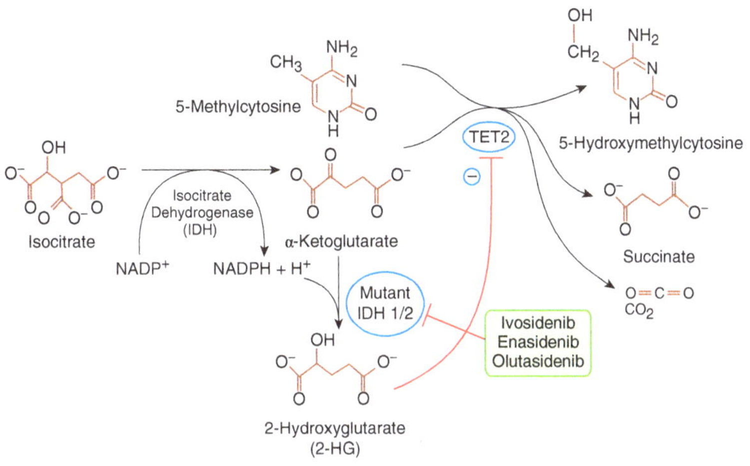

FIGURE 12.11 IDH and TET2 mutations and their metabolic and genetic consequences.

IDH catalyzes the decarboxylation of isocitrate to α-ketoglutarate (α-KG). IDH1 mediates this reaction in the cytosol and IDH2 mediates this reaction in the mitochondria. The mutated IDH cannot catalyze the normal decarboxylation of isocitrate to α-KG reaction and instead catalyzes the reduction of α-KG to 2-hydroxyglutarate (2-HG). 2-HG is normally present in very low concentration within the cell and its accumulation leads to suppression of the epigenetic enzyme ten-eleven translocation 2 (TET2). Suppression of TET2 inhibits DNA demethylation, gene activation, and cell differentiation. The result is hypermethylation, blockage of differentiation, and enhanced cell survival. TET2 mutation has similar effects.

Mutated IDH1 and IDH2 lead to gain-of-function activity in some myeloid malignancies (e.g., AML, MDS, MPN), brain tumors (e.g., adult-type diffuse gliomas including IDH-mutant astrocytoma, IDH-mutant oligodendroglioma), chondrosarcoma, intrahepatic cholangiocarcinoma, and angioimmunoblastic T-cell lymphoma.

AML, acute myeloid leukemia; MDS, myelodysplastic syndrome; MPN, myeloproliferative neoplasm; NADP, nicotinamide adenine dinucleotide phosphate.

The IDH1 inhibitor ivosidenib is used in both newly diagnosed in combination with azacitidine and relapsed or refractory IDH1-mutated AML. Furthermore, ivosidenib is also used in locally advanced or metastatic cholangiocarcinoma that has progressed after chemotherapy.

The IDH2 inhibitor enasidenib is used in relapsed or refractory or refractory IDH2-mutated AML.

Olutasidenib A is an IDH1 inhibitor indicated for the treatment of adult patients with relapsed or refractory AML with a susceptible IDH1 mutation.

Both of the IDH inhibitors (IDH1 and IDH2) have a black box warning for differentiation syndrome (fever, volume overload, hypotension, and rash), and while rare, this can be treated with steroids.

Bruton Tyrosine Kinase and BTK Inhibitors

Bruton tyrosine kinase (BTK) was first discovered as the gene responsible for the development of Bruton agammaglobulinemia. BTK is a downstream target of the B-cell receptor (BCR), for which constitutive BCR signaling is a feature of several B-cell neoplasms.

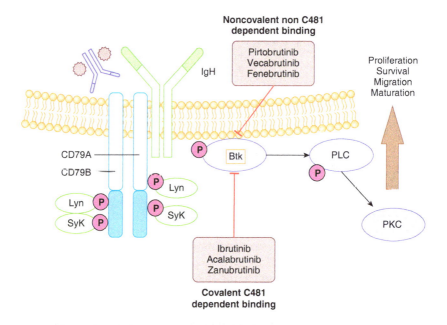

FIGURE 12.12 **The B-cell receptor (BCR) and Bruton tyrosine kinase (BTK).**
Antigen binding to the BCR triggers phosphorylation of CD79a and CD79b, which leads to phosphorylation of spleen tyrosine kinase (SYK) and ultimately to phosphorylation and activation of BTK. There are two key tyrosine (Y) phosphorylation sites, Y223 and Y551 (in the kinase domain). During BCR signaling, phosphorylation by SYK at Y551 initiates autophosphorylation of Y223 and activation of BTK. This activation of BTK initiates activation of phospholipase C (PLC) and protein kinase C (PKC), which ultimately results in proliferation, survival, migration, and maturation.

The fundamental role of BTK activation in BCR signaling offered strong biological rationale for BTK inhibition as a targeted therapeutic strategy in B-cell malignancies.

Ibrutinib, as the first generation, and acalabrutinib and zanubrutinib, as the second generation BTK inhibitors covalently binds to cysteine (C) 481 and inhibit BTK. Noncovalent BTKi (not yet approved) offer a therapeutic alternative for patients with B-cell malignancies, including those who are intolerant to or have disease progression during treatment with a covalent BTKi.

Ibrutinib

BTK inhibitors ibrutinib, acalabrutinib, and zanubrutinib (as well as afatinib and neratinib [indicated for the extended adjuvant treatment of adult patients with early stage HER2-overexpressed/amplified breast cancer, to follow adjuvant trastuzumab-based therapy]) are type VI (covalent-binding via nucleophilic attack of sulfur in cysteine to α/β unsaturated ketone [blue circle]) protein kinase inhibitors.

Resistance to the irreversible type VI inhibitors often involves mutation of a cysteine residue where the inhibitor binding occurs.

- Ibrutinib is the first generation BTK inhibitor indicated for the treatment of adult patients with:
  ○ Mantle cell lymphoma (MCL) who have received at least one prior therapy [560 mg PO qday]
  ○ Marginal zone lymphoma (MZL) who require systemic therapy and have received at least one prior anti-CD20-based therapy [560 mg PO qday]
  ○ Chroni lymphocyctic leukemia (CLL)/Small lymphocytic lymphoma (SLL) [420 mg PO qday]
  ○ CLL/SLL [420 mg PO qday]
  ○ CLL/SLL with 17p deletion [420 mg PO qday]
  ○ Waldenström's macroglobuliemia (WM) [420 mg PO qday]
  ○ Chronic graft versus host disease (cGVHD) after failure of one or more lines of systemic therapy [420 mg PO qday] (also for pediatric patients age 1 year and older)
- WARNINGS AND PRECAUTIONS
  ○ Serious and opportunistic infections including early-onset invasive fungal infections, in particular invasive aspergilosis with frequent cerebral involvement
  ○ Hemorrhage
  ○ Second primary malignancies
  ○ Atrial fibrillation and flutter

Acalabrutinib is approved for patients with mantle cell lymphoma (MCL) who have received at least one prior therapy and those with chronic lymphocytic leukemia (CLL)/small lymphocytic leukemia (SLL).

Zanubrutinib is approved for treatment of patients with MCL who have received at least one prior therapy, Waldenström macroglobulinemia (WM), or relapsed or refractory marginal zone lymphoma (MZL) who have received at least one anti-CD20-based regimen

Both acalabrutinib and zanubrutinib show lower rates of cardiovascular side effects compared to the first-generation ibrutinib. Two randomized Phase 3 studies compared second-generation BTKi with ibrutinib. In the ELEVATE RR study, acalabrutinib was non-inferior to ibrutinib for efficacy, with lower rates of atrial fibrillation, hypertension, and bleeding. In the ALPINE study in which patients were randomized 1:1 to either ibrutinib or zanubrutinib, at a median follow-up of ~30 months, zanubrutinib was superior to ibrutinib with respect to progression-free survival (PFS) among 652 patients (hazard ratio for disease progression or death, 0.65; 95% CI 0.49 to 0.86; p = .002 [78.4% in the zanubrutinib group and 65.9% in the ibrutinib group]). The safety profile of zanubrutinib was better than that of ibrutinib, with fewer cardiac events, including fewer cardiac events leading to treatment discontinuation or death.

PHOSPHATIDYINOSITOL KINASE 3

The phosphatidylinositol kinase 3 (PI3K) pathway is a non-tyrosine non-serine/threonine kinase.

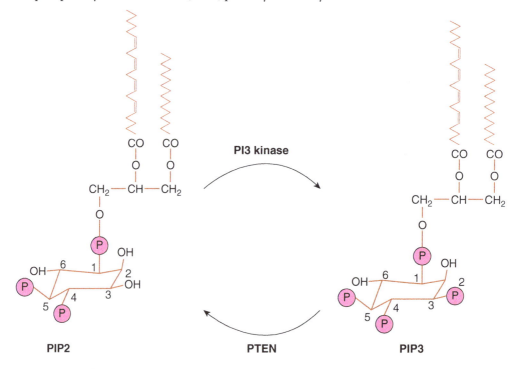

FIGURE 12.13 Phosphatidylinositol (4,5)-bisphosphate (PIP2) phosphorylation (by PI3K) to phosphatidylinositol (3,4,5)-trisphosphate (PIP3) and dephosphorylation back to PIP2.

PI3K is downstream of many growth promoting molecules and leads to activation of protein kinase B (PKB, also known as Akt) and activation of Akt mediates cellular proliferation and survival. Constitutive activation of PI3K/Akt pathways have been found in many different cancers.

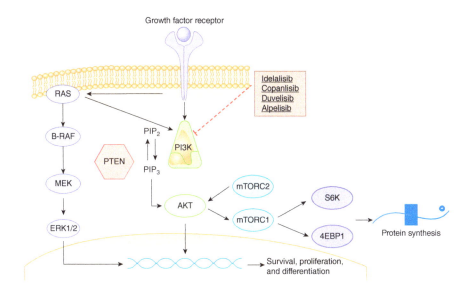

FIGURE 12.14 PI3K/AKT/mTOR pathway.

ERK, extracellular signal-regulated kinase; MEK, mitogen-activated extracellular signal-regulated kinase; PIP2, phosphatidylinositol 4,5-bisphosphate; PIP3, phosphatidylinositol 3,4,5-trisphosphate; PTEN, phosphatase and tensin homolog; RAS rat sarcoma virus.

While there are active attempts in targeting PI3K in many cancers, PI3K inhibitors are used in the treatment of non-Hodgkin lymphoma. Despite initial FDA approvals for the treatment of follicular lymphoma for PI3K inhibitors duvelisib, idelalisib, and umbralisib, these approvals have since been withdrawn due to safety concerns. Idelalisib and duvelisib are still available for treatment of chronic lymphocytic leukemia (CLL)/small lymphocytic leukemia (SLL).

There are significant class-effect safety concerns with the use of PI3K inhibitors including *severe and fatal hepatotoxicity, severe diarrhea and colitis, pneumonitis, and intestinal perforations as well as drug reaction with eosinophilia and systemic symptoms (DRESS) and toxic epidermal necrolysis (TEN).*

Copanlisib retains its usage for relapsed follicular lymphoma after two lines of therapy and is associated with hypertension and hyperglycemia. As copanlisib targets different isoforms of PI3K, it is suggested to have a lower association with severe hepatotoxicity, colitis, and pneumonitis compared to other PI3K inhibitors.

Alpelisib (PI3K-α inhibitor) is approved by the FDA for use in combination with endocrine therapy fulvestrant for treatment of HR^+ (hormone receptor positive) and $HER2/neu^-$ breast cancer.

mTOR Inhibitors

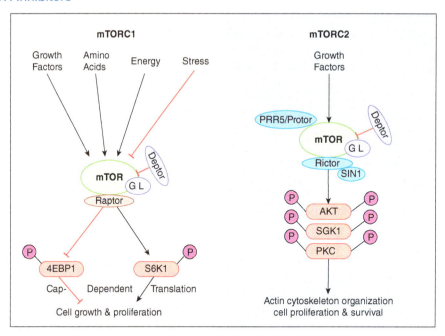

FIGURE 12.15 mTORC1 and mTORC2 structures and functions.
The mTOR comprises two protein complexes called the mammalian target of rapamycin complex 1 (mTORC1) and mTORC2. mTORC1 consists of mTOR, raptor, GβL and deptor. mTORC2 consists of mTOR, rictor, GβL, PRR5, deptor, and SIN1. mTORC1 incorporates signals from growth factors, nutrients, and energy supply to stimulate cell growth when energy is sufficient and mainly regulates cell growth and metabolism. mTORC2 mainly controls cell proliferation and survival.

Clinically available mTOR inhibitors include

- Sirolimus: for prophylaxis of organ rejection in patients ≥13 years old receiving renal transplant and for treatment of patients with lymphangioleiomyomatosis
- Temsirolimus: for treatment of advanced renal cell carcinoma (RCC)
- Everolimus: for treatment of
  ○ Postmenopausal HR⁺, HER2⁻ breast cancer in combination with exemestane after failure of an aromatase inhibitor
  ○ Progressive PNET and progressive, well-differentiated, nonfunctional NET of GI or lung origin (unresectable, locally advanced, or metastatic)
  ○ Advanced RCC after failure of sunitinib or sorafenib
  ○ Renal angiomyolipoma and tuberous sclerosis complex (TSC), not requiring immediate surgery
  ○ Pediatric and adult patients with TSC who have subependymal giant cell astrocytoma (SEGA) that requires therapeutic intervention but cannot be curatively resected

Lipid panel should be monitored closely during treatment with everolimus.

GI, gastrointestinal; HER2, human epidermal growth factor receptor-2; HR⁺, hormone receptor positive; PKC, protein kinase C; PNET, pancreatic neuroendocrine tumor; PRR5, proline-rich protein 5; SGK1, serum- and glucocorticoid-induced protein kinase 1.

JANUS KINASE/SIGNAL TRANSDUCER AND ACTIVATOR OF TRANSCRIPTION

The Janus kinase (JAK)/signal transducer and activator of transcription (STAT) signal transduction pathway is a complex network of receptors and proteins involving four different JAK proteins and seven different STAT proteins. Its native function is involved in the immune response to viral infections.

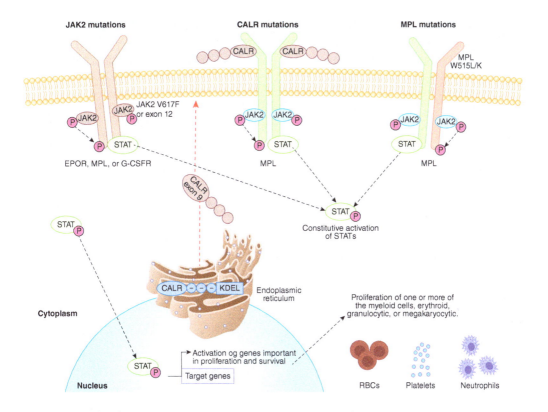

FIGURE 12.16 JAK/STAT pathway.
Binding of ligands (e.g., erythropoietin) to JAK receptors leads to receptor dimerization, phosphorylation, and STAT dissociation. Activated STAT proteins heterodimerize or homodimerize and translocate from the cytosol to the cell nucleus and affect transcription. The JAK-STAT pathway is involved in development, immunity, and cell death. Mutations in this pathway are found in a number of cancers, such as leukemia, lymphoma, breast cancer, prostate cancer, and melanoma.

EPOR, erythropoietin receptor; G-CSFR, granulocyte colony-stimulating factor receptor; JAK, Janus kinase; RBCs, red blood cells; STAT, signal transducer and activator of transcription.

The single nucleotide JAK2-V617F mutation is found in the majority of patients with polycythemia vera (PV) and leads to erythropoietin-independent red blood cell production. The small molecular inhibitor ruxolitinib inhibits JAK1 and JAK2 and is used for the treatment of myeloproliferative neoplasms (MPNs), such as PV and primary myelofibrosis regardless of the presence of a JAK2 mutation and for the treatment of steroid refractory graft-versus-host disease. Abrupt discontinuation of ruxolitinib may lead to a rapid rebound of symptoms and the development of ruxolitinib withdrawal syndrome, and as such, ruxolitinib should be tapered rather than abruptly stopped.

Fedratinib is a selective JAK2 inhibitor that is currently used in the treatment of high-risk myelofibrosis. Development of Wernicke encephalopathy with the usage of fedratinib was reported; hence, thiamine levels should be monitored.

Pacritinib is another selective JAK2 inhibitor for the treatment of myelofibrosis that can be used for patients with platelet count <50,000/μL. Usage of pacritinib has been associated with increased rates of bleeding, cardiovascular events, thrombosis, secondary malignancies, and increased risk of infections.

Other JAK inhibitors (tofacitinib, baricitinib, and upadacitinib) are approved for the treatment of rheumatoid arthritis.

EPIDERMAL GROWTH FACTOR RECEPTOR AND HUMAN EPIDERMAL GROWTH FACTOR RECEPTOR

There are four members of the ErbB or human epidermal growth factor receptor (HER) family of receptors. All members have tyrosine kinase domains (TKDs) on the cytoplasmic side of the cell membrane. Binding of the ligands to HER induces homodimerization or heterodimierzation of the receptors. Dimerization results in phosphorylation of the TKDs and induces several intracellular signaling cascades. This leads to cellular survival, proliferation, and angiogenesis. Epidermal growth factor receptor (EGFR) is also known as ErbB1 or Her1. EGFR mutations negate the need for ligand binding and lead to autophosphorylation of TKDs.

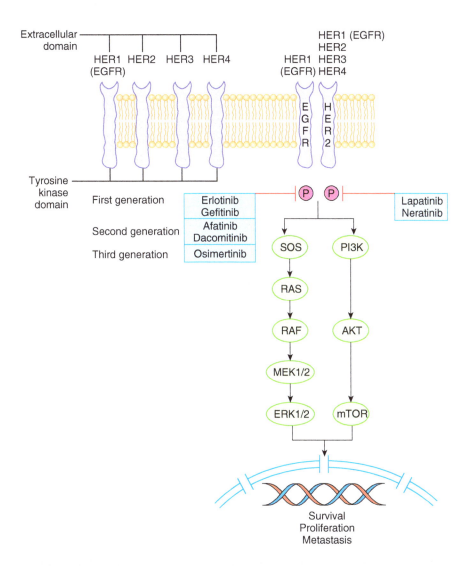

FIGURE 12.17 **EGFR and HER and their inhibitors.**

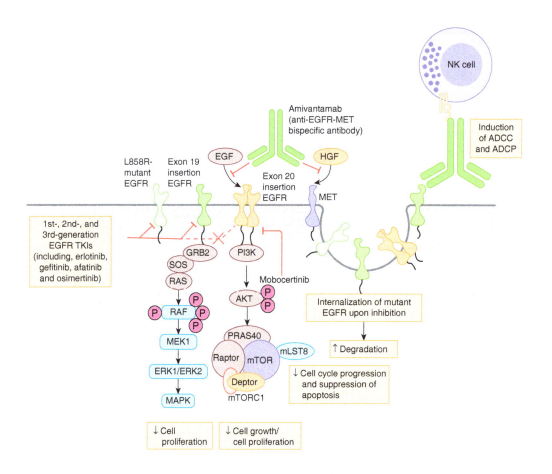

FIGURE 12.18 EGFR signaling and mutations.
EGFR was first found to be overexpressed in lung cancer and EGFR inhibitors were developed to target this abnormality. During clinical development, EGFR mutations were serendipitously found in a group of patients who were non-smokers and who had an extraordinary response to EGFR inhibition. This led to the characterization of EGFR mutations (most commonly resulting in exon 19 deletions and exon 21 L858R).

ADCC, antibody-dependent cellular cytotoxicity; ADCP, antibody-dependent cellular phagocytosis; EGF, epidermal growth factor; EGFR, epidermal growth factor receptor; ERK, extracellular signal-regulated kinase; GRB2, growth factor receptor binding protein 2; HGF, hepatocyte growth factor; MAPK, mitogen-activated protein kinase; MEK, mitogen-activated extracellular signal-regulated kinase; MET, mesenchymal epithelial transition; MLST8, mammalian lethal with SEC13 protein 8; mTOR, mammalian target of rapamycin; NK, natural killer; PI3K, phosphatidylinositol 3-kinase; PRAS40, proline-rich Akt substrate of 40 kD; RAF, rapidly accelerated fibrosarcoma; RAS, rat sarcoma virus; SOS, son of sevenless; TKI, tyrosine kinase inhibitor.

The first-generation reversible EGFR tyrosine kinase inhibitor (TKI), erlotinib, was found to significantly prolong progression-free survival (PFS) compared to platinum doublet chemotherapy in lung cancer. Data from 13 Phase 3 clinical trials of patients treaed with EGFR TKI or platinum-based chemotherapy were described in a meta-analysis from 2,620 patients (1,475 with and 1,114 without EGFR mutation). In patients with EGFR mutation, EGFR TKI was associated with a significantly decreased risk of disease progression in the front-line or subsequent treatments. Erlotinib can also be used in combination with gemcitabine in locally advanced or metastatic pancreatic cancer.

Subsequent development of EGFR inhibitors focused on increasing the binding affinity to mutant EGFR while limiting affinity to wild-type EGFR, which inhibition is thought to be the primary mechanism for EGFR inhibitor-related toxicity. Afatinib, a second-generation irreversible inhibitor was developed to overcome EGFR mutations but was not found to inhibit the most common acquired mutation that mediated resistance to first-generation EGFR mutations (T790M) at clinically relevant doses.

Osimertinib is a third-generation EGFR TKI that was specifically designed to overcome the most common acquired resistance mechanisms, T790M. In advanced EGFR-mutated non-small cell lung cancer (NSCLC), osimertinib demonstrated improved PFS when compared to the first-generation EGFR-TKI therapy (erlotinib or gefitinib) in the first-line setting. Osimertinib was shown to have improved intracranial penetration when compared to earlier generation TKIs and is now used in the first-line setting for metastatic NSCLC with EGFR mutation with intracranial metastasis and as adjuvant therapy after surgical resection of EGFR positive NSCLC with an exon 19 deletion or exon 21 L858R.

Uncommon mutations other than exon 19 deletions and exon 21 L858R mutations are less studied, and treatment is based on smaller studies with afatinib commonly used in this setting. Exon 20 mutations are particularly difficult to treat with traditional EGFR inhibitors as this leads to an inward folding of the EGFR ATP binding pocket and binding is more difficult. Amivantamab-vmjw, which is a bispecific antibody against EGFR and MET as well as mobocertinib, was designed and has been FDA approved for the treatment of exon 20 mutations.

Mobocertinib has a black box warning for development of QTc prolongation and the development of torsades de pointes and may cause cardiac dysfunction.

Afatinib

Afatinib is indicated for first-line treatment of patients with metastatic NSCLC whose tumors have nonresistant (deletion in exon 19 or point mutation in exon 21 [L858R]) and resistant (a second mutation in exon 20 of EGFR [T790M]) EGFR mutations and treatment of patients with metastatic, squamous NSCLC progressing after platinum-based chemotherapy.

Afatinib is another type VI (covalent-binding via nucleophilic attack of sulfur in cysteine to α/β unsaturated ketone [blue circle]) protein kinase inhibitor.

Resistance to the irreversible type VI inhibitor often involves mutation of a cysteine residue where the inhibitor binding occurs.

EGFR, epidermal growth factor receptor; NSCLC, non-small cell lung cancer.

Increased rates of pneumonitis have been found when EGFR inhibitors are used in combination with immune checkpoint inhibitors.

The usage of EGFR inhibitors has been associated with diarrhea, interstitial lung disease, cardiovascular events, keratitis, and bullous skin disorders.

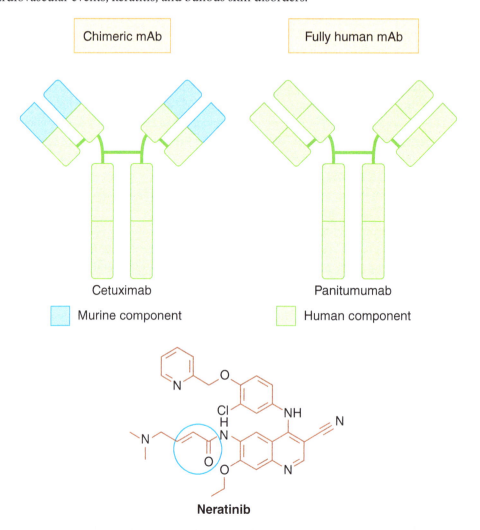

Neratinib

Neratinib is indicated for the extended adjuvant treatment of adult patients with early stage HER2-overexpressed/amplified breast cancer, to follow adjuvant trastuzumab-based therapy. Neratinib has been associated with severe diarrhea. Antidiarrheal prophylaxis with loperamide must be started with the first dose of neratinib and continue during first two cycles (56 days) of treatment.

Neratinib is another type VI (covalent-binding via nucleophilic attack of sulfur in cysteine to α/β unsaturated ketone [blue circle]) protein kinase inhibitors.

Resistance to the irreversible type VI inhibitors often involves mutation of a cysteine residue where the inhibitor binding occurs.

mAb, monoclonal antibody.

Panitumumab and cetuximab are monoclonal antibodies that target wild-type EGFR and are approved in the treatment of colon cancers in patients without a KRAS mutation (KRAS wild-type) and cetuximab is approved in the treatment of squamous cell carcinoma of the head and neck. Both panitumumab and cetuximab have a black box warning for severe infusion reactions. Panitumumab can also cause severe dermatologic toxicities and cetuximab can increase risk of cardiopulmonary arrest and requires optimization of electrolytes.

Lapatinib and neratinib are dual EGFR and HER2 TKIs approved for use in HER2-overexpressed breast cancer. Lapatinib has been associated with severe hepatotoxicity, reduction in ejection fraction, and interstitial lung disease.

ANAPLASTIC LYMPHOMA KINASE

The anaplastic lymphoma kinase (ALK) gene was first identified when it was found to be fused to the nucleophosmin 1 gene (NPM1) in the setting of anaplastic large cell lymphoma. The ALK gene, which is located on chromosome 2, is prone to oncogenesis by forming fusions with several genes.

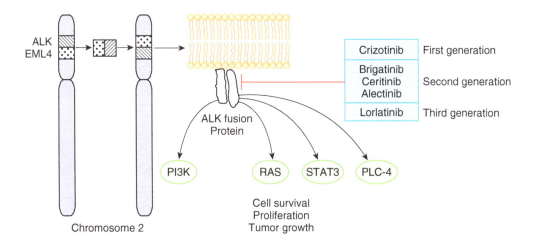

FIGURE 12.19 ALK fusion and alk inhibitors.
The numerous gene fusion partners associated with the ALK gene differ based on the cancer type. Currently, the clinical usage of ALK inhibitors is limited to non-small cell lung cancer (NSCLC) and anaplastic large cell lymphoma in pediatric patients and young adults.

In NSCLC, ALK forms a fusion protein with EML4 and this results in constitutive activation of tyrosine kinase. This fusion protein serves as a driver mutation in 3% to 5% of cases of NSCLC, the overwhelming majority of which are adenocarcinomas.

ALK, anaplastic lymphoma kinase; EML4, echinoderm microtubule-associated protein-like 4; PI3K, phosphatidylinositol 3-kinase; PLC, phospholipase C; RAS, rat sarcoma virus; STAT, signal transducer and activator of transcription.

Crizotinib is a first-generation ALK inhibitor, and it was demonstrated to be superior to chemotherapy. Second-generation ALK inhibitors were designed to increase the potency against ALK resistance mutations and to increase central nervous system (CNS) penetration. Ceritinib was found to be superior to platinum chemotherapy but has not been compared head to head with crizotinib. Other second-generation ALK inhibitors, brigotinib and alectinib, have been compared head to head with crizotinib in the front-line setting and have shown increased PFS. The third-generation ALK inhibitor, lorlatinib, was developed to overcome the ALK G1202R mutation that is not inhibited by the second-generation ALK inhibitors and to increase CNS penetration. While lorlatinib was found to increase PFS compared to crizotinib, it was also found to significantly induce hypercholesterolemia, hypertriglyceridemia, and neurocognitive effects. ALK inhibitors are associated with hepatotoxicity/GI toxicity, interstitial lung disease, and visual disturbances.

ROS1 is a structurally similar proto-oncogene to ALK and ROS1 rearrangements have been found in 1% to 2% of NSCLC cases. Given the structural similarity to ALK, the ALK inhibitor crizotinib has been approved for the treatment of ROS1 rearrangement lung cancer. Entrectinib is a specific inhibitor against ROS1 and neurotrophic tyrosine receptor kinase (NTRK) that has an accelerated approved in both ROS1 rearranged NSCLC and in solid tumors that harbor a NTRK gene fusion. Unlike entrectinib, larotrectinib is only specific for NTRK fusion and has an accelerated approval for the treatment of solid tumors that harbor a NTRK fusion. Both entrectinib and larotrectinib are associated with CNS toxicity and hepatotoxicity, but entrectinib is also associated with congestive heart failure, increased risk of fractures, hyperuricemia, and visual disturbances.

MESENCHYMAL EPITHELIAL TRANSITION

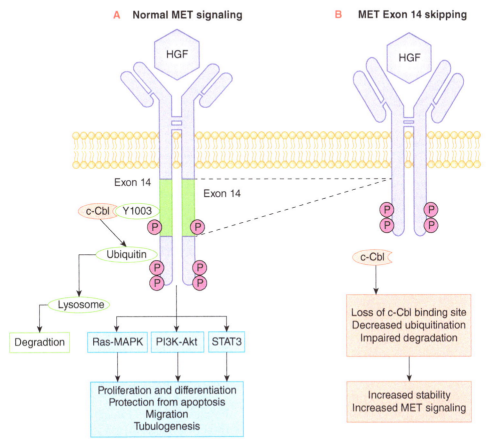

FIGURE 12.20 MET signaling.
The mesenchymal epithelial transition (MET) gene is a proto-oncogene that is a receptor tyrosine kinase that is normally expressed on epithelial cells and is activated by hepatocyte growth factor (HGF). Similar to other receptor tyrosine kinases alterations, alterations of *MET* lead to increased activation of the receptor tyrosine kinase promoting cellular survival and proliferation. *MET* alterations can be classified as either exon 14 skipping mutations or *MET* amplifications. MET exon 14 skipping mutation leads to a shorter variant of the MET protein which is more stable and less susceptible to degradation.

MAPK, mitogen-activated protein kinase; PI3K, phosphatidylinositol 3-kinase; STAT, signal transducer and activator of transcription.

Capmatinib and tepotinib have both received accelerated approvals for the treatment of NSCLC with MET exon 14 skipping mutations. Both capmatinib and tepotinib are associated with interstitial lung disease and hepatotoxicity, while capmatinib is associated with the development of photosensitivity reactions.

Mesenchymal epithelial transition (MET) amplifications can occur due to a gain in the copy number of the MET gene resulting in excessive copies of the MET gene. This is measured as a ratio in reference to centromere 7 (CEN7). While studies are underway for the MET amplified NSCLC, there are no currently FDA-approved treatments for this indication.

VASCULAR ENDOTHELIAL GROWTH FACTOR RECEPTOR

Axitinib, cabozanitinib, lenvatinib, pazopanib, sorafenib, and sunitinib are FDA approved in advanced clear cell renal cell carcinoma treatment.

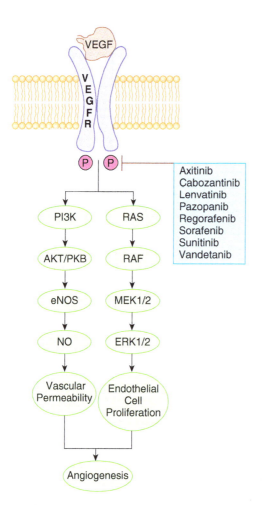

Axitinib
Cabozantinib
Lenvatinib
Pazopanib
Regorafenib
Sorafenib
Sunitinib
Vandetanib

FIGURE 12.21 VEGF and VEGF inhibitors.
Vascular endothelial growth factors (VEGFs) are signaling proteins (or ligands) for VEGF receptors (VEGFRs) and are important for angiogenesis.

Targeting angiogenesis is thought to prevent metastasis and to limit the acquisition of nutrients to the tumor itself. VEGFR dimerization induces intracellular signaling cascades, and VEGFR mutations negate the need for ligand binding to active tyrosine kinase domains.

VEGF receptor mutations are found in several solid tumor malignancies including colon cancer, gastric cancer, kidney cancer, liver cancer, sarcoma, and thyroid cancer. Small molecule VEGF inhibitors are mostly multikinase inhibitors.

Serious adverse effects of these medications include those related to blood vessel regulatory functions, such as hypertension, bleeding, thrombosis, and poor wound healing.

eNOS, endothelial nitric oxide synthase; ERK, extracellular signal-regulated kinase; MEK, mitogen-activated extracellular signal-regulated kinase; NO, nitric oxide; PI3K, phosphatidylinositol 3-kinase; PKB, protein kinase B; RAF, rapidly accelerated fibrosarcoma; RAS, rat sarcoma virus; VEGFR, vascular endothelial growth factor receptor.

REARRANGED DURING TRANSFECTION

The rearranged during transfection gene (RET) is a proto-oncogene receptor tyrosine kinase that is normally a part of normal kidney development and the enteric nervous system. The RET gene was found to be the genetic cause of multiple endocrine neoplasia 2 (MEN2). RET alterations (mutations or rearrangements) are found in both papillary thyroid cancer and medullary thyroid cancer. In NSCLC, RET alterations occur through RET rearrangements and the formation of a fusion protein. Currently, there are two RET inhibitors, selpercatinib and pralsetinib, that are approved both against the RET fusion proteins and RET mutations in RET altered thyroid cancer and RET fusion NSCLC. Both selpercatinib and pralsetinib are associated with hepatotoxicity, hypertension, bleeding, poor wound healing, and QT prolongation. Pralsetinib has an additional risk for interstitial lung disease.

FIBROBLAST GROWTH FACTOR RECEPTOR

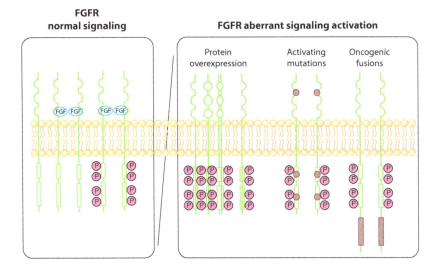

FIGURE 12.22 FGFR aberrant signaling activation.
Fibroblast growth factor receptors (FGFRs) are a family of four (FGFR1–4) receptor tyrosine kinase receptors that are important for embryonic development and play an important role in angiogenesis. FGFR alterations can occur as mutations, gene rearrangements, or amplifications. FGFR2 fusions are found in 10% to 20% of intrahepatic cholangiocarcinoma and results in constitutive FGFR2 signaling.

There are currently three oral FGFR inhibitors, pemigatinib, infigratinib, and futibatinib, which are approved by the FDA for the treatment of relapsed, unresectable locally advanced or metastatic intrahepatic cholangiocarcinoma.

Pemigatinib and infigratinib are FGFR1–3 inhibitors while futibatinib is an irreversible FGFR1–4 inhibitor. Activating mutations and gene rearrangements in FGFR3 have been most frequently found in urothelial cancers. FGFR3 can be targeted by erdafitinib, which has been approved by the FDA for the treatment of urothelial carcinoma with FGFR2 or FGFR3 alterations that has progressed after platinum-containing chemotherapy.

FGFR inhibitors as a class are associated with hyperphosphatemia and can cause ocular toxicity and all require regular ophthalmologic monitoring while on treatment.

MITOGEN-ACTIVATED PROTEIN KINASE PATHWAY

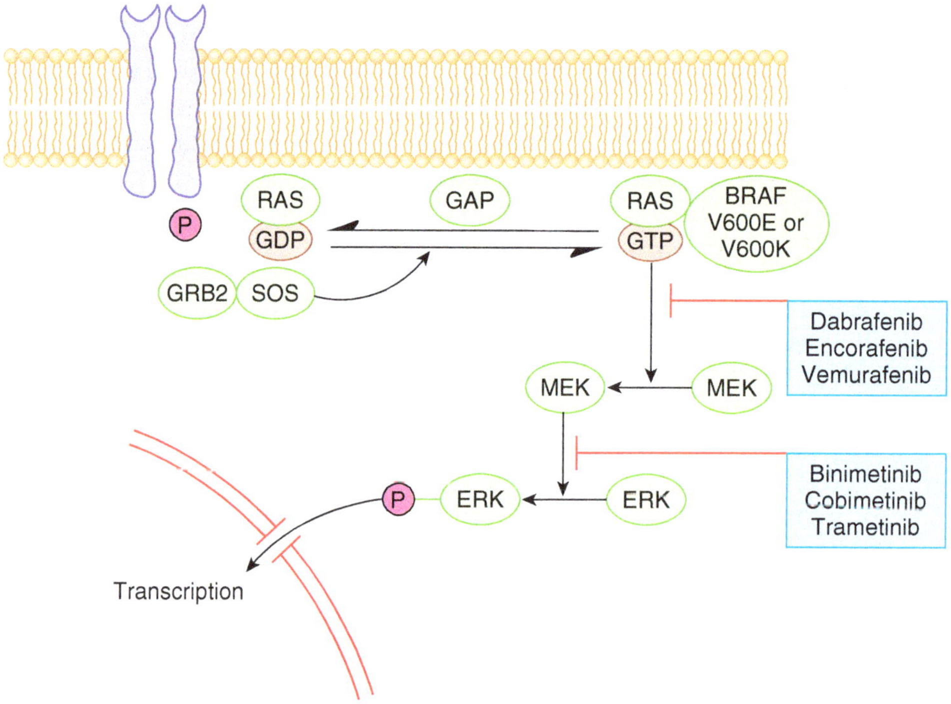

FIGURE 12.23 MAPK/ERK signaling pathway and its inhibitors.

The Ras/Raf/Mek/Erk or mitogen-activated protein kinase (MAPK)/extracellular signal-related kinase (ERK) pathways are complex cell signaling pathways that depend on phosphorylation cascades to regulate transcription.

The common driver mutation BRAF V600E is found in several cancers, such as melanoma, non-small cell lung cancer, thyroid cancer, hairy cell leukemia, Langerhans cell histiocytosis, and ameloblastoma.

GAP, GTPase activating protein; GDP, guanosine diphosphate; GRB2, growth factor receptor binding protein 2; GTP, guanosine triphosphate; MEK, mitogen-activated extracellular signal-regulated kinase; RAS, rat sarcoma virus; SOS, son of sevenless.

BRAF inhibitor monotherapy is associated with acquired resistance, most commonly via reactivation of the MAPK pathway. Combining BRAF and MEK inhibitor therapy allows for more complete inhibition of the MAPK pathway. Currently, there are three combinations of BRAF and MEK inhibitors that are currently FDA approved and widely used: dabrafenib+trametinib, encorafenib+binimetinib, vemurafenib+cobimetinib. All three combinations have been found to improve PFS and overall survival (OS) compared to vemurafenib monotherapy (BRAF inhibitor) among patients with treatment-naïve metastatic V600E- or V600K-mutated melanoma. The usage of BRAF inhibitor encorafenib in BRAF V600E mutated colon cancer has also been approved by the FDA combined with cetuximab in the treatment of progressive metastatic colon cancer.

KIRSTEN RAT SARCOMA VIRUS INHIBITOR

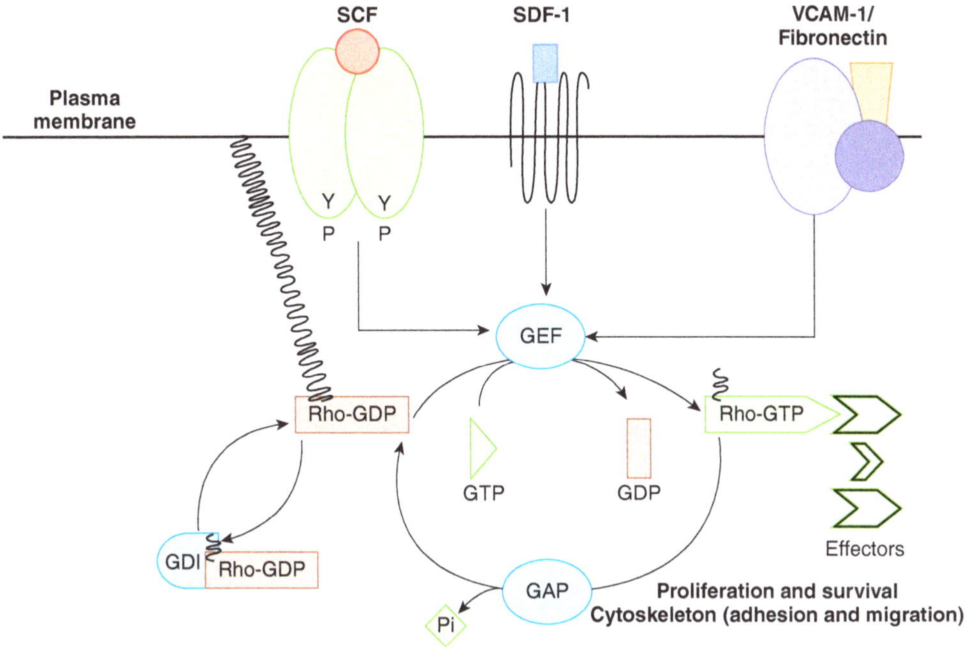

FIGURE 12.24 **The Rho GTPase cycle.**

Most Rho GTPases cycle between an active (GTP-bound) and an inactive (GDP-bound) conformation. In the active state, they interact with one of over 60 target proteins (effectors) and affect many aspects of cell biology. The cycle is highly regulated by three classes of protein: in mammalian cells, around 60 GEFs catalyse nucleotide exchange and mediate activation; more than 70 GAPs stimulate GTP hydrolysis, leading to inactivation; and four GDIs extract the inactive GTPase from membranes. Rho/Rac GTPases integrate signals from multiple surface receptors involved in hematopoietic stem/progenitor cell engraftment and retention. Stromal derived factor-1α (SDF-1α) and its receptor, the G-protein-coupled seven-span transmembrane receptor, CXCR4, play key roles in hematopoietic stem/progenitor cell trafficking and repopulation: after initial phase of tethering and rolling of hematopoietic stem/progenitor cell to the endothelium the second phase of engraftment involves the subsequent interaction of specific hematopoietic stem/progenitor cell surface receptors, such as $\alpha_4\beta_1$-integrin receptors with VCAM-1 and fibronectin in the extracellular matrix, and interactions with growth factors which are soluble or membrane- or matrix-bound; playing an important and independent role in hematopoietic stem/progenitor cell mobilization is the interaction between SCF and its receptor tyrosine kinase, c-kit. SCF/c-kit interaction plays a critical role in G-CSF-mediated mobilization.

GAP, GTPase-activating protein; GDI, guanine nucleotide dissociation inhibitor; GDP, guanosine diphosphate; GEF, guanine nucleotide exchange factor; GTP, guanosine triphosphate; SCF, stem cell factor; VCAM-1, vascular cell adhesion molecule 1.

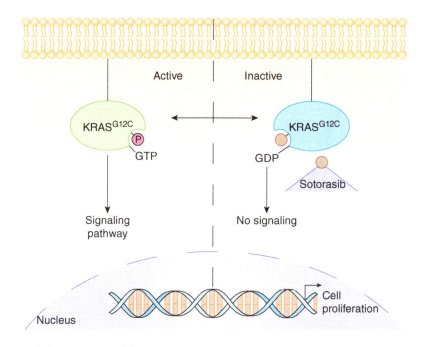

FIGURE 12.25 KRAS activation.
Kirsten rat sarcoma virus (KRAS) is a variant of the RAS family (other members being Harvey rat sarcoma virus [HRAS] and neuroblastoma rat sarcoma virus [NRAS]) of oncogenes that are commonly mutated in many cancers. RAS proteins act downstream of receptor tyrosine kinases and upon signaling from receptor tyrosine kinases, RAS signaling leads to cellular proliferation and survival. KRAS had originally been thought to be undruggable mostly because of its small size, lack of binding pockets, and its usage of guanosine triphosphate (GDP) over adenosine triphosphate (ATP).
  Common KRAS mutations include G12, G13, and Q61.

Note: KRAS p.G12C mutation occurs in approximately 1% to 2% of pancreatic cancers.

Kirsten rat sarcoma virus (KRAS) had not been able to be targeted until the development of sotorasib, which is able to specifically inhibit KRAS G12C where it is able to covalently bind to KRAS G12C and lead to trapping of KRAS in an inactive state. Sotorasib currently has accelerated approval by the FDA after it was studied in NSCLC with a KRAS G12C mutation after patients had received one prior line of therapy and were found to have a response rate of 36%. Sotorasib showed promising efficacy in patients with advanced pancreatic adenocarcinoma who had received a median of two lines (range, 1 to 8) of prior therapy and resulted in ~20% response rate with the median PFS of 4 months and the median OS of was ~7 months. Sotorasib is associated with the development of hepatotoxicity and interstitial lung disease.

CHAPTER SUMMARY

A deep understanding of the molecular pathways described in this chapter provides a foundation for hematologists and medical oncologists to comprehend the currently available armamentarium and clinical applications of commonly used targeted therapies. Newer, more potent drugs are in development and will continue to exploit alterations in these pathways that allow cancer cells to arise, proliferate, and metastasize. Combination therapies with multiple targeted agents are used in certain situations to enhance drug efficacy or overcome acquired resistance mechanisms that allow tumor cells to bypass and surmount the action of targeted therapies. Targeted therapies can be highly effective because these therapies limit damage to noncancerous cells and reduce toxicity, as compared to traditional cytotoxic chemotherapy. As our understanding of molecular changes in tumorigenesis grows and more specific and effective treatments for cancers driven by molecular alterations are developed, the targeted therapy armamentarium will continue to increase in diversity and specificity for tumors driven by molecular derangements.

CLINICAL PEARLS

- BCR-ABL inhibitors in CML and ALL are well tolerated and produce durable responses. Patients with progressive disease after early generation BCR-ABL inhibitor treatment should undergo testing for T315I resistance mutation and can be treated with ponatinib.
- Targetable (or actionable) mutations in AML include FLT3, IDH1, and IDH2 with clinically available inhibitors to be used as monotherapy or in combination both in front-line setting as well as for relapsed or refractory disease.
- Osimertinib is an EGFR TKI with superior intracranial penetration and strongly inhibits the resistant T790M mutation.
- Lorlatinib is the only ALK inhibitor that is able to inhibit G1202R resistance mutation but is associated with the development of hypertension, hypertriglyceridemia, and CNS toxicity.
- FGFR inhibitors are used in locally advanced/metastatic cholangiocarcinoma and urothelial carcinoma and as a class are associated with hyperphosphatemia and ocular toxicity.

MULTIPLE-CHOICE QUESTIONS

1. A 48-year-old woman never smoker presents to her primary care physician with 3 months of a nonproductive cough and associated unintentional weight loss that has not subsided despite adequate antibiotic treatment for community-acquired pneumonia. A CT scan of the chest shows a right lower lobe 4.8 × 3.7 cm spiculated lung mass with associated mediastinal lymphadenopathy. The patient underwent endobronchial biopsy of the mass and mediastinal lymph nodes. Pathology is positive for adenocarcinoma of lung origin. EGFR mutational analysis from the tissue is

positive for exon 19 deletion by next-generation sequencing. Brain MRI shows a single 1.3×1.7 right parietal lobe ring-enhancing lesion consistent with metastatic disease. The patient is without neurologic symptoms. What is the next step in the management?

A. Neurosurgical excision of the brain lesion
B. Stereostatic radiosurgery of the brain lesion
C. Platinum doublet combination
D. Erlotinib
E. Osimertinib

2. A 59-year-old Irish American woman is diagnosed with metastatic cutaneous melanoma. After discussion at a multidisciplinary conference, the patient is deemed not to be a candidate for surgical metastatectomy. The recommendation is for systemic treatment. Molecular analysis of the tumor reveals a BRAF V600E mutation. She is not interested in immunotherapy. Which of the following is the next best step?

A. Interferon α
B. Cisplatin, vinblastine, dacarbazine
C. Dabrafenib plus trametinib
D. Observation

3. A previously healthy 37-year-old man presented with leukocytosis and peripheral blasts. He was diagnosed with AML with normal karyotype. Mutational analysis revealed FLT3-ITD mutation with 32% allelic burden. He underwent 7 + 3 with midostaurin induction therapy. Upon count recovery, a repeat bone marrow biopsy and aspiration showed refractory leukemia and a repeat mutational analysis confirmed persistent FLT3-ITD mutation. How would you treat him?

A. Reinduction with 7 + 3 chemotherapy
B. Midostaurin single agent
C. Allogeneic stem cell transplantation
D. Gilteritinib

4. A 78-year-old woman with excellent performance status and history of low-risk myelodysplastic syndrome presented with worsening shortness of breath, petechiae, and fatigue. Blood count showed anemia, thrombocytopenia, and peripheral blasts. The patient refused a bone marrow biopsy citing pain and fear of needles. A peripheral blood mutational analysis showed an IDH2 mutation and a normal karyotype. The patient received six cycles of decitabine without improvement in blood counts and with persistence of peripheral blasts. What is the best next step?

A. 7 + 3 induction chemotherapy
B. Hospice referral
C. Enasidenib
D. Supportive care

5. A 73-year-old man has been on active surveillance for CLL for the past 5 years. He presents for routine follow-up and reports increasing fatigue, pallor, and lymph node swelling. Physical examination reveals increased splenomegaly. Laboratory values show a white blood cell count of 150,000/µL (84,000/µL 3 months ago), hemoglobin is 10.5 g/dL, and platelets are 75,000/µL. Previously, lymph node biopsy revealed del(17p)/TP53. What is the next best step?

    A. Ibrutinib
    B. Bone marrow aspiration and biopsy
    C. Bendamustine and rituximab (BR)
    D. Fludarabine, cyclophosphamide, and rituximab (FCR)

6. A 56-year-old woman with a 60 pack-year smoking history after having a seizure is diagnosed with metastatic adenocarcinoma of the lung. She was found to have a PD-L1 of 30% and next-generation sequencing revealed a KRAS G12C mutation. She undergoes whole brain radiation due the presence of brain metastases and is treated with carboplatin, pemetrexed, and pembrolizumab but she is found to have progressive disease. She mentions that she is tired of intravenous infusions and would like an oral option. What is the next best step?

    A. Pembrolizumab and ipilimumab
    B. Docetaxel
    C. Sotorasib
    D. Osimertinib

7. A 67-year-old woman has been recently diagnosed with primary myelofibrosis. Mutational testing found that she was negative for a JAK2 V617F and MPL mutation, but she was found to have a type 2 CALR mutation. She is in the office complaining of worsening abdominal pain, fatigue, and intermittent pruritus. Her lab tests show a white blood cell count of 3,000/µL (absolute neutrophil count [ANC] 1,200/µL), hemoglobin 10.1 g/dL, and platelet count 75,000/µL. Physical exam is notable for splenomegaly 14 cm below the costal margin. What is the next best step in management?

    A. Hydroxyurea
    B. Ruxolitinib
    C. 7 + 3 therapy
    D. Eltrombopag

8. A 52-year-old man with diabetes is recently diagnosed with metastatic urothelial carcinoma of the bladder. He receives cisplatin and gemcitabine initially but is found to have progressive disease. In the second-line setting he receives pembrolizumab, which he responds to for 6 months, but he again has progressive disease. He is started on erdafitinib but he develops difficulty with vision and is diagnosed with central serous chorioretinopathy. What is the most likely cause of this?

    A. Erdafitinib
    B. Diabetes
    C. Accidental eye trauma
    D. Pembrolizumab

9. A 59-year-old man with past medical history significant for hypertension, hyperlipidemia, hypothyroidism, and asthma is scheduled to start everolimus for his stage IV pancreatic neuroendocrine tumor (PNET) with several liver metastases. His disease has progressed after 15 months of treatment with monthly Sandostatin that controlled his disease prior to progression. Which of the following tests will need to be monitored most closely during treatment with everolimus?

   A. Urine protein-to-creatinine ratio
   B. Lipid panel
   C. Thyroid-stimulating hormone (TSH) and free thyronine (T4)
   D. Coronary artery calcium score

ANSWERS TO MULTIPLE-CHOICE QUESTIONS

1. **E.** Osimertinib is approved for the first-line treatment of patients with metastatic NSCLC whose tumors have EGFR exon 19 deletions or exon 21 L858R mutations, as detected by an FDA-approved test. The efficacy of osimertinib was demonstrated in a randomized, multicenter, double-blind, active controlled trial (FLAURA [NCT02296125]). Patients with central nervous system (CNS) metastases not requiring steroids and with stable neurologic status for at least 2 weeks after completion of definitive surgery or radiotherapy were eligible. Of these 200 patients, 41 had measurable CNS lesions according to RECIST guidelines v1.1. CNS overall response rate in osimertinib arm ($n = 22$) was 77% (95% CI 55, 92) with 18% complete response compared with 63% in gefitinib or erlotinib arm (95% CI 38, 84) with 0% complete response.

2. **C.** Dabrafenib, in combination with trametinib, is indicated for (1) the treatment of patients with unresectable melanoma with BRAF V600E or V600K mutations, (2) the adjuvant treatment of patients with melanoma with BRAF V600E or V600K mutations and involvement of lymph node(s) following complete resection, (3) the treatment of patients with metastatic NSCLC with BRAF V600E mutation, (4) the treatment of patients with locally advanced or metastatic anaplastic thyroid cancer with BRAF V600E mutation and with no satisfactory locoregional treatment options. The presence of mutations should be detected by an FDA-approved test.

3. **D.** Single-agent oral gilteritinib improved response and survival compared with parenteral salvage chemotherapy in patients with FLT3 mutant-positive relapsed or refractory (R/R) AML. Compared with salvage chemotherapy, gilteritinib was generally associated with lower toxicity during the first 30 days of treatment, which facilitated outpatient administration of the drug. Gilteritinib allowed many patients ($n = 63$) to undergo hematopoietic stem cell transplantation (HSCT). The relative contribution of HSCT to the observed survival benefit from gilteritinib appears small. Results from the ADMIRAL study had practice-changing implications that established a new treatment paradigm for FLT3 mutant R/R AML.

4. **C.** Enasidenib is an IDH2 inhibitor indicated by the treatment of adult patients with R/R AML with an IDH2 mutation as detected by an FDA-approved test. The efficacy

of enasidenib was evaluated in an open-label, single-arm, multicenter clinical trial (NCT01915498) of 199 adult patients with R/R AML and an IDH2 mutation who were assigned to receive 100 mg daily dose. The complete remission (CR) rate was 19%. The complete remission with partial hematologic recovery (CRh), defined as less than 5% of blasts in the bone marrow, no evidence of disease, and partial recovery of peripheral blood counts (platelets ≥50,000/μL and ANC ≥500/μL), was 4%. The median duration of CR+CRh was 8.2 months.

5. **A.** Ibrutinib is approved for the treatment of adult patients with (a) CLL/SLL, (b) CLL/SLL with 17p deletion, (c) Waldenström macroglobulinemia, (d) marginal zone lymphoma (MZL) who require systemic therapy and have received at least one prior anti-CD20-based therapy, (e) mantle cell lymphoma (MCL) who have received at least one prior therapy, and (f) chronic graft-versus-host disease (cGVHD) after failure of one or more lines of systemic therapy.

6. **C.** Sotorasib currently has accelerated approval in patients with NSCLC with a KRAS G12C mutation that has progressed after platinum-based therapy. Sotorasib was studied in the Phase 2 study of 126 patients with an overall response rate of 36% and a median duration of response of 11.1 months.

7. **B.** Ruxolitinib is a JAK1/JAK2 inhibitor and is used in the treatment of myeloproliferative neoplasms (MPNs). There is no requirement for patients to harbor a JAK2 V617F mutation as MPNs are characterized by increased JAK signaling. Ruxolitinib is able to improve splenomegaly and reduce constitutional symptoms and was the first oncologic drug approved based on quality of life metrics.

8. **A.** Erdafitinib is a FGFR1–4 inhibitor and is associated with the development of ocular side effects, which occurred in 62% of patients during the Phase 2 trial. While on erdafitinib patients need to have routine ophthalmologic evaluations and monitoring and if the patients develop central serous retinopathy, erdafitinib should be discontinued until resolution or permanently if symptoms are not resolved after 4 weeks.

9. **B.** Everolimus modulates the expression of lipid metabolism enzymes such as lipoprotein lipase (LPL), which hydrolyzes lipoprotein-bound triglyceride and allows uptake and storage of triglycerides. Hence, everolimus can disturb the ability for adipose tissue to clear lipids from plasma. For patients who are going to receive everolimus, lipid levels should be checked at baseline, monitored 4 weeks after commencement, and followed at 6-month intervals thereafter to avoid complications such as pancreatitis.

SELECTED REFERENCES

Abou-Alfa GK, Sahai V, Hollebecque A, et al. Pemigatinib for previously treated, locally advanced or metastatic cholangiocarcinoma: A multicentre, open-label, phase 2 study. Lancet Oncol. 2020;21(5):671–84. https://doi.org/10.1016/S1470-2045(20)30109-1

Amado RG, Wolf M, Peeters M, et al. Wild-type KRAS is required for panitumumab efficacy in patients with metastatic colorectal cancer. J Clin Oncol. 2008;26(10):1626–34. https://doi.org/10.1200/JCO.2007.14.7116

Bahleda R, Meric-Bernstam F, Goyal L, et al. Phase I, first-in-human study of futibatinib, a highly selective, irreversible FGFR1-4 inhibitor in patients with advanced solid tumors. Ann Oncol. 2020;31(10):1405–12. https://doi.org/10.1016/j.annonc.2020.06.018

Baselga J, Bradbury I, Eidtmann H, et al. Lapatinib with trastuzumab for HER2-positive early breast cancer (NeoALTTO): A randomised, open-label, multicentre, phase 3 trial. Lancet. 2012;379(9816):633–40. https://doi.org/10.1016/S0140-6736(11)61847-3

Blackwell KL, Burstein HJ, Storniolo AM, et al. Overall survival benefit with lapatinib in combination with trastuzumab for patients with human epidermal growth factor receptor 2-positive metastatic breast cancer: Final results from the EGF104900 study. J Clin Oncol. 2012;30(21):2585–92. https://doi.org/10.1200/JCO.2011.35.6725

Bonner JA, Harari PM, Giralt J, et al. Radiotherapy plus cetuximab for squamous-cell carcinoma of the head and neck. N Engl J Med. 2006;354(6):567–78. https://doi.org/10.1056/NEJMoa053422

Brown JR, Eichhorst B, Hillmen P, et al. Zanubrutinib or ibrutinib in relapsed or refractory chronic lymphocytic leukemia. N Engl J Med. 2023;388(4):319–32. https://doi.org/10.1056/NEJMoa2211582

Burger JA, Tedeschi A, Barr PM, et al. Ibrutinib as initial therapy for patients with chronic lymphocytic leukemia. N Engl J Med. 2015;373(25):2425–37. https://doi.org/10.1056/NEJMoa1509388

Byrd JC, Hillmen P, Ghia P, et al. Acalabrutinib versus ibrutinib in previously treated chronic lymphocytic leukemia: Results of the first randomized phase III trial. J Clin Oncol. 2021;39(31):3441–52. https://doi.org/10.1200/JCO.21.01210

Camidge DR, Kim HR, Ahn MJ, et al. Brigatinib versus crizotinib in ALK-positive non-small-cell lung cancer. N Engl J Med. 2018;379(21):2027–39. https://doi.org/10.1056/NEJMoa1810171

Cervantes F, Vannucchi AM, Kiladjian JJ, et al. Three-year efficacy, safety, and survival findings from COMFORT-II, a phase 3 study comparing ruxolitinib with best available therapy for myelofibrosis. Blood. 2013;122(25):4047–53. https://doi.org/10.1182/blood-2013-02-485888

Chan A, Delaloge S, Holmes FA, et al. Neratinib after trastuzumab-based adjuvant therapy in patients with HER2-positive breast cancer (ExteNET): A multicentre, randomised, double-blind, placebo-controlled, phase 3 trial. Lancet Oncol. 2016;17(3):367–77. https://doi.org/10.1016/S1470-2045(15)00551-3

Chanan-Khan A, Cramer P, Demirkan F, et al. Ibrutinib combined with bendamustine and rituximab compared with placebo, bendamustine, and rituximab for previously treated chronic lymphocytic leukaemia or small lymphocytic lymphoma (HELIOS): A randomised, double-blind, phase 3 study. Lancet Oncol. 2016;17(2):200–11. https://doi.org/10.1016/S1470-2045(15)00465-9

Chia PL, Mitchell P, Dobrovic A, John T. Prevalence and natural history of ALK positive non-small-cell lung cancer and the clinical impact of targeted therapy with ALK inhibitors. Clin Epidemiol. 2014;6:423–32. https://doi.org/10.2147/CLEP.S69718

Choueiri TK, Escudier B, Powles T, et al. Cabozantinib versus everolimus in advanced renal-Cell carcinoma. N Engl J Med. 2015;373(19):1814–23. https://doi.org/10.1056/NEJMoa1510016

Choueiri TK, Halabi S, Sanford BL, et al. Cabozantinib versus sunitinib as initial targeted therapy for patients with metastatic renal cell carcinoma of poor or intermediate risk: The alliance A031203 CABOSUN trial. J Clin Oncol. 2017;35(6):591–7. https://doi.org/10.1200/JCO.2016.70.7398

Cortes JE, Kim DW, Pinilla-Ibarz J, et al. A phase 2 trial of ponatinib in Philadelphia chromosome-positive leukemias. N Engl J Med. 2013;369(19):1783–96. https://doi.org/10.1056/NEJMoa1306494

Dasmahapatra G, Patel H, Dent P, et al. The Bruton tyrosine kinase (BTK) inhibitor PCI-32765 synergistically increases proteasome inhibitor activity in diffuse large-B cell lymphoma (DLBCL) and mantle cell lymphoma (MCL) cells sensitive or resistant to bortezomib. Br J Haematol. 2013;161(1):43–56. https://doi.org/10.1111/bjh.12206

Dimopoulos MA, Tedeschi A, Trotman J, et al. Phase 3 trial of ibrutinib plus rituximab in Waldenstrom's macroglobulinemia. N Engl J Med. 2018;378(25):2399–410. https://doi.org/10.1056/NEJMoa1802917

DiNardo CD, Stein EM, de Botton S, et al. Durable remissions with ivosidenib in IDH1-mutated relapsed or refractory AML. N Engl J Med. 2018;378(25):2386–98. https://doi.org/10.1056/NEJMoa1716984

Doebele RC, Drilon A, Paz-Ares L, et al. Entrectinib in patients with advanced or metastatic NTRK fusion-positive solid tumours: Integrated analysis of three phase 1–2 trials. Lancet Oncol. 2020;21(2):271–82. https://doi.org/10.1016/S1470-2045(19)30691-6

Douillard JY, Siena S, Cassidy J, et al. Randomized, phase III trial of panitumumab with infusional fluorouracil, leucovorin, and oxaliplatin (FOLFOX4) versus FOLFOX4 alone as first-line treatment in patients with previously untreated metastatic colorectal cancer: The PRIME study. J Clin Oncol. 2010;28(31):4697–705. https://doi.org/10.1200/JCO.2009.27.4860

Dreyling M, Jurczak W, Jerkeman M, et al. Ibrutinib versus temsirolimus in patients with relapsed or refractory mantle-cell lymphoma: An international, randomised, open-label, phase 3 study. Lancet. 2016;387(10020):770–8. https://doi.org/10.1016/S0140-6736(15)00667-4

Dreyling M, Santoro A, Mollica L, et al. Phosphatidylinositol 3-kinase inhibition by copanlisib in relapsed or refractory indolent lymphoma. J Clin Oncol. 2017;35(35):3898–905. https://doi.org/10.1200/JCO.2017.75.4648

Drilon A, Laetsch TW, Kummar S, et al. Efficacy of larotrectinib in TRK fusion-positive cancers in adults and children. N Engl J Med. 2018;378(8):731–9. https://doi.org/10.1056/NEJMoa1714448

Drilon A, Siena S, Dziadziuszko R, et al. Entrectinib in ROS1 fusion-positive non-small-cell lung cancer: Integrated analysis of three phase 1–2 trials. Lancet Oncol. 2020;21(2):261–70. https://doi.org/10.1016/S1470-2045(19)30690-4

Dummer R, Ascierto PA, Gogas HJ, et al. Encorafenib plus binimetinib versus vemurafenib or encorafenib in patients with BRAF-mutant melanoma (COLUMBUS): A multicentre, open-label, randomised phase 3 trial. Lancet Oncol. 2018;19(5):603–15. https://doi.org/10.1016/S1470-2045(18)30142-6

Escudier B, Eisen T, Stadler WM, et al. Sorafenib in advanced clear-cell renal-cell carcinoma. N Engl J Med. 2007;356(2):125–34. https://doi.org/10.1056/NEJMoa060655

Flinn IW, Hillmen P, Montillo M, et al. The phase 3 DUO trial: Duvelisib vs ofatumumab in relapsed and refractory CLL/SLL. Blood. 2018;132(23):2446–55. https://doi.org/10.1182/blood-2018-05-850461

Furman RR, Sharman JP, Coutre SE, et al. Idelalisib and rituximab in relapsed chronic lymphocytic leukemia. N Engl J Med. 2014;370(11):997–1007. https://doi.org/10.1056/NEJMoa1315226

Gainor JF, Curigliano G, Kim DW, et al. Pralsetinib for RET fusion-positive non-small-cell lung cancer (ARROW): A multi-cohort, open-label, phase 1/2 study. Lancet Oncol. 2021;22(7):959–69. https://doi.org/10.1016/S1470-2045(21)00247-3

Heissig B, Hattori K, Dias S, et al. Recruitment of stem and progenitor cells from the bone marrow niche requires MMP-9 mediated release of kit-ligand. Cell. 2002;109(5):625–37. https://doi.org/10.1016/s0092-8674(02)00754-7

Hoelzer D. Advances in the management of Ph-positive ALL. Clin Adv Hematol Oncol. 2006;4(11):804–5.

Jagasia M, Perales MA, Schroeder MA, et al. Ruxolitinib for the treatment of steroid-refractory acute GVHD (REACH1): A multicenter, open-label phase 2 trial. Blood. 2020;135(20):1739–49. https://doi.org/10.1182/blood.2020004823

James C, Ugo V, Le Couédic JP, et al. A unique clonal JAK2 mutation leading to constitutive signalling causes polycythaemia vera. Nature. 2005;434(7037):1144–8. https://doi.org/10.1038/nature03546

Javle M, Roychowdhury S, Kelley RK, et al. Infigratinib (BGJ398) in previously treated patients with advanced or metastatic cholangiocarcinoma with FGFR2 fusions or rearrangements: Mature results from a multicentre, open-label, single-arm, phase 2 study. Lancet Gastroenterol Hepatol. 2021;6(10):803–15. https://doi.org/10.1016/S2468-1253(21)00196-5

Kantarjian H, Shah NP, Hochhaus A, et al. Dasatinib versus imatinib in newly diagnosed chronic-phase chronic myeloid leukemia. N Engl J Med. 2010;362(24):2260–70. https://doi.org/10.1056/NEJMoa1002315

Kopetz S, Grothey A, Yaeger R, et al. Encorafenib, binimetinib, and cetuximab in BRAF V600E-mutated colorectal cancer. N Engl J Med. 2019;381(17):1632–43. https://doi.org/10.1056/NEJMoa1908075

Lapidot T, Kollet O. The essential roles of the chemokine SDF-1 and its receptor CXCR4 in human stem cell homing and repopulation of transplanted immune-deficient NOD/SCID and NOD/SCID/B2m(null) mice. Leukemia. 2002;16(10):1992–2003. https://doi.org/10.1038/sj.leu.2402684

Larkin J, Ascierto PA, Dréno B, et al. Combined vemurafenib and cobimetinib in BRAF-mutated melanoma. N Engl J Med. 2014;371(20):1867–76. https://doi.org/10.1056/NEJMoa1408868

Lee CK, Davies L, Wu YL, et al. Gefitinib or erlotinib vs chemotherapy for EGFR mutation-positive lung cancer: Individual patient data meta-analysis of overall survival. J Natl Cancer Inst. 2017;109(6). https://doi.org/10.1093/jnci/djw279

Lévesque JP, Hendy J, Winkler IG, et al. Granulocyte colony-stimulating factor induces the release in the bone marrow of proteases that cleave c-KIT receptor (CD117) from the surface of hematopoietic progenitor cells. Exp Hematol. 2003;31(2):109–17. https://doi.org/10.1016/s0301-472x(02)01028-7

Loriot Y, Necchi A, Park SH, et al. Erdafitinib in locally advanced or metastatic urothelial carcinoma. N Engl J Med. 2019;381(4):338–48. https://doi.org/10.1056/NEJMoa1817323

Lynch TJ, Bell DW, Sordella R, et al. Activating mutations in the epidermal growth factor receptor underlying responsiveness of non-small-cell lung cancer to gefitinib. N Engl J Med. 2004;350(21):2129–39. https://doi.org/10.1056/NEJMoa040938

Manning G, Whyte DB, Martinez R, et al. The protein kinase complement of the human genome. Science. 2002;298(5600):1912–34. https://doi.org/10.1126/science.1075762

Mascarenhas J, Hoffman R, Talpaz M, et al. Pacritinib vs best available therapy, including ruxolitinib, in patients with myelofibrosis: A randomized clinical trial. JAMA Oncol. 2018;4(5):652–9. https://doi.org/10.1001/jamaoncol.2017.5818

Montesinos P, Recher C, Vives S, et al. Ivosidenib and azacitidine in IDH1-mutated acute myeloid leukemia. N Engl J Med. 2022;386(16):1519–31. https://doi.org/10.1056/NEJMoa2117344

Moore MJ, Goldstein D, Hamm J, et al. Erlotinib plus gemcitabine compared with gemcitabine alone in patients with advanced pancreatic cancer: A phase III trial of the National Cancer Institute of Canada Clinical Trials Group. J Clin Oncol. 2007;25(15):1960–6. https://doi.org/10.1200/JCO.2006.07.9525

Motzer R, Alekseev B, Rha SY, et al. Lenvatinib plus pembrolizumab or everolimus for advanced renal cell carcinoma. N Engl J Med. 2021;384(14):1289–300. https://doi.org/10.1056/NEJMoa2035716

Motzer RJ, McCann L, Deen K. Pazopanib versus sunitinib in renal cancer. N Engl J Med. 2013;369(20):1970. https://doi.org/10.1056/NEJMc1311795

Motzer RJ, Rini BI, Bukowski RM, et al. Sunitinib in patients with metastatic renal cell carcinoma. JAMA. 2006;295(21):2516–24. https://doi.org/10.1001/jama.295.21.2516

Nowell P, Hungerford DA. A minute chromosome in human chronic granulocytic leukemia. Science. 1960;132:1497.

Noy A, de Vos S, Thieblemont C, et al. Targeting Bruton tyrosine kinase with ibrutinib in relapsed/refractory marginal zone lymphoma. Blood. 2017;129(16):2224–32. https://doi.org/10.1182/blood-2016-10-747345

O'Brien SG, Guilhot F, Larson RA, et al. Imatinib compared with interferon and low-dose cytarabine for newly diagnosed chronic-phase chronic myeloid leukemia. N Engl J Med. 2003;348(11):994–1004. https://doi.org/10.1056/NEJMoa022457

Paik PK, Felip E, Veillon R, et al. Tepotinib in non-small-cell lung cancer with MET exon 14 skipping mutations. N Engl J Med. 2020;383(10):931–43. https://doi.org/10.1056/NEJMoa2004407

Pardanani A, Harrison C, Cortes JE, et al. Safety and efficacy of fedratinib in patients with primary or secondary myelofibrosis: A randomized clinical trial. JAMA Oncol. 2015;1(5):643–51. https://doi.org/10.1001/jamaoncol.2015.1590

Park K, Haura EB, Leighl NB, et al. Amivantamab in EGFR exon 20 insertion-mutated non-small-cell lung cancer progressing on platinum chemotherapy: Initial results from the CHRYSALIS phase I study. J Clin Oncol. 2021;39(30):3391–402. https://doi.org/10.1200/JCO.21.00662

Perl AE, Martinelli G, Cortes JE, et al. Gilteritinib or chemotherapy for relapsed or refractory FLT3-mutated AML. N Engl J Med. 2019;381(18):1728–40. https://doi.org/10.1056/NEJMoa1902688

Peters S, Camidge DR, Shaw AT, et al. Alectinib versus crizotinib in untreated ALK-positive non-small-cell lung cancer. N Engl J Med. 2017;377(9):829–38. https://doi.org/10.1056/NEJMoa1704795

Réa D, Mauro MJ, Boquimpani C, et al. A phase 3, open-label, randomized study of asciminib, a STAMP inhibitor, vs bosutinib in CML after 2 or more prior TKIs. Blood. 2021;138(21):2031–41. https://doi.org/10.1182/blood.2020009984

Reungwetwattana T, Nakagawa K, Cho BC, et al. CNS response to osimertinib versus standard epidermal growth factor receptor tyrosine kinase inhibitors in patients with untreated EGFR-mutated advanced non-small-cell lung cancer. J Clin Oncol. 2018;36(33):3290–7. https://doi.org/10.1200/JCO.2018.78.3118

Rini BI, Escudier B, Tomczak P, et al. Comparative effectiveness of axitinib versus sorafenib in advanced renal cell carcinoma (AXIS): A randomised phase 3 trial. Lancet. 2011;378(9807):1931–9. https://doi.org/10.1016/S0140-6736(11)61613-9

Rini BI, Wilding G, Hudes G, et al. Phase II study of axitinib in sorafenib-refractory metastatic renal cell carcinoma. J Clin Oncol. 2009;27(27):4462–8. https://doi.org/10.1200/JCO.2008.21.7034

Robert C, Karaszewska B, Schachter J, et al. Improved overall survival in melanoma with combined dabrafenib and trametinib. N Engl J Med. 2015;372(1):30–9. https://doi.org/10.1056/NEJMoa1412690

Saglio G, Kim DW, Issaragrisil S, et al. Nilotinib versus imatinib for newly diagnosed chronic myeloid leukemia. N Engl J Med. 2010;362(24):2251–9. https://doi.org/10.1056/NEJMoa0912614

Shaw AT, Bauer TM, de Marinis F, et al. First-line lorlatinib or crizotinib in advanced ALK-positive lung cancer. N Engl J Med. 2020;383(21):2018–29. https://doi.org/10.1056/NEJMoa2027187

Shaw AT, Ou SH, Bang YJ, et al. Crizotinib in ROS1-rearranged non-small-cell lung cancer. N Engl J Med. 2014;371(21):1963–71. https://doi.org/10.1056/NEJMoa1406766

Skoulidis F, Li BT, Dy GK, et al. Sotorasib for lung cancers with KRAS p.G12C mutation. N Engl J Med. 2021;384(25):2371–81. https://doi.org/10.1056/NEJMoa2103695

Solomon BJ, Mok T, Kim DW, et al. First-line crizotinib versus chemotherapy in ALK-positive lung cancer. N Engl J Med. 2014;371(23):2167–77. https://doi.org/10.1056/NEJMoa1408440

Soria JC, Ohe Y, Vansteenkiste J, et al. Osimertinib in untreated EGFR-mutated advanced non-small-cell lung cancer. N Engl J Med. 2018;378(2):113–25. https://doi.org/10.1056/NEJMoa1713137

Soria JC, Tan DSW, Chiari R, et al. First-line ceritinib versus platinum-based chemotherapy in advanced ALK-rearranged non-small-cell lung cancer (ASCEND-4): A randomised, open-label, phase 3 study. Lancet. 2017;389(10072):917–29. https://doi.org/10.1016/S0140-6736(17)30123-X

Stein EM, DiNardo CD, Pollyea DA, et al. Enasidenib in mutant IDH2 relapsed or refractory acute myeloid leukemia. Blood. 2017;130(6):722–31. https://doi.org/10.1182/blood-2017-04-779405

Stone RM, Mandrekar SJ, Sanford BL, et al. Midostaurin plus chemotherapy for acute myeloid leukemia with a FLT3 mutation. N Engl J Med. 2017;377(5):454–64. https://doi.org/10.1056/NEJMoa1614359

Subbiah V, Hu MI, Wirth LJ, et al. Pralsetinib for patients with advanced or metastatic RET-altered thyroid cancer (ARROW): A multi-cohort, open-label, registrational, phase 1/2 study. Lancet Diabetes Endocrinol. 2021;9(8):491–501. https://doi.org/10.1016/S2213-8587(21)00120-0

Subbiah V, Wolf J, Konda B, et al. Tumour-agnostic efficacy and safety of selpercatinib in patients with RET fusion-positive solid tumours other than lung or thyroid tumours (LIBRETTO-001): A phase 1/2, open-label, basket trial. Lancet Oncol. 2022;23(10):1261–73. https://doi.org/10.1016/S1470-2045(22)00541-1

Van Cutsem E, Köhne CH, Hitre E, et al. Cetuximab and chemotherapy as initial treatment for metastatic colorectal cancer. N Engl J Med. 2009;360(14):1408–17. https://doi.org/10.1056/NEJMoa0805019

Vannucchi AM. Ruxolitinib versus standard therapy for the treatment of polycythemia vera. N Engl J Med. 2015;372(17):1670–1. https://doi.org/10.1056/NEJMc1502524

Wang M, Rule S, Zinzani PL, et al. Acalabrutinib in relapsed or refractory mantle cell lymphoma (ACE-LY-004): A single-arm, multicentre, phase 2 trial. Lancet. 2018;391(10121):659–67. https://doi.org/10.1016/S0140-6736(17)33108-2

Wang ML, Rule S, Martin P, et al. Targeting BTK with ibrutinib in relapsed or refractory mantle-cell lymphoma. N Engl J Med. 2013;369(6):507–16. https://doi.org/10.1056/NEJMoa1306220

Williams DA, Rios M, Stephens C, Patel VP. Fibronectin and VLA-4 in haematopoietic stem cell-microenvironment interactions. Nature. 1991;352(6334):438–41. https://doi.org/10.1038/352438a0

Williams DE, Fletcher FA, Lyman SD, de Vries P. Cytokine regulation of hematopoietic stem cells. Semin Immunol. 1991;3(6):391–6.

Wolf J, Seto T, Han JY, et al. Capmatinib in MET exon 14-mutated or MET-amplified non-small-cell lung cancer. N Engl J Med. 2020;383(10):944–57. https://doi.org/10.1056/NEJMoa2002787

Wu YL, Tsuboi M, He J, et al. Osimertinib in resected EGFR-mutated non-small-cell lung cancer. N Engl J Med. 2020;383(18):1711–23. https://doi.org/10.1056/NEJMoa2027071

Yang JC, Schuler M, Popat S, et al. Afatinib for the treatment of NSCLC harboring uncommon EGFR mutations: A database of 693 cases. J Thorac Oncol. 2020;15(5):803–15. https://doi.org/10.1016/j.jtho.2019.12.126

Zhou C, Ramalingam SS, Kim TM, et al. Treatment outcomes and safety of mobocertinib in platinum-pretreated patients with EGFR exon 20 insertion-positive metastatic non-small cell lung cancer: A phase 1/2 open-label nonrandomized clinical trial. JAMA Oncol. 2021a;7(12):e214761. https://doi.org/10.1001/jamaoncol.2021.4761

Zhou K, Zou D, Zhou J, et al. Zanubrutinib monotherapy in relapsed/refractory mantle cell lymphoma: A pooled analysis of two clinical trials. J Hematol Oncol. 2021b;14(1):167. https://doi.org/10.1186/s13045-021-01174-3

CHAPTER 13

Hormonal Therapies Alone and in Combinations for Treatment of Breast Cancer

AMY M. FULTON • KATHERINE H. R. TKACZUK

DEDICATION

This chapter is dedicated to our colleague, mentor, and friend, the late Angela Hartley Brodie, PhD. Angela was a pioneer in developing novel approaches to breast cancer therapy. She led the field in proposing that inhibition of the aromatase enzyme, CYP19A1, would provide a novel and effective means to block estrogen-mediated stimulation of breast cancer by inhibiting the peripheral conversion of androgens to estrogens. This hypothesis led to the identification of several aromatase inhibitors (anastrozole, letrozole, and exemestane) that are used clinically to improve the outcomes of women with breast cancer worldwide.

INTRODUCTION

The breast epithelium is a hormonally responsive tissue that is stimulated by 17β-estradiol to proliferate (Figure 13.1). In the premenopausal woman, luteinizing hormone–releasing hormone (LHRH) in the hypothalamus acts on the pituitary gland to stimulate release of gonadotropins (follicle-stimulating hormone [FSH] and luteinizing hormone [LH]) that stimulate the ovary to produce estrogens and progesterone. After menopause, as ovarian function declines, the peripheral conversion of androgens to estrogens is catalyzed by the aromatase enzyme CYP19A1, a member of the cytochrome P450 superfamily. In premenopausal women, estradiol is produced in the ovaries, while in postmenopausal women the ovarian function ceases. Estradiol production continues "peripherally" in a number of extragonadal sites, including breast, bone, fat, liver, vascular smooth muscle, and various sites in the brain with the aid of an aromatase enzyme, which takes part in peripheral conversion of androgens (androstenedione and testosterone) to estrogens (estrone and estradiol; Figure 13.2). Of note, three major forms of estrogen are present in females: estrone (E1), estradiol (E2), and estriol (E3). E2 is the most potent estrogen in the premenopausal state, while E1 is more important after menopausal ovarian failure, when it is synthesized in adipose and other tissues (Figure 13.2).

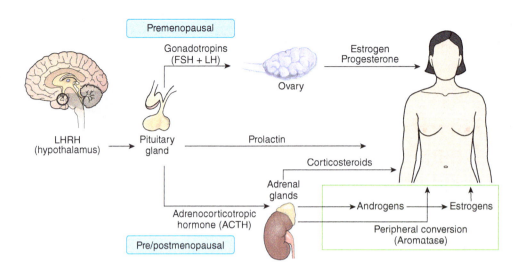

FIGURE 13.1 **Hormones affecting the breast.**
Estrogen stimulates proliferation of normal and malignant breast epithelium. The hypothalamus secretes LHRH that acts on the pituitary gland in premenopausal women to release the gonadotropins FSH and LH that subsequently induce the ovary to produce estrogens and progesterone. In both pre- and postmenopausal women, the pituitary gland stimulates the adrenal gland through ACTH to produce androgens in peripheral tissues that are converted (via aromatase enzyme) to estrogens. Estrogens act through two types of nuclear receptors (ERα and ERβ) as well as the cell membrane receptors (GPER and ER-X). Both classes of estrogen receptors are expressed in the periphery and brain, with cell- and tissue-specific distributions.

ERα, estrogen receptor alpha; ERα, estrogen receptor beta; FSH, follicle-stimulating hormone; GPER, G protein–coupled estrogen receptor; LH, luteinizing hormone; LHRH, luteinizing hormone–releasing hormone.

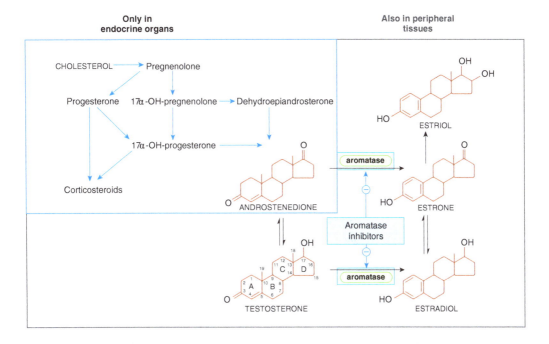

FIGURE 13.2 Estrogen biosynthesis from cholesterol precursors in endocrine organs through androstenedione and in peripheral tissues by aromatase-mediated conversion to estrone, estradiol, and estriol.

ESTROGEN RECEPTOR IN BREAST CANCER

Estrogen receptor (ER)–positive breast cancer (BC) is the most common phenotype of invasive breast cancer. Approximately 70% of newly diagnosed invasive breast carcinomas are hormone receptor (HR)–positive and are therefore considered sensitive to hormonal therapies. Thus, hormonal and endocrine therapies play an important role in the prevention and treatment of breast cancer. Based on the American Society of Clinical Oncology/College of American Pathologists (ASCO/CAP) guidelines, the breast tumor is considered HR$^+$ if ER and/or progesterone receptor (PR) is ≥1% by immunohistochemistry (IHC) staining. Recently, the ASCO/CAP Expert Panel acknowledged that there are limited data on endocrine therapy benefit for patients with breast cancers with 1% to 10% of cells staining ER$^+$, and breast cancers with these results should be reported using a new reporting category of ER$^+$ low. A meta-analysis of response to neoadjuvant chemotherapy (NeoCT) in patients with ER$^+$ low tumors, suggests that ER$^+$ low BCs have outcomes like ER$^-$ BCs in terms of disease-free survival (DFS) and overall survival (OS). ER$^+$ low expression had a predictive role for response to NeoCT; there is need for prospective trials investigating the molecular background and the most appropriate treatment strategies for ER$^+$ low BC. HR$^+$ breast cancer can also be HER2$^+$, but only approximately 20% of breast cancers overall are HER2$^+$. ER is one of the first pharmacologic targets ever described in oncology and to date has remained a key therapeutic target for the therapy of ER$^+$ breast cancer (Figures 13.3 and 13.4).

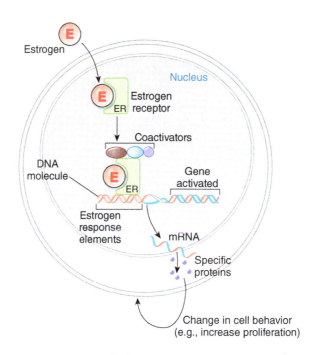

FIGURE 13.3 **Molecular effect of estrogen on the estrogen receptor (ER).**
Estrogen mediates cellular responses in both normal and malignant breast cells
by passive diffusion into the cell, binding to nuclear hormone receptors ERα
and ERβ, and forming a complex with several cofactors/coactivators and RNA
polymerases. This complex acts as a transcription factor, binding to specific
sequences on the DNA and resulting in increased transcription of both ER and
other ER-regulated genes, which leads to changes in cell behavior including
an increase in proliferation. The role of ERβ in breast cancer remains to be
established, in part due to the presence of multiple ERβ isoforms and because
the function of ERβ is partially dependent on the presence or absence of
ERα. Likewise, the functions of plasma membrane–bound G protein–coupled
estrogen receptor (GPER) in breast cancer are less well defined. Therefore, the
rest of the chapter will focus only on ERα as a functional target in breast cancer.

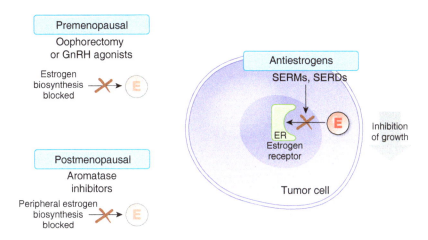

FIGURE 13.4 Estrogen-dependent tumor growth.
There are two general approaches to interfere with ER-mediated growth stimulation; either estrogen actions on ER can be interrupted or estrogen synthesis can be inhibited surgically or pharmacologically. The therapeutic choice is based on a number of factors. In premenopausal women, estrogen production occurs primarily in the ovaries and can be blocked by surgical oophorectomy or pharmacologically by administering GnRH agonists, or by radiation to the ovaries. In postmenopausal women, peripheral estrogen production, via aromatase enzyme, can be blocked pharmacologically by using highly specific oral agents, aromatase inhibitors, or estrogen effect on the ER can be blocked by selective estrogen receptor modulators (SERMs) or degraders (SERDs). GnRH, gonadotropin-releasing hormone.

SELECTIVE ESTROGEN RECEPTOR MODULATORS

Selective estrogen receptor modulators (SERMs) such as tamoxifen have both antagonist and agonist ER functions depending on the site of action (Figure 13.5). SERM tissue specificity is multifactorial and is dependent on different affinity of ligands (e.g., SERMs) for ER subtypes (alpha or beta), which, in turn, are differentially and heterogeneously expressed in target tissues. SERM binding induces conformational changes in the ER and binding to various cofactors that can result in differential target gene activation (Figures 13.6 and 13.7). Tamoxifen functions as an *antagonist* of the ER in breast cancer cells, inhibiting translocation and nuclear binding of the ER, and ultimately altering transcriptional and posttranscriptional events leading to clinical tumor regression. The therapeutic effect of tamoxifen depends on active metabolites and cytochrome P450 2D6 (CYP2D6)–mediated formation of its metabolites (endoxifen and others). When the activity levels of tamoxifen metabolites were measured using an estrogen response element reporter assay, the strongest ER inhibition was found for (Z)-endoxifen and (Z)-4-hydroxytamoxifen (inhibitory concentration 50 (IC50) 3 and 7 nmol/L, respectively). In the treatment of metastatic breast cancer, (MBC), ongoing exposure to Tamoxifen eventually leads to resistance, stimulation of tumor growth, and lack of benefit. tamoxifen is an ER *agonist* in the endometrium and can cause endometrial proliferation, increasing the risk of endometrial cancer (relative risk [RR] 2.5, age ≥50 years, RR = 4), deep venous thrombosis (RR = 1.6), stroke (RR = 1.59) and pulmonary embolism (RR = 3), while

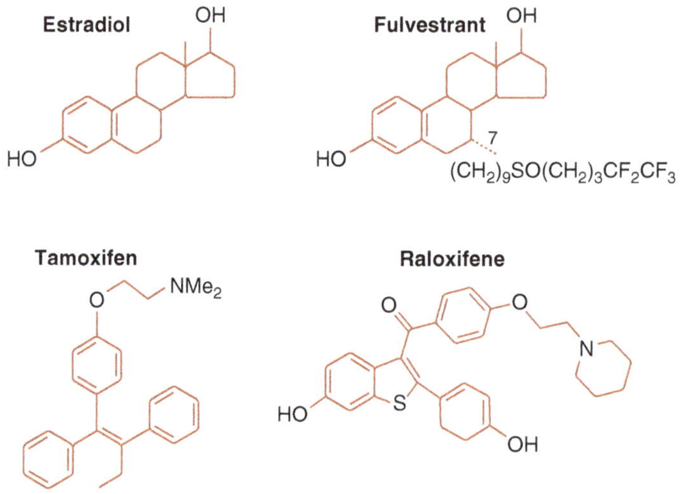

FIGURE 13.5 Structures of antiestrogenic molecules.
Antiestrogens used clinically have two slightly different modes of action.
Selective estrogen receptor modulators (SERMs), such as tamoxifen, toremifene
and raloxifene, block estrogen receptor in the tumor and breast tissue but
have a weak estrogenic effect in other tissues such as uterus. Alternatively,
fulvestrant, the estrogen receptor inactivator or degrader or selective estrogen
receptor degrader (SERD), has a "pure" antiestrogenic effect in the tumor.

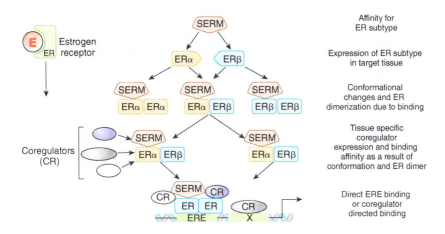

FIGURE 13.6 Cellular (nuclear and nonnuclear) mechanisms of estrogen action.
(a) Estrogen (E)–estrogen receptor (ER) complex binds directly to DNA (estrogen responsive element [ERE]) and recruits additional factors (e.g., coactivators, chromatin remodelers) involved in transcriptional regulation. (b) E–ER complex can also bind indirectly through a tethering mechanism to AP1 or SP1 binding sites (GC) to regulate transcription. (c) Growth factors (e.g., IGF, EGF) can phosphorylate ER through membrane growth factor receptor (GFR)–mediated intracellular signaling pathways (P) to regulate gene expression in the absence of ligand (nuclear action). (d) Estrogen also binds and activates membrane ERα or GPR30, inducing the intracellular signaling pathway (nonnuclear action).

AP1, activator protein; EGF, epidermal growth factor; IGF, insulin-like growth factor; GPR30, G protein–coupled receptor 30; SERM, selective estrogen receptor modulator; SP1, specificity protein 1.

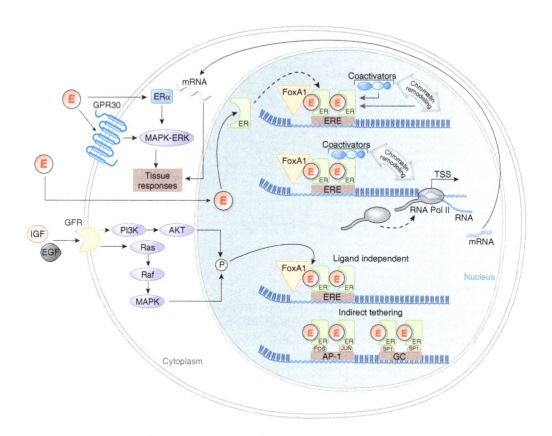

FIGURE 13.7 Selective estrogen receptor modulators (SERMs; e.g., tamoxifen). SERM tissue specificity depends on numerous factors: (a) SERMs have differential and specific affinity for estrogen receptor (ER) subtypes; (b) ER subtypes are differentially expressed in target tissues and can be heterogeneously expressed in a particular tissue; (c) SERM binding induces specific conformational changes in ER that influence dimerization and binding to various cofactors that can determine resultant target gene (X) activation or repression; (d) cofactors (i.e., activators and repressors) are differentially expressed in target tissues; and (e) ER-SERM complexes can bind directly to an ERE or be directed to bind other transcriptional motifs as a result of binding to various cofactors.

AKT, AP-1, activator protein; EGF, epidermal growth factor; ER, estrogen receptor; ERE, estrogen responsive element; ERK, extracellular signal-regulated kinase; FoxA1, forkhead box protein A1; GFR, glomerular filtration rate; GPR30, G protein–coupled receptor 30; IGF, insulin-like growth factor; MAPK, mitogen-activated protein kinase; mRNA, messenger RNA; Raf, rapidly accelerated fibrosarcoma; Ras, rat sarcoma; TSS, transcription start site.

lowering the risk of bone fractures, including hip fractures, by approximately 45%. Common tamoxifen-attributed side effects are hot flashes (64%), vaginal dryness (35%), sleep problems (36%), weight gain (6%), and depression, irritability, or mood swings (6%). In the clinical practice, tamoxifen is utilized in the *prevention* of HR⁺ breast cancer (P1 prevention trial) with the relative risk reduction of invasive and noninvasive BC of 49% and for *treatment* of early and advanced HR⁺ breast cancer, Tamoxifen can be combined with ovarian suppression with gonadotropin-releasing hormone (GnRH) agonists. In contrast, another SERM toremifene is only FDA (U.S. Food and Drug Administration) approved for treatment of advanced HR⁺

breast cancer, while raloxifene is indicated for the prevention of breast cancer in women at high risk for developing breast cancer (STAR prevention trial). All three agents are dosed orally daily and can be taken for extended periods, depending on the indication.

AROMATASE INHIBITORS

Aromatase inhibitors (AIs) inhibit aromatase, the enzyme that converts androgens (androstenedione/testosterone) to estrogens (estrone/estradiol; Figure 13.8). Aromatase is found predominantly in peripheral tissues (e.g., skin, muscle, fat) and leads to low, but stable levels of estrogen. In the context of functioning ovaries, AIs reduce estrogen-mediated negative feedback to the hypothalamus and pituitary gland, leading to gonadotropin secretion and *increased* ovary-derived estrogen. Thus, it is important to **never** use AIs in premenopausal women unless ovarian function suppression (OFS) with a GnRH agonist is utilized concurrently (TEXT and SOFT trials).

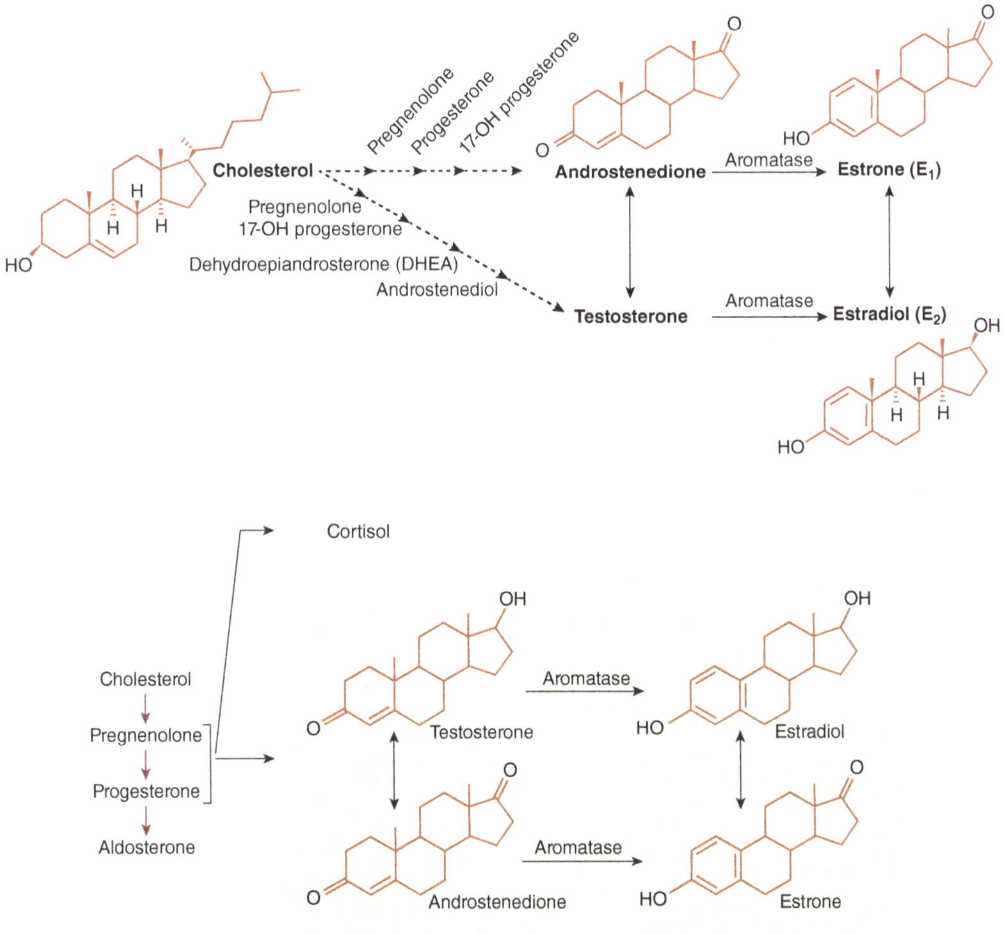

FIGURE 13.8 Steroid biosynthesis and aromatase enzyme.
In the pathway from cholesterol precursor to testosterone or androstenedione, aromatase catalyzes the formation of estradiol from testosterone or estrone from the androstenedione precursor.

AIs are categorized into nonsteroidal (e.g., anastrozole, letrozole) and steroidal (e.g., exemestane; Figure 13.9). Both classes of AIs are used clinically and considered equally effective for treatment of early and advanced HR⁺ breast cancer. AIs are dosed once daily orally, for extended durations of time: in early-stage breast cancer for up to 10 years (MA.17R trial) and in advanced breast cancer until progression of disease (National Comprehensive Cancer Network [NCCN] guidelines).

Aromatase Inhibitors

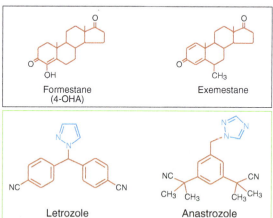

Steroidal

- Substrate analogs interact with steroid binding site
- Enzyme inactivation
- Irreversible
- Good selectivity
- Highly potent

Nonsteroidal

- Reversible inhibitors interact with heme region
- Good selectivity
- Highly potent

Formestane (4-OHA)   Exemestane

Letrozole   Anastrozole

FIGURE 13.9 Aromatase inhibitors (AIs).
AIs prevent the peripheral tissue conversion of testosterone or androstenedione to estradiol and estrone. AIs are either steroidal-based, for example, formestane and exemestane, or nonsteroidal-based, for example, letrozole and anastrozole, and both types are considered clinically equivalent.

Formestane is not active orally and was available only as an intramuscular depot injection. Formestane was approved by the U.S. Food and Drug Administration but the injectable form that was used in Europe in the past has been withdrawn from the U.S. market.

SELECTIVE ESTROGEN RECEPTOR DEGRADERS

Fulvestrant is the only FDA-approved agent in this class that binds to the ER in a competitive mode with affinity comparable to estradiol and downregulates the ER protein in breast cancer cells (Figure 13.10). Fulvestrant was initially FDA approved as 250 mg intramuscular (IM) injection every 4 weeks, after it was shown to be noninferior to anastrozole in postmenopausal women with HR⁺ advanced BC who progressed on first-line endocrine therapy (ET), but with this dose regimen the steady-state plasma fulvestrant concentrations were not reached for several months, putting patients at risk for early disease progression. For this reason, a "high-dose" (500 mg IM) fulvestrant regimen with loading over 1 month (500 mg IM on days 0, 14, 28) then 500 mg IM every 28 days was later established as the recommended dosing schedule. This loading dose approach enabled fast steady-state plasma levels of fulvestrant to be achieved within the first month of treatment. The new "high-dose" fulvestrant regimen was well tolerated and was shown to be superior for progression-free survival (PFS) and OS compared with the original dosing in the Phase 3 double-blind placebo-controlled

CONFIRM trial. This trial enrolled postmenopausal women with advanced HR⁺ BC who relapsed while on adjuvant ET or progressed after first-line ET for advanced disease. This new fulvestrant dose also showed superior efficacy to AIs in HR⁺ advanced BC in subsequent randomized controlled trials. The fulvestrant fIRst-line STudy (FIRST) compared endocrine treatments in an open label, randomized Phase 2 trial of fulvestrant (500 mg) versus anastrozole (1 mg/day) in first-line treatment of HR⁺ MBC and showed a significant increase in median PFS favoring fulvestrant over anastrozole (23.4 vs. 13.1 months, hazard ratio [HR] 0.66, $p = .01$) and a 34% reduction in risk of progression (HR 0.66; $p = .01$). Best overall response to subsequent therapy and clinical benefit rate for subsequent ET was similar between the treatment groups. A post hoc unplanned analysis showed that the HR (95% CI) for OS was 0.70 ($p = .04$; with median OS, 54.1 vs. 48.4 months), respectively, favoring fulvestrant over anastrozole as first-line treatment of advanced HR⁺ BC.

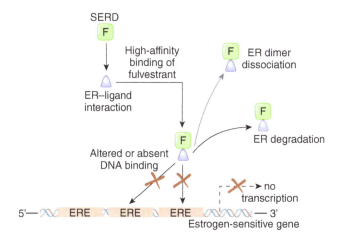

FIGURE 13.10 Selective estrogen receptor degrader (SERD).
Fulvestrant is a SERD that binds to estrogen receptor (ER) with high affinity and downregulates ER protein, preventing binding to estrogen responsive element (ERE) on the DNA.

In the United States fulvestrant is indicated for treatment of HR⁺ HER2⁻ MBC in postmenopausal women not previously treated with hormone therapy (first line) or with disease progression following hormone therapy (second line) or in combination with cyclin-dependent kinase (CDK) 4/6 inhibitors, palbociclib, or abemaciclib for the treatment of HR⁺, HER2⁻ MBC with disease progression after ET.

A large, randomized trial was done to assess if the combination of two hormonal agents with different mechanisms of action is beneficial in treatment of HR⁺ MBC with the AI anastrozole, which inhibits ER synthesis, while fulvestrant binds and accelerates degradation of ER receptors. The investigators hypothesized that the combination of the two agents might be more effective than anastrozole alone in patients with HR⁺ MBC. Postmenopausal women in first-line setting were randomly assigned, in a 1:1 ratio, to anastrozole (1 mg; group 1), with crossover to fulvestrant alone strongly encouraged at progression, or anastrozole/fulvestrant in combination (group 2). Patients were stratified according to prior or no prior receipt of adjuvant tamoxifen therapy. Fulvestrant was administered at a dose of 500 mg on day 1 and 250 mg on days 14 and 28 and monthly thereafter. The primary endpoint was PFS, with OS as a prespecified secondary outcome. The median PFS was 13.5 months in anastrozole alone and 15.0 months in anastrozole/fulvestrant group (HR for progression or death with combination therapy, 0.80; $p = .007$ by the log-rank test). The combination therapy was generally more effective than anastrozole alone in all subgroups, with no significant interactions. OS was longer with combination therapy (median, 41.3 vs. 47.7 months [anastrozole vs. anastrozole/fulvestrant]; HR for death, 0.81; $p = .05$ by the log-rank test), approximately 41% of the patients in anastrozole alone group crossed over to fulvestrant after progression. The rates of grade 3 or higher toxic effects did not differ significantly between the two groups.

Despite the small (PFS/OS) benefit noted in this trial with the combination of anastrozole/fulvestrant versus anastrozole alone, this approach is not considered standard of care. Except for the GnRH ovarian suppression with AI or selective estrogen receptor degrader (SERD) or SERM combinations in premenpausal women, in postmenopausal women the preferred approach is to sequence single-agent hormonal therapies in treatment of HR⁺ MBC. Moreover, the new preferred approaches in treatment of HR⁺/HER2⁻ MBC in first and second line include combinations of hormonal agents and CDK 4/6 inhibitors.

Several oral SERDs are currently in clinical trials in first and later line therapy of advanced HR⁺/HER2⁻ BC.

OVARIAN FUNCTION SUPPRESSION

In premenopausal women, estrogen production occurs in the ovaries and is driven by the intact hypothalamic–pituitary–gonadal (HPG) axis. Hypothalamic GnRH is the central regulator of the production and release of the pituitary gonadotropins, the LH, and FSH that regulate gonadal functions and the production of sex steroids. GnRH agonists bind to GnRH receptors (GnRHRs) and mimic the activity of the natural decapeptide. Administration of GnRH agonist, after an initial stimulation of gonadotropins causing the "flare effect," is followed by suppression of the activity of the pituitary–gonadal axis, through downregulation of GnRHRs.

Ovarian function suppression (OFS) is used in the treatment of early and advanced HR⁺ breast cancer as a form of hormonal treatment. OFS is the practice of making premenopausal women postmenopausal by eliminating ovarian function via surgical oophorectomy, providing radiation to the ovaries, or medically using GnRH analogs such as goserelin, leuprolide, and triptorelin. NCCN guidelines for treatment of early and advanced HR⁺ breast cancer in premenopausal women include OFS as an effective form of anticancer therapy; OFS can be combined with other hormonal agents, SERMs, SERDS, or AIs.

Two large, prospective randomized trials—TEXT (Tamoxifen and Exemestane Trial) and SOFT (Suppression of Ovarian Function Trial)—were conducted to assess the benefit of OFS in premenopausal women with HR⁺ early-stage breast cancer. In TEXT, all women received OFS by GnRH agonist triptorelin from the start of adjuvant therapy; after at least 6 months of triptorelin treatment, women could opt for bilateral oophorectomy or ovarian irradiation. Adjuvant chemotherapy was optional and, if administered, was started concurrently with triptorelin. In TEXT 2,672 premenopausal women were randomly assigned to 5 years of exemestane + OFS or tamoxifen + OFS. Randomization was stratified for intended use of adjuvant chemotherapy and lymph node status. SOFT aimed to determine the value of adding OFS to tamoxifen or exemestane in two cohorts of premenopausal women: those who remained premenopausal after completion of (neo)adjuvant chemotherapy and those for whom adjuvant tamoxifen without chemotherapy was considered suitable treatment. In SOFT 3,066 women were randomly assigned to 5 years of exemestane + OFS or tamoxifen + OFS or tamoxifen alone (three study arms). In SOFT randomization was stratified according to prior use of chemotherapy, lymph node status, and intended initial method of OFS (if randomly assigned to OFS). Based on the results of these trials premenopausal women with HR$^+$ early-stage breast cancer and high recurrence risk, defined by clinicopathologic characteristics, may experience improvement of 10% to 15% in 5-year BC-free interval (BCFI) with exemestane + OFS versus tamoxifen alone. An improvement of at least 5% may be achieved for women at intermediate risk but improvement is minimal for those at lowest risk.

In the adjuvant setting OFS can be started concurrently with adjuvant chemotherapy as done in TEXT while tamoxifen or exemestane hormone therapy are added after completion of adjuvant chemotherapy. If no adjuvant chemotherapy is planned GnRH analog such as triptorelin, leuprolide (Lupron), or goserelin (Zoladex) should be initiated first while the AI is started 6 weeks later (two doses of GnRH), this approach assures adequate OFS before the AI therapy is initiated. The use of depot GnRH agonists (dosed every 3–6 months) for OFS in premenopausal women is not recommended due to the concern for inadequate sustained OFS.

The TEXT and SOFT trials assessed the benefit of OFS in premenopausal women with HR$^+$ early-stage BC; in SOFT women were randomized to one of three treatment arms, tamoxifen alone or OFS/tamoxifen or OFS/exemestane, while in TEXT, the randomization included two arms OFS/tamoxifen or OFS/exemestane. In both trials adjuvant hormonal therapy was continued for 5 years. Premenopausal women with high-risk clinicopathologic factors, who were also more likely to receive adjuvant chemotherapy, had improved BC-specific outcomes ranging from 5% to 15% absolute difference in BCFI with OFS/exemestane compared with OFS/tamoxifen or tamoxifen alone. The clinicopathologic characteristics with greatest contribution to the higher composite measure of recurrence risk were young age (<35 years), four or more positive lymph nodes, and grade 2 to 3 tumor; not unexpectedly, patients with these tumor features also had higher chance of receiving adjuvant or neoadjuvant chemotherapy in these trials. Importantly the OncotypeDX or similar secondary tumor genomic tests were not available and not utilized in the decision-making regarding the benefit and use of adjuvant chemotherapy in the TEXT and SOFT trials.

COMBINATIONS OF HORMONAL THERAPIES WITH NEW TARGETED AGENTS

In patients with HR$^+$ early and advanced breast cancer, AIs, SERMs, and SERDs can be combined with other nonhormonal agents such as mTOR inhibitors, cyclin-dependent kinases (CDK) 4 and 6 inhibitors, *PIK3CA* inhibitors, and HER2 targeted agents (see following sections for discussion of these agents). Preclinically and in prospective clinical trials these combinations have been shown to be more effective than single-agent hormonal therapies.

HR$^+$/HER2$^+$ Breast Cancer: HER2 Targeted Agents

For HR$^+$/HER2$^+$ early and advanced BC, hormonal and HER2 targeted therapy combinations are routinely used based on improved efficacy of the combinations targeting both ER and HER2 receptors.

In the adjuvant setting hormonal therapies (tamoxifen, AIs or OFS/AIs or tamoxifen) are initially given together with monoclonal antibodies (see also Chapter 17), trastuzumab alone or trastuzumab/pertuzumab combination, to complete the 12 months of antiHER2 therapy, followed by the continuation of the initial hormonal therapy for 5 or 10 years. Similarly, neratinib, an orally bioavailable HER2 tyrosine kinase inhibitor (see also Chapter 12), is indicated for extended adjuvant therapy of HER2$^+$ breast cancer after completion of 12 months of HER2 directed therapy with trastuzumab (Extenet trial). In this setting neratinib is combined with hormonal therapies when appropriate. In the metastatic setting, although chemotherapy/antiHER2 combinations are often considered and preferred in the first-line setting, combination therapies targeting the ER and HER2 have significant activity and lower toxicity and are considered an acceptable first-line treatment option for some patients with ER$^+$/HER2$^+$ MBC (NCCN guidelines); the nonchemotherapy option may be particularly desirable for older or debilitated patients who are not candidates for chemotherapy.

PI3 Kinase Pathway and *PIK3CA* Inhibitors

Mammalian target of rapamycin (mTOR) is a serine/threonine protein kinase belonging to the family of phosphatidylinositol 3-kinases (PI3Ks) that regulate cellular metabolism, growth, and protein translation (**Figure 13.11**).

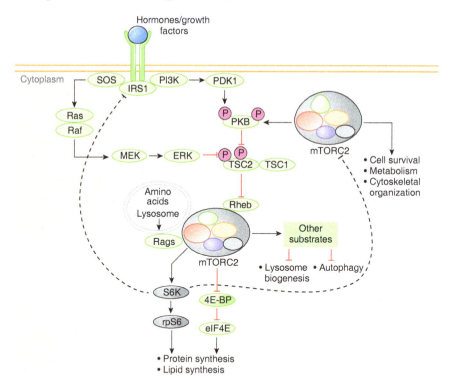

FIGURE 13.11 PI3 kinase pathway. The PI3K/PTEN/AKT/mTORC1 kinase cascade interacts with the estrogen receptor and is often aberrantly expressed in breast cancer driving cell proliferation. https://doi.org/10.1056/NEJMoa1813904

BP, binding protein; ERK, extracellular signal-regulated kinase; IRS1, insulin-receptor substrate 1; MEK, mitogen-activated extracellular signal-regulated kinase; mTORC1, mammalian target of rapamycin complex 1; PDK1, 3-phosphoinositide-dependent kinase 1; PI3K, phosphatidylinositol 3-kinase; PKB, protein kinase B; Raf, rapidly accelerated fibrosarcoma; Ras, rat sarcoma; SOS, son of sevenless protein; TSC, tuberous sclerosis complex.

Source: Adapted from Andre F, Cirrielos E, Rubovsky G, et al., N Engl J Med, 2019.

Rapamycin and modified rapamycin (rapalogs), including sirolimus, temsirolimus, everolimus, and ridaforolimus, may enhance the effectiveness of hormone-based therapies in patients with HR$^+$ breast cancer that has become resistant to endocrine therapies. In HR$^+$, endocrine-resistant advanced breast cancer (Bolero-2 trial), a combination of an mTOR inhibitor (everolimus) and an AI (exemestane) improved PFS (approximately doubled), compared to exemestane plus placebo in patients previously treated with nonsteroidal AI, but no OS benefit was seen. Similar improvements in PFS were noted with the combination of tamoxifen plus everolimus in patients with hormone-resistant breast cancer whose disease failed prior treatment with an AI.

Activation of the PI3K pathway via *PIK3CA* mutations occurs in approximately 28% to 46% of HR$^+$/HER2$^-$ MBC and has been associated with poorer prognosis and chemotherapy resistance. Alpelisib is an orally bioavailable, selective, PI3K inhibitor that is 50 times more potent against PI3K alpha than other isoforms. In preclinical models, alpelisib showed a dual mechanism of action by inhibiting PI3K and inducing p110 alpha degradation in a dose-dependent manner.

In SOLAR-1 trial, alpelisib/fulvestrant combination demonstrated clinically meaningful efficacy in patients in HR$^+$/HER2$^-$ *PIK3CA* mutated MBC following prior AI-based treatment. Based on the SOLAR-1 trial alpelisib is FDA indicated in combination with fulvestrant for the treatment of postmenopausal women, and men, with HR$^+$/HER2$^-$, *PIK3CA*-mutated, advanced or MBC following progression on or after an endocrine-based regimen.

The SOLAR-1 was a placebo controlled, randomized trial of alpelisib/fulvestrant or placebo/fulvestrant in men and postmenopausal women with HR$^+$/HER2$^-$ MBC after progression on or after AI. The addition of alpelisib to fulvestrant treatment in patients with confirmed *PIK3CA* mutation provided statistically significant and clinically meaningful improvement in PFS. In these patients the PFS at a median follow-up of 20 months was 11.0 versus 5.7 months (HR for progression or death, 0.65; $p < .001$). The overall response rate (ORR) in patients with *PIK3CA*-mutated cancer was doubled with the addition of alpelisib to fulvestrant (26.6% vs. 12.8%). The median OS was 39.3 versus 31.4 months; while the OS results did not cross the prespecified efficacy boundary, the median OS in patients with visceral metastases (lung and/or liver) was more pronounced in favor of the combination of alpelisib/fulvestrant (37.2 vs 22.8 months, respectively). Additionally, the median times to chemotherapy were longer for the combination of alpelisib/fulvestrant versus fulvestrant alone (23.3 vs 14.8 months, respectively). In SOLAR-1 trial the most frequent grade 3 or 4 adverse events for the alpelisib/fulvestrant versus fulvestrant were hyperglycemia (36.6% vs. 0.7%), rash (9.9% vs. 0.3%), and grade 3 diarrhea (6.7% vs 0.3%, respectively). More patients discontinued alpelisib compared to placebo due to adverse events (25.0% and 4.2%, respectively). The investigators concluded that although the OS analysis did not cross the prespecified boundary for statistical significance, there was a 7.9-month numeric improvement in median OS for the alpelisib/fulvestrant combination treatment compared to fulvestrant alone in patients with *PIK3CA*-mutated, HR$^+$/HER2$^-$ MBC and these results further support the PFS prolongation observed with alpelisib/fulvestrant in this population, which has otherwise overall poor prognosis due to a *PIK3CA* mutation.

Poly (Adenosine Diphosphate Ribose) Polymerase Inhibitors

Poly (ADP-ribose) polymerases (PARPs) are important enzymes in the DNA damage repair mechanisms. PARP activation is promoted by DNA damage, PARP synthesizes a polymer

(ADP-ribose polymer) that induces the assembly of DNA repair complexes at sites of damage. Synthetic PARP inhibitors (PARPi) block the repair of DNA damage typically repaired by the homologous recombination, resulting in chromosomal instability, cell cycle arrest and subsequent apoptosis. PARPi efficacy is notable in tumors that are defective in the *BRCA1* or *BRCA2* genes via the so-called "synthetic lethality." PARPi cause an increase in DNA single-strand breaks (SSBs) then converted during replication to irreparable toxic DNA double-strand breaks (DSBs) in *BRCA1* or *BRCA2* defective cancer cells. PARP and PARPi are also discussed in Chapter 9. Clinical trials have shown that PARPi are more effective in the treatment of cancers in patients who are carriers of germline *BRCA* (gBRCA) mutations including patients with gBRCA mutated breast cancer.

Olaparib and talazoparib are oral PARPi with promising antitumor activity in gBRCA mutated early (olaparib) and MBC (olaparib, talazoparib). In the metastatic setting olaparib and talazoparib are the two PARPi that are currently FDA approved for treatment of gBRCA-associated HER2⁻ MBC to be used as single agents; in this setting they are typically not combined with hormonal therapies or chemotherapy.

Olaparib was also studied as adjuvant therapy in women with gBRCA mutated early-stage BC. OlympiA is a Phase 3, double-blind, randomized trial in patients with HER2⁻ early BC with *BRCA1* or *BRCA2* germline pathogenic or likely pathogenic variants and high-risk clinicopathologic factors who completed standard of care local treatment and neoadjuvant or adjuvant chemotherapy. Patients were randomly assigned (1:1) to 1 year of oral olaparib or placebo. The primary endpoint was invasive disease–free survival (IDFS); 1,836 patients were randomized. With a median follow-up of 2.5 years, the 3-year IDFS was 85.9% in the olaparib group versus 77.1% in the placebo group (95% HR for IDFS or death, 0.58; $p < .001$). The 3-year distant disease–free survival (DDFS) was 87.5% in the olaparib group and 80.4% in the placebo group, a 7.1% difference. Numerically fewer deaths occurred in the olaparib arm, but this difference was initially not statistically different. A 2022 update of the OlympiA trial noted ongoing benefit from the olaparib adjuvant therapy: olaparib significantly improved OS versus placebo (HR 0.68; $p = .009$), crossing the significance boundary (4-year OS 89.8% vs. 86.4% [diff. 3.4%]), with sustained improvements in IDFS and DDFS (IDFS HR 0.63, 4-year IDFS 82.7% vs. 75.4% [diff. 7.3%]; DDFS HR 0.61, 4-year DDFS 86.5% vs. 79.1% [diff. 7.4%]). Olaparib benefit was consistent across all subgroups, including HR⁺ patients (all HR <1.0). No new safety signals were reported; adverse events remained consistent with olaparib's safety profile. Grade 3 adverse events in >1% of olaparib patients were anemia (8.7%), neutropenia (4.9%), leukopenia (3.0%), fatigue (1.8%), and lymphocytopenia (1.3%). No new cases or excess of myelodysplastic syndrome or acute myeloid leukemia were reported for olaparib.

For patients with early-stage, HR⁺/HER2⁻with high risk of recurrence and gBRCA1 or *BRCA2* pathogenic or likely pathogenic variants, 1 year of adjuvant olaparib (PARPi) concurrently with hormonal therapy should be offered as adjuvant therapy to those considered to be at high risk of recurrence.

Based on the OlympiA trial patients with ER/PR/HER2⁻ (triple negative) BC and with any residual disease post neoadjuvant chemotherapy or if pT ≥2 cm or any pLN+ if adjuvant chemotherapy was offered were eligible. Patients with HR⁺⁺/HER2⁻ BC must have had at least four involved axillary LNs (pN2) before adjuvant chemotherapy; if neoadjuvant chemotherapy was offered patients must have had residual disease with a clinical/pathologic stage

(CPS), ER status, and tumor grade (CPS+EG) score ≥3. The CPS+EG scoring system estimates relapse probability based on clinical and pathologic stage (CPS) and ER status and histologic grade (EG); scores range from 0 to 6, with higher scores indicating worse prognosis.

Cyclin-Dependent Kinase 4/6 Inhibitors

As discussed in Chapter 9, CDK4 and 6 are serine/threonine protein kinases that phosphorylate and inhibit members of the retinoblastoma (RB) family to regulate cell cycle during the G1/S transition (**Figure 13.12**). Phosphorylation of RB1 allows dissociation of the transcription factor E2F, leading to cell cycle progression. Cancer cells overcome RB-dependent growth inhibition by CDK4- and CDK6-mediated inactivation of RB.

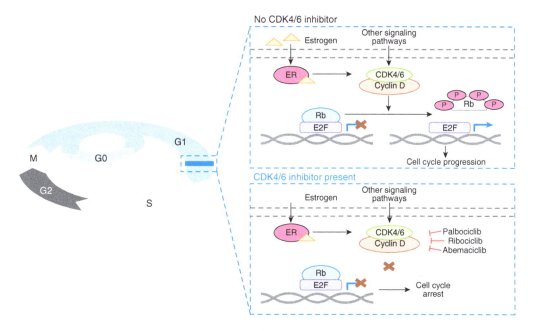

FIGURE 13.12 Interaction of estrogen receptor, CDK4/6, and mTOR signaling pathways.
In addition to estrogen-stimulated growth, breast cancers commonly express epidermal growth factor receptors that activate PI3K/AKT/mTOR signaling. In advanced breast cancer, AIs are combined with inhibitors of either mTOR or with the downstream CDK4/6 kinases that regulate cell cycle progression, cell metabolism, and protein synthesis.

CDK, cyclin-dependent kinases; ER, estrogen receptor; mTOR, mammalian target of rapamycin; PI3K, phosphatidylinositol 3-kinase.
Source: Adapted from Andre F, Cirrielos E, Rubovsky G, et al., N Engl J Med, 2019.

Advanced Breast Cancer ER⁺/HER2⁻

In advanced HR⁺, HER2⁻ breast cancers, CDK4/6 selective inhibitors (palbociclib, ribociclib, and abemaciclib) in combination with endocrine therapies (AIs or fulvestrant) significantly improve (approximately double) PFS compared to endocrine therapies alone. The OS benefit was also noted when CDK4/6 inhibitors (ribociclib or abemaciclib) were combined with AIs or fulvestrant in first- and second-line setting in patients with advanced HR$^+$/HER2$^-$ breast cancer.

Ribociclib

Ribocilib, an orally bioavailable inhibitor of CDK 4 and 6, is FDA indicated for the treatment of adult patients with HR$^+$/HER2$^-$ MBC in combination with an aromatase inhibitor as initial endocrine-based therapy fulvestrant as initial endocrine-based therapy or following disease progression on endocrine therapy in postmenopausal women or in men.

In MONALEESA 2 trial of letrozole/ribocilib versus letrozole/placebo median OS was 63.9 versus 51.4 months (HR for death, 0.76; two-sided p = .008). The MONALEESA-7 (Mammary Oncology Assessment of LEE011's [Ribociclib's] Efficacy and Safety–7) trial showed significantly longer OS with ribociclib/endocrine therapy than with endocrine therapy alone among premenopausal or perimenopausal patients with HR$^+$/HER2$^-$ MBC (HR for death, 0.71; p = .00973), and a significant OS benefit was noted in the ribociclib/fulvestrant group as compared with the placebo/fulvestrant group, with a 28% difference in the RR of death (HR for death, 0.72) in the MONALEESA 3. The reported extended OS follow-up in MONALEESA 3, median OS was 12 months longer in patients with HR$^+$/HER2$^-$ MBC treated with ribociclib/fulvestrant compared with fulvestrant monotherapy.

Abemaciclib

Abemaciclib is an orally bioavailable, potent, and selective small-molecule inhibitor of CDK4 and CDK6 that is 14 times more potent against CDK4 than CDK6 in enzymatic assays. Abemaciclib is currently the only FDA-approved inhibitor of CDK4 and CDK6 for the treatment of patients with HR$^+$/HER2$^-$ MBC as monotherapy for endocrine refractory disease based on the MONARCH 1 trial. Abemaciclib is also indicated in combination with endocrine therapy for treatment of HR$^+$/HER2$^-$ MBC as initial first-line therapy with an AI based on the MONARCH 3 trial and after progression on endocrine therapy with fulvestrant based on the MONARCH 2 trial. Additionally, abemaciclib is the only CD4K/6 inhibitor that is also indicated for adjuvant therapy of early stage, high risk for recurrence, ER$^+$/HER2$^-$ breast cancer.

MONARCH 2 was a Phase 3 randomized, double-blind study of abemaciclib or placebo in combination with fulvestrant in patients with HR$^+$/HER2$^-$ MBC who progressed on endocrine therapy. In this study compared to fulvestrant/placebo the abemaciclib/fulvestrant combination significantly improved median PFS (16.4 vs. 9.3 months; HR 0.553; p <.001); ORR (measurable disease, 48.1% vs. 21.3%; p <.001) and the absolute difference in median OS was 9.4 months (median 46.7 vs 37.3 months, HR 0.757; p =.01). The OS improvement was consistent across all stratification factors, with evidence of benefit observed in patient populations generally considered to be more difficult to treat, such as patients with visceral disease (HR 0.675) and primary resistance to prior ET (HR 0.686). Additionally, the time to second disease progression (median, 23.1 vs. 20.6 months), time to chemotherapy (median, 50.2 vs. 22.1 months), and the chemotherapy-free survival (median, 25.5 vs. 18.2 months) were all significantly improved in the abemaciclib arm versus placebo arm, allowing patients to remain off chemotherapy for longer periods of time, which is considered a significant quality of life benefit.

MONARCH 3 was randomized, Phase 3, double-blind study of abemaciclib/placebo combined with nonsteroidal AI (anastrozole or letrozole) in postmenopausal women with HR$^+$, HER2$^-$ MBC with no prior systemic therapy. The addition of abemaciclib to AI in first-line setting had significantly increased median PFS when compared to the placebo/AI arm (28.18 vs. 14.76 months; HR 0.540; p = .000002), higher ORR (61.0% vs. 45.5%, measurable disease, p = .003), and greater median duration of response (27.39 vs. 17.46 months). The most frequent grade ≥3 adverse events in the abemaciclib versus placebo arms were neutropenia (23.9% vs. 1.2%), diarrhea (9.5% vs. 1.2%), and leukopenia (8.6% vs. 0.6%). Abemaciclib with nonsteroidal AI was an effective initial treatment with an acceptable safety profile for HR$^+$, HER2$^-$ MBC.

Palbociclib

Three large prospective clinical trials assessed the benefit of the combination of palbociclib with hormonal therapies in patients with HR$^+$/HER2$^-$ MBC.

PALOMA-3 was a randomized placebo-controlled trial in patients with HR$^+$/HER2$^-$ MBC who progressed or relapsed on endocrine therapy to receive palbociclib/fulvestrant or placebo/fulvestrant. The median OS was 34.9 versus 28.0 months (HR for death, 0.8; p = 0.09; absolute difference, 6.9 months); however, this difference was not statistically significant; of note 16% of the patients in the placebo/fulvestrant group crossed over to the CDK4/6 inhibitor. In patients with prior sensitivity to endocrine therapy, the median OS was longer (39.7 vs. 29.7 months, HR 0.72; absolute difference, 10.0 months). The median time to chemotherapy was longer for patients in the palbocicilb arm (17.6 vs. 8.8 months, HR 0.58; p <.001).

PALOMA-2 was a double-blind, randomized study in postmenopausal women with HR$^+$/HER2$^-$ MBC, with first-line treatment palbociclib/letrozole or placebo/letrozole (2:1 randomization). The median PFS was 24.8 versus 14.5 months (HR for disease progression or death, 0.58; p <.001). With a median follow-up of 90 months, the median OS was 53.9 months in the palbociclib/letrozole arm and 51.2 months in the placebo/letrozole arm (HR 0.956, p = not significant). Patients in the combination arm had numerically longer OS, but the results were not statistically significant. The frequency of side effects was higher in the palbociclib group, most common grade ≥3 adverse events were neutropenia (66.4% vs. 1.4%), leukopenia (24.8% vs. 0%), anemia (5.4% vs.1.8%), and fatigue (1.8% vs. 0.5%). The febrile neutropenia was rare, 1.8% in the palbociclib/letrozole group and the rates of permanent discontinuation of any study treatment due to adverse events were 9.7% versus 5.9%, respectively.

PALOMA-1 is an open-label randomized 1:1 Phase 2 trial in patients with ER$^+$/HER2$^-$ MBC treated with palbociclib/letrozole or letrozole as first-line therapy. The median PFS was significantly increased in the combination arm compared to letrozole alone (20.2 mos vs. 10.2 months, HR .488) and this led to the accelerated approval of the palbocliclib/letrozole combination by the FDA. PALOMA-1 was a two-part study: Part 1 enrolled unselected postmenopausal women with HR$^+$/HER2$^-$ while Part 2 enrolled HR$^+$/HER2$^-$ patients additionally screened for CCND1 amplification and/or loss of p16; 165 patients were randomized; 66 were in Part 1 and 99 were in Part 2. Median OS was reported as 37.5 versus 34.5 months (HR .897; p = .281) for all patients, and the median OS results were also not significant for Part 1 or Part 2 of this study. In summary in the PALOMA-1, the combination of palbociclib/letrozole was shown to significantly prolong PFS compared with letrozole alone and provided a statistically *nonsignificant trend* toward an improvement in OS.

TABLE 13.1 CDK4/6 Hormone Therapy Trials in HR$^+$/HER2$^-$ Advanced and Early-Stage Breast Cancer

STUDY	PHASE	DESIGN/LINE OF THERAPY	TREATMENT	PFS (MONTHS)	OS (MONTHS)
PALOMA 1	Phase 2	Randomized, first line	Palbociclib/ letrozole vs. letrozole	20.2 vs. 10.2, HR = .488	37.5 vs. 34.5, HR .897, p = .281 (NS)
PALOMA 2	Phase 3, double blind, placebo controlled	Randomized, first line	Palbociclib/ letrozole vs. placebo/ letrozole	24.8 vs. 14.5, HR = .58; p < .001	53.9 vs. 51.2, HR .956, p = NS
PALOMA 3	Phase 3 placebo controlled	Randomized, second line	Palbociclib/ fulvestrant vs. placebo/ fulvestrant		34.9 vs. 28.0, HR .8; p = .09 (NS)
MONARCH 1	Phase 2, single arm study	Nonrandomized, late line, hormone resistant	Abemaciclib 200 mg BID	6.0	17.7
MONARCH 2	Phase 3 double blind placebo controlled	Randomized, second line	Abemaciclib or placebo/ fulvestrant	16.4 vs. 9.3, HR .553; p <.001	46.7 vs. 37.3; HR 0.757; p = .01
MONARCH 3	Phase 3, double blind	Randomized, first line	Abemaciclib/ placebo or nonsteroidal AI (anastrozole or letrozole	28.1 vs. 14.7, HR .540; p = .000002	67.1 vs. 54.5; HR .754; p =.0301
monarchE	Phase 3 adjuvant	Open label, randomized High-risk early-stage BC, HR$^+$/HER2$^-$	Abemaciclib/ ET or ET	IDFS (2-year IDFS 92.2% vs. 88.7%, p = .01; HR .75)	DDFS (HR .69, nominal p < .0001)
MONALEESA-2	Phase 3 postmenopausal	Randomized, first line	Letrozole/ ribociclib vs. letrozole/ placebo	25.3 vs. 16, HR .568; log-rank p = 9.63 × 10^{-8}	63.9 vs. 51.4, (HR .76; two-sided p = .008)

(continued)

TABLE 13.1 CDK4/6 Hormone Therapy Trials in HR⁺/HER2⁻ Advanced and Early-Stage Breast Cancer (*continued*)

STUDY	PHASE	DESIGN/LINE OF THERAPY	TREATMENT	PFS (MONTHS)	OS (MONTHS)
MONALEESA-3	Phase 3 Postmenopausal	Randomized, first or second line	Fulvestrant/ ribociclib vs. fulvestrant/ placebo	First line 33.6 vs. 19.2	At 42 months of follow-up 57.8% vs. 45.9%, HR, .72; $p = .00455$
MONALEESA-7	Phase 3, pre/ perimenopausal	Randomized	Ribociclib/ goserelin/ tamoxifen or AI vs. goserelin/ tamoxifen or AI		Estimated OS at 42 months, 70.2% vs. 46.0%, HR for death, .71; $p = .00973$

AI, aromatase inhibitor; BC, breast cancer; DDFS, distant disease–free survival; ET, endocrine therapy; HR, hazard ratio; HR+, hormone receptor positive; HER2, human epidermal growth factor receptor-2; IDFS, invasive disease–free survival; NS, not significant; OS, overall survival; PFS, progression-free survival.

Early-Stage Breast Cancer

Abemaciclib is the only CDK4/6 inhibitor that is FDA approved for the adjuvant treatment of high-risk HR⁺/HER2⁻ breast cancer, after completion of neoadjuvant/adjuvant chemotherapy, surgery, and radiation. Both ASCO and NCCN guidelines panels endorse 2 years of abemaciclib (150 mg twice daily) with hormonal therapy (tamoxifen or AI or ovarian suppression/AI or tamoxifen) for treatment of early-stage BC with a high risk of recurrence and a Ki-67 proliferation score of ≥20% as determined by an FDA-approved tumor tissue test.

MonarchE is a Phase 3, open-label trial that randomized (1:1) 5,637 patients to adjuvant ET for ≥5 years with or without abemaciclib for 2 years. Cohort 1 enrolled patients with four or more positive axillary lymph nodes (ALNs), or one to three positive ALNs and either grade 3 disease or tumor ≥5 cm. Cohort 2 enrolled patients with one to three positive ALNs and centrally determined high Ki-67 index (≥20%). The primary endpoint was IDFS in the intent-to-treat population (cohorts 1and 2). Secondary endpoints were IDFS in patients with high Ki-67, distant disease–free survival (DRFS), OS, and safety. The first analysis showed a 29% reduction in the risk of developing an IDFS event with abemaciclib/ET compared with ET alone [HR .71, $p = .0009$]. Subsequent follow-up analysis, with 27 months median follow-up and 90% of patients off treatment, showed maintained benefit for the combination of abemaciclib/ET versus ET; IDFS risk reduction was 30% (HR .70, $p < .0001$) and the DRFS risk reduction was 31% (HR .69, nominal $p < .0001$). The absolute improvements in 3-year IDFS and DRFS rates were 5.4% and 4.2%, respectively. The Ki-67 index was prognostic, but not predictive of the abemaciclib benefit, as the benefit was consistent regardless of Ki-67 index. Safety data were consistent with the known abemaciclib risk profile. Additionally, the treatment benefit of abemaciclib extended beyond the 2-year treatment period.

Based on the analysis of monarchE trial abemaciclib for 2 years plus hormonal therapy for ≥5 years may be offered to the broader patient population with resected, HR$^+$/ER2$^-$, LN-positive, early BC at high risk of recurrence, defined as having four or more positive axillary lymph nodes, or one to three positive axillary LNs and one or more of the following factors: histologic grade 3, tumor size ≥5 cm, or Ki-67 index ≥20%. Exploratory analyses of monarchE suggested similar abemaciclib benefit regardless of Ki-67 status, but due to small numbers of Ki-67 low tumors, the investigators commented that the potential benefits of abemaciclib in Ki-67 low tumors must be weighed against the potential side effects of treatment and the cost of the therapy.

CHAPTER SUMMARY

The estrogen receptor (ER) was one of the first specific therapeutic targets identified in cancer and remains the key target for ER$^+$ breast cancers that represent ~70% of invasive breast cancer diagnoses. ER drives the transcription of a number of estrogen-regulated genes, resulting in malignant cell proliferation. There are multiple FDA-approved approaches to subverting ER actions that are context-dependent (Table 13.2). These include removing the primary source of estrogen by oophorectomy, radiation of the ovaries, or pharmacologically by using injections of GnRH analogs monthly (goserelin, triptorelin, leuprolide acetate), blocking the actions of estrogen on the ER using SERMs (tamoxifen, toremifene, raloxifene), or preventing ER-mediated signaling by degrading ER with SERDs (fulvestrant). These agents, alone or in combination with GnRH analogs if premenopausal, are indicated for prevention and treatment of early and advanced ER$^+$ breast cancer.

TABLE 13.2 Hormonal Agents and Combinations for Prevention and Treatment of ER$^+$ and/or PR$^+$ (HR$^+$) Breast Cancer

PREMENOPAUSAL	POSTMENOPAUSAL
PREVENTION	
Tamoxifen (5 years)	Tamoxifen (5 years)
	Raloxifene (5 years)
	AIs (5 years)
ADJUVANT THERAPY	
Tamoxifen (up to 10 years)	AI (up to 10 years)
OFS (GnRH)/tamoxifen (5 years)	Tamoxifen → AI (10 years)
OFS (GnRH) aromatase inhibitor (5 years)	AI → Tamoxifen (10 years)
	Tamoxifen (up to 10 years)
Abemaciclib/HT (high risk) Olaparib/HT if gBRCA 1 or 2 positive	Abemaciclib/HT (high risk) Olaparib/HT if gBRCA 1 or 2 positive

(continued)

TABLE 13.2 Hormonal Agents and Combinations for Prevention and Treatment of ER+ and/or PR+ (HR+) Breast Cancer (*continued*)

PREMENOPAUSAL	POSTMENOPAUSAL
ADVANCED BREAST CANCER*	
OFS/AI or OFS/SERD or OFS/SERM	AI or SERD or SERM
OFS/AI/CDK4/6 inhibitor	AI/CDK4/6 inhibitor
OFS/SERD/CDK4/6 inhibitor	SERD/CDK4/6 inhibitor
OFS/AI/mTOR inhibitor or OFS/SERD/alpelisib if *PIK3CA* positive	AI/mTOR inhibitor or SERD/alpelisib if *PIK3CA* positive
OFS and megestrol acetate, OFS and ethinyl estradiol (if hormone resistant)	Megestrol acetate, ethinyl estradiol (if hormone resistant)
If ER+ and/or PR+/HER2+ always add anti-HER2 therapy (trastuzumab or lapatinib/trastuzumab) to AI or SERM or SERD, while anti-HER2/CDK4/6 inhibitor/hormonal therapy combinations are in clinical trials	If ER+ and/or PR+/HER2+ always add anti-HER2 therapy (trastuzumab or lapatinib/trastuzumab) to AI or SERM or SERD, while anti-HER2/CDK4/6 inhibitor/ hormonal therapy combinations are in clinical trials

*Note that premenopausal women are receiving OFS or ablation.

AI, aromatase inhibitor; CDK, cyclin-dependent kinases; ER, estrogen receptor, HER2, human epidermal growth factor receptor-2; GnRH, gonadotropin-releasing hormone; HT, hormonal therapy; mTOR, mammalian target of rapamycin; OFS, ovarian function suppression; PR, progesterone receptor; SERD, selective estrogen receptor degrader; SERM, selective estrogen receptor modulator.

Novel combinations of hormonal agents with CDK4/6 inhibitors (palbociclib, ribociclib, and abemaciclib), mTOR blockers (everolimus), or *PIK3CA* blocker (alpelisib) are indicated for treatment of hormone-sensitive and -resistant advanced breast cancer. In advanced HR+, HER2− breast cancer, CDK4/6 selective inhibitors in combination with endocrine therapies (AIs or fulvestrant) approximately doubled PFS compared to endocrine therapies alone. The OS benefit was also noted with some of these combinations in first- and second-line setting. In HR+, endocrine-resistant advanced breast cancer, combinations of an mTOR inhibitor (everolimus) and AI (exemestane) or mTOR/SERM (tamoxifen) approximately doubled PFS, but no OS benefit was noted. More recently a *PIK3CA* inhibitor alpelisib was added to the hormonal therapy combinations when *PIK3CA* mutation is present in tumor. When both ER and HER2 targets are present combinations of hormonal therapies and anti-HER2 therapies (antibodies or tyrosine kinase inhibitors) are indicated Additionally, other novel compounds such as entinostat (histone deacetylase [HDAC] inhibitor) and venetoclax (BCL2 inhibitor) are being studied in hormone-resistant, HER2−, advanced breast cancer in combination with hormonal therapies, while triplet therapy, including ER blockade with anti–HER2 therapy and with CDK4/6 inhibitor, is under investigation in advanced ER+/HER2+ breast cancer

CLINICAL PEARLS

- CDK 4/6 inhibitors can be associated with hematologic toxicities, mainly neutropenia, which is reversible with temporary drug discontinuation.
- Aromatase inhibitor action results in decreased estrogen-mediated negative feedback to the pituitary, which, in turn, results in increased gonadotropin secretion and increased ovary-derived estrogen production. Therefore, aromatase inhibitors should not be used in premenopausal women unless menopause is induced chemically (GnRH agonists) or surgically (oophorectomy).
- PARP inhibitors are utilized in treatment of gBRCA1 and 2 associated HR$^+$ early and advanced breast cancer.
- The novel combinations are significantly delaying progression of HR$^+$/HER2$^-$, advanced breast cancer and certainly improving patients' quality of life, while studies are ongoing in early-stage hormone-sensitive breast cancer with these combinations to assess clinical benefit in the neoadjuvant and adjuvant setting.

MULTIPLE-CHOICE QUESTIONS

1. A 37-year-old woman was diagnosed with T2/N1/M0, ER-50%, PR-50%, HER2 3+ (by IHC) invasive ductal carcinoma of her left breast while she was 24 weeks pregnant. She underwent modified radical mastectomy and axillary lymph node dissection and presents to your office for further adjuvant recommendations. What would you recommend for adjuvant systemic therapy?

   A. Start docetaxel, carboplatin, trastuzumab, and pertuzumab (TCHP) immediately, during pregnancy.
   B. Start docetaxel and carboplatin during the pregnancy, and doxorubicin and cyclophosphamide (AC) followed by trastuzumab/pertuzumab after delivery.
   C. Start doxorubicin and cyclophosphamide (AC) every 2 weeks with Neulasta support for four cycles during the pregnancy, and trastuzumab + pertuzumab + paclitaxel after delivery.
   D. Start trastuzumab + pertuzumab immunotherapy during pregnancy, and chemotherapy after delivery.
   E. Do not start any treatment until after delivery.

2. The following figure illustrates the cellular mTOR pathway. Estrogen and other growth factors activate mTOR complex 1 (mTORC1) through the SOS/Ras/Raf–MEK–ERK (MAPK) or the IRS1/PI3K–PDK1–PKB pathways or both. mTORC2 also contributes to the activation of protein kinase B (PKB) through the direct phosphorylation of its turn motif as well as its hydrophobic motif. These pathways impinge on the tuberous sclerosis complex (TSC), which serves as a GTPase activator protein for the small G protein Rheb. Upon inhibitory phosphorylation evoked by upstream kinases, such as PKB, the activity of TSC is suppressed, promoting the accumulation

of GTP-bound Rheb, which, in turn, activates mTORC1 on the surface of lysosomes. Which of the following is correct about the clinical indications of mTOR inhibitors?

A. Sirolimus is FDA approved for treatment of advanced renal cell carcinoma.
B. Rapamycin, in combination with an AI, is FDA approved for treatment of ER^+/ PR^+, $HER2^-$, metastatic breast cancer as the third-line treatment.
C. Everolimus is FDA approved for treatment of postmenopausal women with advanced HR^+ $HER2^-$ breast cancer in combination with exemestane after failure of treatment with letrozole or anastrozole.
D. Everolimus is FDA approved for treatment of adults with advanced hepatocellular carcinoma after failure of treatment with sorafenib.
E. Sirolimus is FDA approved for treatment of chronic graft-versus-host disease.

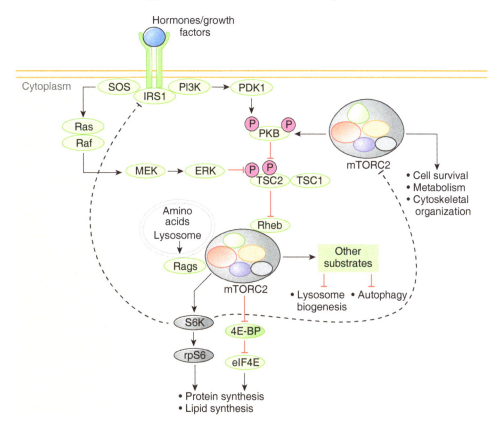

3. A 49-year-old woman with diagnosis of ER^+ ductal carcinoma in situ (DCIS) is planning to receive tamoxifen after lumpectomy surgery. The oncologist discussed the potential adverse events of tamoxifen. Which one of the following is NOT correct about tamoxifen's adverse events?

A. It can cause vaginal dryness.
B. It increases the probability of ocular toxicity, including keratopathy, maculopathy, and cataract.
C. It increases the risk of thromboembolism, including stroke and pulmonary embolism.

D. It increases the risk of aggressive, high-grade endometrial cancers.

E. It increases the risk of depression.

4. A 52-year-old premenopausal woman was recently diagnosed with stage 1, grade 1, ER⁺/PR⁺, HER2⁻, oncotype Dx RS-6, invasive ductal carcinoma, underwent right lumpectomy with sentinel lymph node biopsy, and received a short course of adjuvant breast radiation. Additionally, she was recommended adjuvant therapy with tamoxifen 20 mg daily for 5 years. Soon after starting tamoxifen, she developed severe vasomotor symptoms including frequent hot flashes and diaphoresis. Which one of the following agents would you recommend for treatment of her vasomotor symptoms?

A. Fluoxetine

B. Paroxetine

C. Sertraline

D. Intermediate dose estradiol once weekly

E. Venlafaxine

5. A 60-year-old postmenopausal women with history of stage 2 breast cancer, previously treated with adjuvant tamoxifen for 5 years, completed several years ago, developed mild lower back pain and rib pain, and was diagnosed with a biopsy confirmed metastatic strongly ER⁺ PR⁺ HER2-1+ negative breast carcinoma. Staging PETCT shows multiple bone metastases, several small lung nodules, and mediastinal adenopathy. She is clinically fairly asymptomatic, states that her back pain is improved with Tylenol, which she takes occasionally; she is 100% functional and continues to work. Complete blood count with differential and comprehensive metabolic panel are within normal limits except for slightly elevated alkaline phosphatase; cancer antigen (CA) 15-3 test is elevated. Which of the following would you recommend to immediately start?

A. Aggressive multiagent chemotherapy to quickly control the metastatic disease

B. Letrozole

C. Fulvestrant

D. Ribociclib and letrozole

E. Zometa

6. A 37-year-old premenopausal woman was diagnosed with stage 2 T2N1M0, ER⁺/PR⁻/HER2⁻ 1+ or negative/Ki-67 50%, invasive ductal carcinoma of her right breast; after lumpectomy/sentinel lymph node biopsy, OFS with triptorelin every 4 weeks was initiated; 1 week before chemotherapy, she then received adjuvant chemotherapy, with ddAC for four cycles, followed by 12 weeks of paclitaxel followed by adjuvant radiation therapy to the involved breast. She presents to your office for further recommendations regarding adjuvant therapy. Which of the following would you recommend?

A. Continued OFS for 5 years

B. Continued OFS and exemestane for 5 years

    C. Continued OFS + exemestane for 5 years, and abemaciclib for 2 years

    D. Zometa for 5 years

    E. Continued OFS + tamoxifen for 5 years

7. A 35-year-old premenopausal woman is diagnosed with a large palpable (5.5 cm), $ER^+/PR^-/HER2^-$, Ki 67 55%, invasive ductal carcinoma of her right breast; on CBE she also has palpable ipsilateral axillary adenopathy; systemic staging shows no distant metastases, and her clinical staging is cT3N2M0. She is planned for neoadjuvant chemotherapy with ddAC-weekly paclitaxel. She will see a fertility specialist before chemotherapy is started. What are your recommendations for hormonal therapy for this patient?

    A. Start tamoxifen concurrently with chemotherapy.

    B. Start OFS 1 week before chemotherapy, continue for 5 years; start exemestane and abemaciclib after chemotherapy is completed.

    C. Start OFS before chemotherapy and continue for 5 years.

    D. Start OFS before chemotherapy, then stop when chemotherapy completed and start tamoxifen and abemaciclib.

    E. Discontinue OFS after chemotherapy to see if postmenopausal; if yes, start exemestane.

8. You are managing a 55-year-old postmenopausal woman with family history of breast cancer on paternal side, who was diagnosed with lymph node positive (4 LN+ for metastases) $ER^+/PR^+ +/HER2^-$, Ki-67 40%, invasive ductal carcinoma of her left breast. After discussion she agreed to genetic testing, and was found to be positive for gBRCA2 mutation. She decided to have bilateral mastectomy and completed adjuvant chemotherapy and postmastectomy radiation therapy. Which additional adjuvant systemic therapy is appropriate for this patient?

    A. No further therapy is needed; she did everything possible already to prevent BC recurrence.

    B. Adjuvant apecitabine chemotherapy for eight cycles

    C. Adjuvant pembrolizumab for 12 months

    D. Adjuvant letrozole for 5–10 years, and olaparib for 1 year

    E. Adjuvant olaparib for 1 year

9. You are planning to treat a 55-year-old postmenopausal female patient with $HR^+/HER2^-/PIK3CA$ positive MBC with alpelisib and fulvestrant. Which one of the following is the most common serious adverse event grade 3 or higher of alpelisib?

    A. Rash

    B. Diarrhea

    C. Hyperglycemia

    D. Nausea

    E. Fatigue

ANSWERS TO MULTIPLE-CHOICE QUESTIONS

1. **C.** Anthracyclines, such as doxorubicin and cyclophosphamide, can be used in the second and third trimesters. Trastuzumab inhibits human epidermal growth receptor-2 (HER2) protein. HER2 plays a role in embryonic development. Trastuzumab exposure during pregnancy may result in oligohydramnios and oligohydramnios sequence (pulmonary hypoplasia, skeletal malformations, and neonatal death). A systematic review of 16 studies (50 pregnancies) suggested that "taxanes may potentially play a promising role in the optimal therapeutic strategy of patients with breast cancer diagnosed during pregnancy" (Zagouri et al., 2013). Carboplatin may cause fetal harm if administered during pregnancy.

2. **C.** A randomized, double-blind, multicenter study (NCT00863655) of everolimus in combination with exemestane versus placebo in combination with exemestane was conducted in 724 postmenopausal women with ER^+, $HER2^-$, advanced breast cancer with recurrence or progression following prior therapy with letrozole or anastrozole. After a median follow-up of approximately 40 months, there was no statistically significant difference in OS between the two groups. However, median PFS was higher in the everolimus group compared with the placebo group (7.8 months, 95% CI 6.9, 8.5 vs. 3.2 months, 95% CI 2.8, 4.1) with hazard ratio .45 (95% CI, 0.38, 0.54, $p < .0001$).

3. **D.** Tamoxifen increases the risk of endometrial cancers (hazard ratio of 1.7 per 1,000 data). However, the endometrial cancers are mostly low-grade and stage I tumors. The greatest cumulative risk of endometrial cancer occurs after 5 years of tamoxifen. The tumors are usually early stage and well differentiated; however, the development of high-risk endometrial cancer is reported. The rest of the choices are included in adverse event profile of tamoxifen.

4. **E.** Concomitant use of tamoxifen with some of the selective serotonin reuptake inhibitors (SSRIs) may result in decreased tamoxifen efficacy. CYP2D6 inhibitors (e.g., fluoxetine, paroxetine, sertraline) interfere with transformation of tamoxifen to the active metabolite endoxifen. Weak CYP2D6 inhibitors such as venlafaxine and citalopram have minimal effect on the conversion to endoxifen.

5. **D.** Treatment of ER^+/$HER2^-$ MBC with CDK4/6 inhibitors/hormonal therapy, as first-line therapy is an established and recommended therapy based on multiple randomized clinical trials (Monaleesa/Monarch/Paloma). These combinations have significantly improved (doubled) PFS, and OS (ribociclib/abemaciclib).

6. **C.** This young premenopausal woman has high-risk HR^+/$HER2^-$ breast cancer, with an elevated Ki67, per MonarchE trial; this patient is expected to have a 29% reduction in the risk of developing an IDFS event with abemaciclib/endocrine therapy (ET) compared with ET. After 27 months median follow-up and 90% of patients off treatment, this benefit of the abemaciclib/ET versus ET persisted, with the IDFS risk reduction of 30% ($p < .0001$) and the DRFS risk reduction of 31% ($p < .0001$). The absolute improvements in 3-year IDFS and DRFS rates were 5.4% and 4.2%, respectively. The Ki-67 index was prognostic, but not predictive, of the abemaciclib benefit,

as the benefit was consistent regardless of Ki-67 index. Additionally, the treatment benefit of abemaciclib extended beyond the 2-year treatment period.

7. **D.** The Tamoxifen and Exemestane Trial (TEXT)/Suppression of Ovarian Function Trial (SOFT) showed superior outcomes for premenopausal women with HR$^+$ breast cancer treated with adjuvant exemestane + OFS or tamoxifen + OFS compared with tamoxifen alone. Premenopausal women with high-risk clinicopathologic factors, who were also more likely to receive adjuvant chemotherapy, had improved BC specific outcomes ranging from 5% to 15% absolute difference in BCFI with OFS/exemestane compared with OFS/tamoxifen or tamoxifen alone. The clinico pathologic characteristics with greatest contribution to the higher composite measure of recurrence risk were young age (<35 years), four or more positive lymph nodes, and grade 2 to 3 tumor; not unexpectedly, patients with these features also had higher chance of receiving adjuvant or neoadjuvant chemotherapy in these trials. The OncotypeDX and similar secondary tumor genomic tests were not available and not utilized in the decision-making regarding the benefit and use of adjuvant chemotherapy in the TEXT and SOFT trials.

8. **D.** Adjuvant therapy with a PARPi in gBRCA1 or 2 mutated early-stage BC; in OlympiA trial, such patients were randomized to 1 year of placebo or olaparib, and treatment with olaparib significantly improved OS versus placebo (HR .68; p = .009), crossing the significance boundary (4-year OS 89.8% vs. 86.4% [diff. 3.4%]), with sustained improvements in IDFS and DDFS (IDFS HR .63, 4-year IDFS 82.7% vs. 75.4% [diff. 7.3%]; DDFS HR .61, 4-year DDFS 86.5% vs. 79.1% [diff. 7.4%]). Olaparib benefit was consistent across all subgroups, including HR$^+$ patients (all HR <1.0).

9. **C.** The SOLAR-1 was a placebo-controlled, randomized trial of alpelisib/fulvestrant or placebo/fulvestrant in men and postmenopausal women with HR$^+$/HER2$^-$ MBC after progression on or after AI. The addition of alpelisib to fulvestrant treatment in patients with confirmed *PIK3CA* mutation provided statistically significant and clinically meaningful improvement in PFS. In these patients the PFS at a median follow-up of 20 months was 11.0 versus 5.7 months (HR for progression or death, .65; p < .001). The ORR in patients with *PIK3CA*-mutated cancer was doubled with the addition of alpelisib to fulvestrant (26.6% vs. 12.8%). In SOLAR-1 trial the most frequent grade 3 or 4 adverse events for the alpelisib/fulvestrant versus fulvestrant were hyperglycemia (36.6% vs. 0.7%), rash (9.9% vs. 0.3%), and grade 3 diarrhea (6.7% vs 0.3%), respectively.

SELECTED REFERENCES

American Cancer Society. Breast cancer facts and figures 2017–2018. Available from: https://www.cancer.org/content/dam/cancer-org/research/cancer-facts-and-statistics/breast-cancer-facts-and-figures/breast-cancer-facts-and-figures-2017-2018.pdf

Andre F, Cirrielos E, Rubovsky G, et al. Alpelisib for *PIK3CA*-mutated, hormone receptor-positive advanced breast cancer. N Engl J Med. 2019;380:1929–40. https://doi.org/10.1056/NEJMoa1813904

Baselga J, Campone M, Piccart M, et al. Everolimus in postmenopausal hormone-receptor-positive advanced breast cancer. N Engl J Med. 2012;366(6):520–9. https://doi.org/10.1056/NEJMoa1109653

Cui J, Shen Y, Li R. Estrogen synthesis and signaling pathways during aging: From periphery to brain. Trends Mol Med. 2013;19(3):197–209. https://doi.org/10.1016/j.molmed.2012.12.007

Dickler MN, Tolaney SM, Rugo HS, et al. MONARCH 1, a phase II study of abemaciclib,a CDK4 and CDK6 inhibitor, as a single agent, in patients with refractory HR+/HER2– metastatic breast cancer. Clin Cancer Res. 2017 Sep 1;23(17):5218–24. https://doi.org/10.1158/1078-0432.CCR-17-0754

Di Leo A, Jerusalem G, Petruzelka L, et al. Results of the CONFIRM phase III trial comparing fulvestrant 250 mg with fulvestrant 500 mg in postmenopausal women with estrogen receptor–positive advanced breast cancer. J Clin Oncol. 2010 Oct 20;28(30):4594–600. https://doi.org/10.1200/JCO.2010.28.8415

Finn RS, Martin M, Rugo HS, et al. Palbociclib and letrozole in advanced breast cancer. N Engl J Med. 2016;375(20):1925–36. https://doi.org/10.1056/NEJMoa1607303

Freedman AN, Yu B, Gail MH, et al. Benefit/risk assessment for breast cancer chemoprevention with raloxifene or tamoxifen for women age 50 years or older. J Clin Oncol. 2011 Jun 10;29(17):2327–33. https://doi.org/10.1200/JCO.2010.33.0258

Goetz MP, Toi M, Campone M, et al. MONARCH 3: Abemaciclib as initial therapy for advanced breast cancer. J Clin Oncol. 2017;35(32):3638–46. https://doi.org/10.1200/JCO.2017.75.6155

Goss PE, Ingle JN, Pritchard KI, et al. Extending aromatase-inhibitor adjuvant therapy to 10 years. N Engl J Med. 2016;375(3):209–19. https://doi.org/10.1056/NEJMoa1604700

Hamilton KJ, Hewitt SC, Arao Y, Korach KS. Estrogen hormone biology. Curr Top Dev Biol. 2017;125:109–46. https://doi.org/10.1016/bs.ctdb.2016.12.005

Hammond ME, Hayes DF, Dowsett M, et al. American Society of Clinical Oncology/College of American Pathologists guideline recommendations for immunohistochemical testing of estrogen and progesterone receptors in breast cancer. J Clin Oncol. 2010;28(16):2784–95. https://doi.org/10.1200/JCO.2009.25.6529

Hortobagyi GN, Stemmer SM, Burris HA, et al. Overall survival with ribociclib plus letrozole in advanced breast cancer. N Engl J Med. 2022;386(10):942–50. https://doi.org/10.1056/NEJMoa2114663

Im SA, Lu YS, Bardia A, et al. Overall survival with ribociclib plus endocrine therapy in breast cancer. N Engl J Med. 2019;381(4):307–16. https://doi.org/10.1056/NEJMoa1903765

Johnston S, Martin M, Di Leo A, et al. MONARCH 3 final PFS: A randomized study of abemaciclib as initial therapy for advanced breast cancer. Breast Cancer. 2019;5:5. https://doi.org/10.1038/s41523-018-0097-z

Martinkovich S, Shah D, Planey SL, Arnott JA. Selective estrogen receptor modulators: Tissue specificity and clinical utility. Clin Interv Aging. 2014;9:1437–52. https://doi.org/10.2147/CIA.S66690

Mehta RS, Barlow WE, Albain KS, et al. Combination anastrozole and fulvestrant in metastatic breast cancer. N Engl J Med. 2012;367(5):435–44. https://doi.org/10.1056/NEJMoa1201622

Osborne CK, Fuqua SA. Mechanisms of tamoxifen resistance. Breast Cancer Res Treat. 1994;32(1):49–55. https://doi.org/10.1007/BF00666205

Osborne CK, Wakeling A, Nicholson RI. Fulvestrant: An oestrogen receptor antagonist with a novel mechanism of action. Br J Cancer. 2004;90(Suppl 1):S2–6. https://doi.org/10.1038/sj.bjc.6601629

Paakkola NM, Karakatsanisy A, Mauri D, et al. The prognostic and predictive impact of low estrogen receptor expression in early breast cancer: A systematic review and meta-analysis. ESMO Open. 2021;6(6):100289. https://doi.org/10.1016/j.esmoop.2021.100289

Pagani O, Francis PA, Fleming GF, et al. Absolute improvements in freedom from distant recurrence to tailor adjuvant endocrine therapies for premenopausal women: Results from TEXT and SOFT. J Clin Oncol. 2020 Apr 20;38(12):1293–303. https://doi.org/10.1200/JCO.18.01967

Pérez Carrión R, Alberola Candel V, Calabresi F, et al. Comparison of the selective aromatase inhibitor formestane with tamoxifen as first-line hormonal therapy in postmenopausal women with advanced breast cancer. Ann Oncol. 1994;5(Suppl 7):S19–24.

Piccart M, Hortobagyi GN, Campone M, et al. Everolimus plus exemestane for hormone-receptor-positive, human epidermal growth factor receptor-2-negative advanced breast cancer: Overall survival results from BOLERO-2. Ann Oncol. 2014;25(12):2357–62. https://doi.org/10.1093/annonc/mdu456

Regan MM, Francis PA, Pagani O, et al. Absolute benefit of adjuvant endocrine therapies for premenopausal women with hormone receptor–positive, human epidermal growth factor receptor 2-negative early breast cancer: TEXT and SOFT trials. J Clin Oncol. 2016;34(19):2221–31. https://doi.org/10.1200/JCO.2015.64.3171

Robertson JFR, Lindemann JPO, Llombart-Cussac A, et al. Fulvestrant 500 mg versus anastrozole 1 mg for the first-line treatment of advanced breast cancer: Follow-up analysis from the randomized 'first' study. Breast Cancer Res Treat. 2012;136(2):503–11. https://doi.org/10.1007/s10549-012-2192-4

Slamon DJ, Neven P, Chia S, et al. Overall survival with ribociclib plus fulvestrant in advanced breast cancer. N Engl J Med. 2020;382(6):514–24. https://doi.org/10.1056/NEJMoa1911149

Slamon DJ, Neven P, Chia S, et al. Phase III randomized study of ribociclib and fulvestrant in hormone receptor-positive, human epidermal growth factor receptor 2-negative advanced breast Cancer: MONALEESA-3. J Clin Oncol. 2018;36(24):2465–72. https://doi.org/10.1200/JCO.2018.78.9909

Sledge GW Jr, Toi M, Neven P, et al. The effect of abemaciclib plus fulvestrant on overall survival in hormone receptor-positive, ERBB2-negative breast cancer that progressed on endocrine therapy – MONARCH 2, a randomized clinical trial. JAMA Oncol. 2020;6(1):116–24. https://doi.org/10.1001/jamaoncol.2019.4782

Turner NC, Ro J, André F, et al. Palbociclib in hormone-receptor-positive advanced breast cancer. N Engl J Med. 2015;373(3):209–19. https://doi.org/10.1056/NEJMoa1505270

Turner NC, Slamon DJ, Ro J, et al. Overall survival with palbociclib and fulvestrant in advanced breast cancer. N Engl J Med. 2018;379(20):1926–36. https://doi.org/10.1056/NEJMoa1810527

Tutt ANJ, Garber RD, Gelber D, et al. VP1-2022: Prespecified event driven analysis of overall survival (OS) in the OlympiA phase III trial of adjuvant olaparib (OL) in germline *BRCA1/2* mutation (gBRCAm) associated breast cancer. Ann Oncol. 2022 Apr 1;33(5):566–8. https://doi.org/10.1016/j.annonc.2022.03.008

Zagouri F, Sergentanis TN, Chrysikos D, et al. Taxanes for breast cancer during pregnancy: A systematic review. Clin Breast Cancer. 2013;13(1):16–23. https://doi.org/10.1016/j.clbc.2012.09.014

CHAPTER 14

Androgen Receptor Axis Targeting in the Treatment of Prostate Cancer

VINCENT C. O. NJAR ● ARIF HUSSAIN

INTRODUCTION

Prostate cancer (PC) is the second leading cause of cancer-related deaths in men in the United States. Because androgen/androgen receptor signaling plays a pivotal role in the development, proliferation, and metastasis of PC, androgen deprivation therapy (ADT) and blockade of the androgen receptor with antiandrogens are considered the backbone of treatment for various stages of the disease. This chapter highlights the role of androgens and androgen receptor signaling in PC and the impact of several classes of U.S. Food and Drug Administration (FDA)-approved drugs for the treatment of PC such as gonadotropin-releasing hormone (GnRH; also called LHRH, luteinizing hormone–releasing hormone) agonist/antagonist, CYP17 inhibitors, and the antiandrogens.

PROSTATE CANCER AND TREATMENT

The standard of care for advanced disease PC remains antihormonal therapy, which includes (a) androgen deprivation (surgical castration [orchiectomy] or medical castration [LHRH agonist/antagonist, CYP17 inhibitors]) or (b) antiandrogen receptor targeting (Figure 14.1). However, despite relatively robust initial responses in most cases, therapies inevitably fail in nearly all patients. Antihormonal therapy was based on the discovery by Dr. Charles Huggins that metastatic PC responds to lowering of androgen levels, i.e., androgen-ablation, via castration.

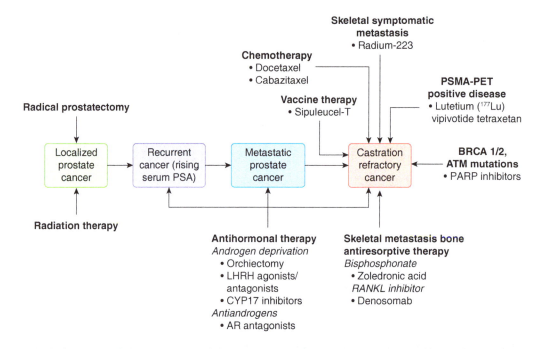

FIGURE 14.1 Prostate cancer progression and treatment.
Localized PC is generally treated with radical prostatectomy (surgical removal of the prostate) or radiation therapy. For patients experiencing rising PSA after local therapies (surgery/radiation) antihormonal therapies can be used, although the optimal timing, duration, and combination of these therapies is not well defined. Androgen deprivation therapy (ADT) and chemotherapy (taxane-based [docetaxel, cabazitaxel], see also Chapter 8) remain the standard treatments for advanced PC.

For castration refractory PC with bone metastasis, bone antiresorptive therapies (bisphosphonates or RANKL inhibitor) are administered to help decrease risk of skeletal related complications, and for those with bone-dominant symptomatic castration-resistant disease radium-223 can be used. More recently, the prostate-specific membrane antigen (PSMA)-directed rad-opharmaceutical lutetium (^{177}Lu) vipivotide tetraxetan has been appioved for PMSA PET (^{68}Ga gozetotide)-positive metastatic castration-resistant PC (mCRPC).

For men with mCRPC harboring mutations in DNA damage response genes, two poly(ADP)ribose polymerase (PARP) inhibitors, olaparib (for *BRCA1, BRCA2, ATM* mutants) and rucaparib (for BRCA1, BRCA1 mutants) have been approved for treatment.

ADP, adenosine diphosphate; AR, androgen receptor; ATM, ataxia-telangiectasia mutated; CYP17, cytochrome P450-C17; LHRH, luteinizing hormone-releasing hormone; PC, prostate cancer; PET, positron emission tomography; PSA, prostate-specific antigen; RANKL, receptor activator of nuclear factor κB ligand.

PROSTATE CANCER AND ANDROGENS BIOSYNTHESIS

PC is the most hormone sensitive of all cancers. The sources of androgens in the prostate are shown in Figure 14.2. Androgens play a vital role in the development, growth, and progression of PC. The testes synthesize about 90% to 95% of the testosterone (T) found in the plasma, with the remaining converted from androgens produced by the adrenal glands. Production from the testes is stimulated when the hypothalamus releases GnRH, which in turn binds to high-affinity receptors on the gonadotropic cells in the anterior pituitary. This stimulates the pituitary gland to release luteinizing hormone (LH), which stimulates testosterone production by the Leydig cells in the testis. Testosterone can be subsequently converted to dihydrotestosterone (DHT) by the enzyme steroid 5α-reductase that is localized primarily in the prostate. In addition, the hypothalamus can also release corticotropin releasing hormone (CRH), which stimulates the anterior pituitary to release ACTH. ACTH stimulates adrenal production and release of the adrenal androgens dehydroepiandrosterone (DHEA), DHEA sulfate, and androstenedione (Δ^4-dione, A4). These inactive precursors are then converted in the prostate to the active androgens testosterone and DHT. It is estimated that conversion of adrenal androgens accounts for as much as 40% of the total DHT present within the prostate.

All steroid hormone synthesis follows the conversion of cholesterol to pregnenolone, which can subsequently progress down the androgen formation pathway, or be converted to progesterone by 3β-hydroxysteroid dehydrogenase (Figure 14.3).

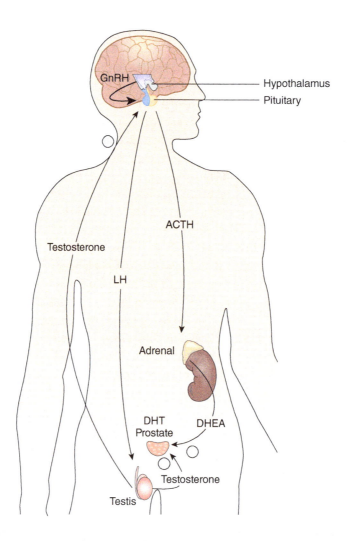

FIGURE 14.2 Sources of androgens in the human prostate.
Hypothalamic GnRH causes the release of LH from the anterior pituitary. LH stimulates the testes to produce testosterone, which is released into the bloodstream. Pituitary ACTH release stimulates the adrenal glands, which secrete the androgen precursor DHEA into the circulation. DHEA is converted into testosterone and then into DHT in the prostate. Each pathway provides similar amounts of androgens.

DHEA, dehydroepiandrosterone; DHT, dihydrotestosterone; GnRH, gonadotropin-releasing hormone; LH, luteinizing hormone.

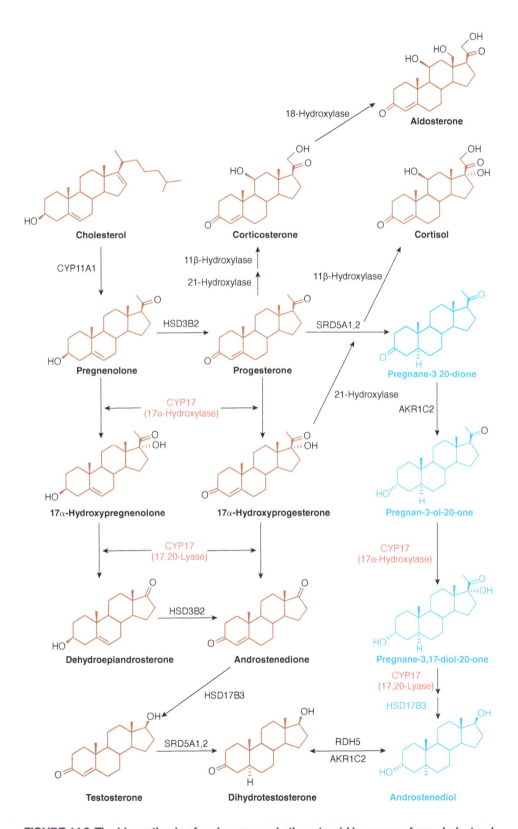

FIGURE 14.3 The biosynthesis of androgens and other steroid hormones from cholesterol.

(*continued*)

FIGURE 14.3 The biosynthesis of androgens and other steroid hormones from cholesterol. (*continued*)

The cytochrome P450 enzyme, 17α-hydroxylase/17,20-lyase (CYP17) catalyzes two key reactions involved in the production of sex steroids, which occur sequentially: the 17α-hydroxylase activity typically converts pregneolone to 17α-hydroxypregnenolone and progesterone to 17α-hydroxyprogesterone, while the C17,20-lyase activity converts 17α-hydroxypregnenolone to DHEA (Δ^5 pathway) and 17α-hydroxyprogesterone to androstenedione (Δ^4 pathway).

The metabolic route of testosterone formation in humans favors pregnenolone as the starting precursor rather than progesterone. The precursor androgens DHEA anandrostenedione may be subsequently transformed to testosterone by other enzymes. Testosterone can then be converted to the more potent DHT by 5α-reductase in target tissue such as the prostate.

Recently, an additional *backdoor pathway* has been described in which DHT synthesis bypasses testosterone as an intermediate **(shown in figure in blue).** It should be noted that CYP17 is still active in the backdoor pathway, and therefore emphasizes its importance as a therapeutic target.

GnRH causes the release of LH from the anterior pituitary. LH stimulates the testes to produce testosterone, which is released into the bloodstream. Pituitary ACTH release stimulates the adrenal glands, which secrete the androgen precursor DHEA into the circulation. DHEA is converted into testosterone and then into DHT in the prostate. Each pathway provides similar amounts of androgens.

DHEA, dehydroepiandrosterone; DHT, dihydrotestosterone; GnRH, gonadotropin-releasing hormone; LH, luteinizing hormone.

ANDROGEN RECEPTOR BIOLOGY AND SIGNALING IN PROSTATE CANCER

The androgen receptor (AR) is an intracellular member of the steroid hormone receptor family of ligand dependent nuclear receptors. When activated by androgens within PC cells, the AR initiates transcription of genes responsible for proliferation, survival, and angiogenesis. When unbound, the receptor resides mainly in the cytoplasm where it is bound to and stabilized by heat shock proteins (e.g., HSP-90, 70, 56, and 23). Binding of the androgens testosterone or the more potent DHT induces a conformational change resulting in dissociation of the receptor from HSP and the formation of homodimers and phosphorylation (Figure 14.4). The dimerized AR then translocates to the nucleus where it binds to a specific sequence of DNA termed the androgen response element (ARE). Once bound to the ARE, the AR recruits multiple coactivators (e.g., NCOA1-3, ARA70, CBP, TIP60 and p300) and cosuppressors (e.g., NCOR). This allows for the binding of RNA polymerase and the initiation of target gene transcription. AR target genes include prostate-specific antigen (PSA), cyclin dependent kinase 8, the p85 catalytic subunit of the phosphatidylinositol 3-kinase (PI3K), and the oncogenic fusion proteins TMPRSS2-ERG1/ETV1, among others. Together these genes initiate cell survival and proliferation.

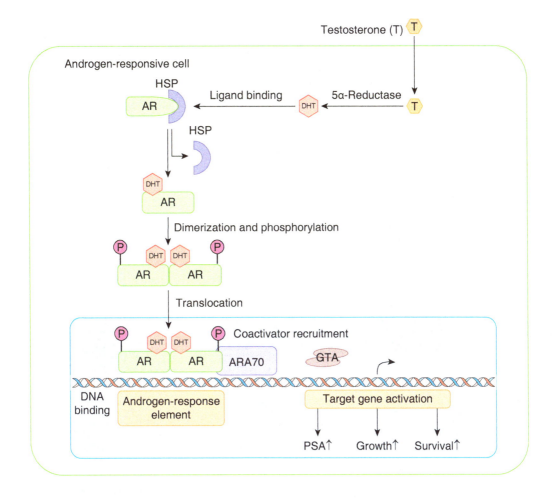

FIGURE 14.4 Molecular mechanism of androgen receptor (AR) activation by dihydrotestosterone (DHT).

Testosterone enters the cell and is converted to DHT by the enzyme 5α-reductase. DHT binding to the AR induces conformational changes in the ligand-binding domain and causes heat shock protein (HSP) dissociation from the AR. The transformed AR undergoes dimerization, phosphorylation, and translocation to the nucleus. The translocated receptor dimer binds to androgen response elements in the DA, thereby activating transcription of AR target genes and ultimately leading to cell proliferation.

ARA, androgen receptor activator; GTA, general transcription activation; PSA, prostate-specific antigen.

THERAPEUTIC STRATEGIES FOR PROSTATE CANCER

Androgen Deprivation Therapy

Because androgens play a vital role in the development, growth, and progression of PC, the major therapeutic strategies include regulation of systemic androgen levels (androgen deprivation therapy, ADT) and prevention of the binding of androgens to the androgen receptor (AR antagonists, antiandrogens; Figure 14.5).

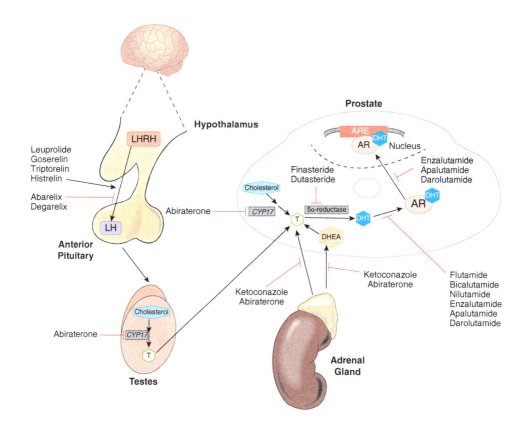

FIGURE 14.5 **Physiologic and anatomic targets of FDA-approved hormonal drugs for prostate cancer.**
LHRH produced by the hypothalamus stimulates production of LH by the anterior pituitary. LH then activates the production of testosterone (T) by the testes. Gonadal testosterone, along with testosterone produced by the adrenal glands and the prostate itself, activates transcription of ARGs. Currently approved therapies for advanced PC target multiple nodes along this physiologic pathway.

AR, androgen receptor; ARE, androgen response element; ARGs, androgen regulated genes; CYP17, cytochrome P450-C17; DHEA, dehydroepiandrosterone; DHT, dihydrotestosterone; FDA, U.S. Food and Drug Administration; LH, luteinizing hormone; LHRH, LH-releasing hormone; PC, prostate cancer.

GnRH Agonists and Antagonists

The most common form of ADT involves chemical suppression of the pituitary gland with GnRH agonists. GnRH agonists in common use for PC include leuprolide, goserelin, triptorelin, histrelin, and nafarelin (**Figure 14.6** and Table 14.1). Long-acting preparations are available in doses that are approved for 3-, 4-, and 6-month administrations. These agents work by overstimulating the anterior pituitary to release LH. This results in a rise ("flare") in serum testosterone levels for 1–2 weeks. The rise in plasma testosterone initiates a negative feedback loop resulting in the cessation of LH release from the anterior pituitary. This results in a near complete inhibition of testicular testosterone production.

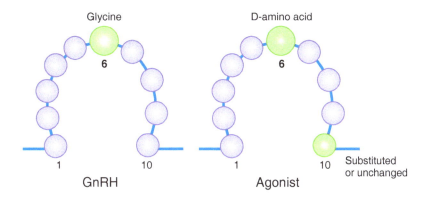

FIGURE 14.6 Schematic structure of gonadotropin-releasing hormone (GnRH) agonist relative to native GnRH.

TABLE 14.1 Clinically Available GnRH Agonists

GENERIC NAME	STRUCTURAL CHANGES RELATIVE TO NATIVE GnRH		BRAND NAME GLYCINE 10
	GLYCINE 6		
Leuprolide	D-Leu	N-ethylamine	Lupron/Eligard
Goserelin	D-Ser(t-Bu)	AzaGly-NH$_2$	Zoladex
Histrelin	D-His(Bzl)	N-ethylamine	Supprelin LA
Nafarelin	D-N-Ala(2)	Gly-NH$_2$	Synarel
Triptorelin	D-Trp	Gly-NH$_2$	Triptodur

Note: These agents share a common configuration; that is, the substitution of glycine 6 by a hydrophobic D-amino acid. In addition, glycine 10 is modified or substituted by an ethyl amide group, but this latter change is not needed for complete super-agonistic activity. Amino acids 1 to 5 need to be conserved for preservation of agonist effect.

GnRH, gonadotropin-releasing hormone.

The early GnRH antagonists cetrorelix and abarelix (no longer marketed), although effective, are now rarely used for PC because of the risk for severe systemic allergic reactions. A newer GnRH antagonist, degarelix, is not associated with systemic allergic reactions and is approved for prostate cancer in the United States. Most recently, an oral LHRH antagonist, relugolix, has also been approved for metastatic castration-sensitive PC. The GnRH antagonists prevent the initial "flare" associated with GnRH agonists.

Inhibitors of 17α-Hydroxylase/17,20-Lyase (CYP17)

Abiraterone is the only CYP17 inhibitor approved for PC therapy in the United States. Abiraterone is approved for metastatic castration-resistant PC preceding or following docetaxel chemotherapy (COU-302, COU-301 trials) as well as for metastatic castration-sensitive PC (LATTITUDE, STAMPEDE trials). Abiraterone inhibition of CYP17A1 reduces the conversion of pregnenolone and progesterone to their 17α-hydroxyl derivatives and reduces the synthesis of DHEA and androstenedione. Thus, circulating levels of testosterone drop to almost-undetectable levels after abiraterone administration. Abiraterone also has some activity as an AR antagonist and inhibitor of other steroid synthetic enzymes and CYP450s.

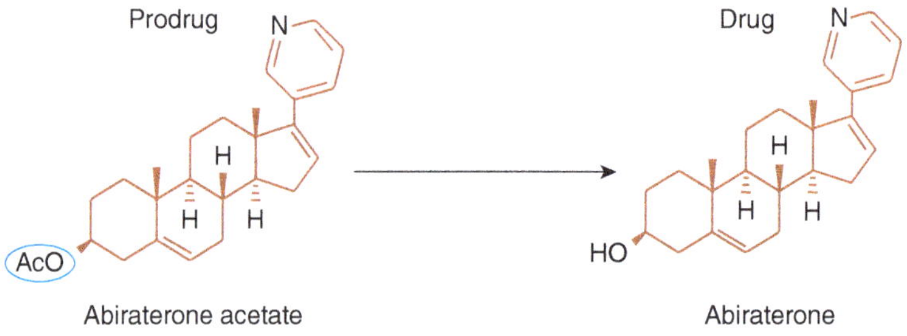

FIGURE 14.7 Chemical structures of abiraterone and its prodrug, abiraterone acetate.
Abiraterone is the active metabolite of abiraterone acetate. With continuous administration, abiraterone increases ACTH levels, resulting in mineralocorticoid excess. Oral abiraterone acetate is administered with prednisone to counteract adrenal suppression. Abiraterone should be taken on an empty stomach. Abiraterone maximum serum concentration and area under the curve are both increased more than 10-fold when a single dose of abiraterone acetate is administered after food compared to a fasted state.

Side effects include hepatotoxicity, joint swelling, hypokalemia, vasomotor symptoms, diarrhea, cough, hypertension, arrhythmia, urinary frequency, dyspepsia, and upper respiratory tract infection. Resistance to abiraterone, like enzalutamide, can occur through selection of tumor cells expressing constitutively active androgen receptor splice variants.

AR Antagonists (Antiandrogens)

AR antagonists are also used as monotherapy or in combination with LHRH agonists. Antiandrogens block both testicular and adrenal androgens and do not cause a testosterone flare and in general are well tolerated. Steroidal antiandrogens such as cyproterone acetate, medroxyprogesterone acetate, and megestrol acetate (**Figure 14.8**) preceded the development of the nonsteroidal agents for PC therapy. Indeed, the unfavorable therapeutic index of the steroidal antiandrogens led to the development and eventual replacement by the safer nonsteroidal agents (**Figure 14.8**).

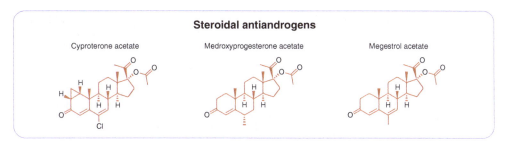

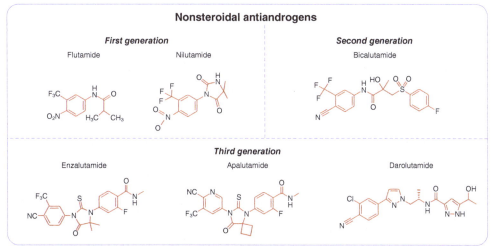

FIGURE 14.8 Chemical structures of steroidal and nonsteroidal antiandrogens. The first-generation nonsteroidal androgens, flutamide and nilutamide, were developed primarily for use in combination with castration to provide complete androgen blockade; however, only modest clinical benefits were observed with the combination of these drugs and castration compared to castration alone.

Bicalutamide, the second-generation nonsteroidal antiandrogen, with a longer half-life of 7 days compared with the first-generation antiandrogens, enabled once daily dosing and replaced flutamide and nilutamide.

With increased knowledge of androgen receptor (AR) structure and biologic functions, a new class of third-generation antiandrogens without agonistic activities has emerged, including enzalutamide, apalutamide, and darolutamide. In addition, these third-generation antiandrogens bind the AR with higher affinity, making them more efficacious than their earlier counterparts. The third-generation antiandrogens have been approved in metastatic prostate cancer and more recently also in nonmetastatic castration-resistant prostate cancer (nmCRPC) at high risk for progressing to metastatic disease.

Enzalutamide

- Enzalutamide is a synthetic nonsteroidal antiandrogen that has five- to eight fold greater binding affinity for the AR compared to bicalutamide. Like other antiandrogens, enzalutamide prevents binding of androgens to the AR and reduces binding of AR to DNA and to AR coactivator proteins. Enzalutamide can also prevent translocation of AR into the cell nucleus and induces cell apoptosis.
- Enzalutamide has improved efficacy and potency compared to older antiandrogens.
- Enzalutamide is given orally once daily with a half-life ($t_{1/2}$) of approximately 6 days. Steady-state levels are achieved in 28 days. CYP2C8 is primarily responsible for the formation of the active metabolite N-desmethyl enzalutamide.
- Enzalutamide prolongs survival of patients with metastatic castration-resistant PC (CRPC) when given in the chemotherapy naïve setting or after docetaxel therapy (PREVAIL, AFFIRM trials). It has also shown a survival benefit when combined with ADT in metastatic castration-sensitive PC (CSPC; ENZAMET, ARCHES trials). Among men with nonmetastatic CRPC at high risk for developing metastasis (such as those with relatively short PSA doubling times), enzalutamide treatment has shown a clinically meaningful and significant ~70% lower risk of metastatic progression or death compared to placebo (PROSPER trial).
- Like other antiandrogens, enzalutamide has negative effects on sexual function. Other notable side effects include gynecomastia, breast pain, fatigue, diarrhea, headache, and hot flashes. Enzalutamide crosses the blood–brain barrier, and seizures occur infrequently in approximately 1% or fewer patients. Resistance to AR inhibitors can develop through mechanisms such as gene rearrangement, mutation, and acquired AR splice variants.

Apalutamide

- Apalutamide emerged from the same class of compounds as enzalutamide. Although it has similar in vitro activity like enzalutamide, its in vivo efficacy in PC xenograft models is superior.
- Apalutamide was approved in 2018 by the FDA based on the success of Phase 3 clinical studies in men with nonmetastatic CRPC (SPARTAN trial). The data showed significantly longer metastases-free survival for apalutamide than for placebo (40.5 vs. 16.2 months, hazard ratio 0.28, 95% CI 0.23–0.35, $p <.0001$).
- Apalutamide was evaluated in metastatic CSPC in combination with ADT; specifically, ADT plus apalutamide was compared to ADT plus placebo in the Phase 3 setting (TITAN trial). The trial met its primary endpoints of radiographic progression-free survival (rPFS) and overall survival (OS). The final analysis of the trial confirmed that despite crossover, apalutamide plus ADT improved OS, delayed castration resistance, maintained health-related quality of life, and had a consistent safety profile in a broad population of patients with metastatic CSPC.

Darolutamide

- Darolutamide is another third-generation antiandrogen, but it has a different chemical structure than apalutamide and enzalutamide, which may explain why it has fewer side effects, including low penetration of the blood–brain barrier.

- Darolutamide significantly improves metastasis-free survival in men with nonmetastatic CRPC, according to a randomized, double-blind, placebo-controlled Phase 3 trial (ARAMIS trial). The trial population comprised 1,509 men with nonmetastatic CRPC with a PSA doubling time of 10 months or less. The trial showed that median metastasis-free survival was 40.4 months in the darolutamide group and 18.4 months in the placebo group (hazard ratio 0.41, 95% CI 0.34–0.50; $p <.001$). Further, darolutamide maintained health-related quality of life by significantly delaying time to deterioration of PC-specific quality of life and disease-related symptoms versus placebo.
- Darolutamide has also been evaluated in the metastatic CSPC setting; specifically, patients received ADT plus docetaxel with or without darolutamide, with primary endpoint being OS (ARASENS trial). The trial met its primary endpoint: adding darolutamide to ADT plus docetaxel improved OS.

CHAPTER SUMMARY

Clearly, significant progress has been achieved in the development of a variety of prostate cancer drug targeting androgen biosynthesis and androgen receptor signaling. In this chapter, we have highlighted all the major clinically used antihormonal prostate cancer drugs, including their advantages and disadvantages. We anticipate that this information will be utilized to select the most appropriate drug(s) to improve the survival and quality of life of patients with prostate cancer.

CLINICAL PEARLS

- Medical or surgical androgen deprivation therapy (ADT) decreases bone mineral density and increases the risk of bone fractures in men with prostate cancer. Daily calcium and vitamin D for all men receiving ADT is recommended.
- Continuous ADT is preferred compared with intermittent androgen deprivation (IAD). This is based on the results from the Intergroup Trial INT 0162 (NCT00002651), which compared intermittent androgen deprivation with continuous ADT for its effect on overall survival (OS) and patient reported outcomes in metastatic hormone-sensitive PC and a serum PSA ≥5 ng/mL. The OS was longer with continuous ADT than with intermittent androgen deprivation (median 5.8 vs. 5.1 years, hazard ratio 1.10, 95% CI 0.99–1.23).
- High-risk or high-volume metastatic hormone-sensitive prostate cancer should be treated with ADT combined with docetaxel or abiraterone rather than ADT alone.
- Adverse events of ADT are (a) sexual dysfunction including loss of libido and erectile dysfunction, (b) osteoporosis and bone fracture, (c) vasomotor symptoms including hot flashes, (d) changes in body composition including loss of lean body mass, increased body fat, and decreased muscle strength, (e) changes in body image including gynecomastia and decreased penile and testicular size, (f) cardiovascular events including venous thromboembolism, arterial embolism, and myocardial infarction, (g) acute kidney injury, (h) anemia, (i) fatigue, and (j) emotional and cognitive changes.

ACKNOWLEDGMENTS

The work was supported in part by the Maryland Department of Health's Cigarette Restitution Fund Program, and the National Cancer Institute Cancer Center Support Grant (CCSG) P30CA134274.

Part of VN's time was supported by the National Cancer Institute of the National Institute of Health under Award Number R01CA22469.

Part of AH's time was supported by a Merit Review Award (I01 BX000545), Medical Research Service, Department of Veterans Affairs, and a Prostate Cancer Foundation (PCF) Precision Oncology Program-Cancer of Prostate (POP CaP) Award #21PILO02.

Multiple-choice questions were created by Professor Ashkan Emadi.

MULTIPLE-CHOICE QUESTIONS

1. A 59-year-old man with no past medical history presents to the ED with severe bone pain and inability to urinate. MRI scan shows several lytic lesions in the ribs, vertebrae, and femur, without evidence of spinal cord compression, but with a significantly enlarged prostate. PSA is 340 ng/mL. What is the best next step for him after performing prostate or bone lesion biopsy?

   A. Radium-223 or strontium-89 or samarium-153
   B. Bicalutamide for 1 week and then leuprolide depot injection
   C. Degarelix
   D. Radical prostatectomy followed by radiation therapy
   E. Docetaxel + prednisone

2. A 55-year-old primary care physician is diagnosed with metastatic prostate cancer. He has read the literature on the clinical outcome of androgen deprivation therapy (ADT) and has some questions. What do you recommend to him and why?

   A. Abiraterone plus ADT, because it has demonstrated a survival advantage for patients with metastatic high-risk castration-sensitive prostate cancer
   B. Either enzalutamide or apalutamide plus ADT, because they have demonstrated improvement in survival in patients with metastatic castration-resistant prostate cancer
   C. Intermittent ADT, because it has shown some benefit with erectile dysfunction and mental health
   D. Bone density measurement every 5 years while on chronic ADT, to diagnose early osteoporosis
   E. Vitamin D 50,000 IU every other week, to prevent bone fracture

3. A 61-year-old man with no significant past medical history presents with back pain. Imaging shows an enlarged prostate and pelvic lymph nodes as well as sclerotic lesions in most of his lumbar spines. His PSA is 180 ng/mL. Biopsy proves prostate adenocarcinoma with Gleason score 8. He has been on flutamide for 2 weeks. What is the best next step?

    A. Add leuprolide
    B. Add leuprolide + prednisone
    C. Add leuprolide + six cycles of docetaxel
    D. Add leuprolide + definitive radiation therapy
    E. Add leuprolide + high-dose finasteride

4. A 71-year-old man with a history of hypertension, hyperlipidemia, and osteoarthritis had been diagnosed with Gleason 8 adenocarcinoma of the prostate with unremarkable CT scan of the abdomen and pelvis. After initial local therapy, he has been taking a GnRH agonist along with bicalutamide. After 13 months, his PSA is now increased to a value of 4.6 ng/mL. He feels well and had no urinary or musculoskeletal symptoms. What is the best next step in management of this patient?

    A. Continue ADT and add docetaxel and prednisone
    B. Add alpha particle emitting agent radium-223
    C. Discontinue bicalutamide
    D. Switch bicalutamide to darolutamide
    E. Add megestrol acetate

5. A mother of a 16-year-old person brings her child with medical history of obesity and diabetes to an oncologist who was referred by the primary care physician. She read on the internet that nafarelin can be used for treatment of prostate cancer. She has several questions and asks about other indications/off-label use of the agent for adolescent/young adult individuals. For which of the following conditions should nafarelin not be prescribed?

    A. Diabetes
    B. Early onset puberty
    C. Uterine fibroids
    D. Endometriosis
    E. Control of ovarian stimulation in in vitro fertilization

6. A 74-year-old man with medical history of hypertension, osteoarthritis, mild cognitive disorder, and hyperlipidemia comes with his family to a genitourinary-focused oncology clinic to discuss the use of enzalutamide for his prostate cancer. His family members are concerned about the adverse events of enzalutamide and particularly with interactions with medications he is currently taking for his other comorbid conditions. What is the best explanation about the pharmacology or clinical benefit of enzalutamide?

    A. At the recommended dosage, enzalutamide causes >20 msec prolongation in the QT interval.
    B. The favorable efficacy of enzalutamide in more than 5,700 patients with castration-resistant prostate cancers (CRPC) or metastatic castration-sensitive

prostate cancer (mCSPC) was demonstrated in five randomized multicenter clinical trials.

C. Enzalutamide is mainly metabolized by aldehyde dehydrogenase; hence, it should not be taken with alcoholic beverages simultaneously.

D. To prevent seizure, patients who are to be treated with enzalutamide should be treated with antiepileptic medications (e.g., levetiracetam [Keppra]) 2 weeks before initiation of enzalutamide.

E. A ~1:1 exposure-response relationship for the efficacy endpoint of overall survival as well as for adverse effects has been observed in patients with prostate cancer who have been treated with enzalutamide.

7. A 66-year-old man with hormone-refractory metastatic prostate cancer measurable by RECIST criteria as well as with rising PSA levels and several new lesions and ECOG (Eastern Cooperative Oncology Group) performance status of 0, who was previously treated with a docetaxel-containing treatment regimen, presents to discuss further chemotherapy options. Patient's neutrophil count is 2,130/μL, platelets 243,000/μL, hemoglobin 10.5 g/dL, creatinine 1.1 × upper limit of normal (ULN), and normal total bilirubin, aspartate transferase (AST), and alanine transferase (ALT). Patient does not have a history of congestive heart failure or myocardial infarction within the last 6 months. He also does not have current or history of uncontrolled cardiac arrhythmias or hypertension. What chemotherapy option has shown clinical benefit in his condition?

A. Mitoxantrone 12 mg/m^2 intravenously every 3 weeks for 10 cycles with prednisone 10 mg orally daily for 10 cycles

B. Carboplatin 300 mg/m^2 intravenously on day 1 every 4 weeks for six cycles

C. Liposomal doxorubicin 20 mg/m^2 intravenously on day 1 every 3 weeks for six cycles

D. Cabazitaxel 20 mg/m^2 intravenously every 3 weeks with prednisone 10 mg orally daily for 10 cycles

8. A 59-year-old man is diagnosed with metastatic high-risk castration-sensitive prostate cancer. His oncologist plan to start him on abiraterone acetate 1,000 mg orally once daily with prednisone 5 mg orally once daily. The patient and his wife have questions on how to take abiraterone acetate with food. What does the physician should recommend?

A. Do not eat food 2 hours before and 1 hour after taking abiraterone and swallow the tablets whole with water.

B. Eat abiraterone with fatty food to increase its gastrointestinal absorption.

C. Eat abiraterone with fatty food to decrease hepatotoxicity.

D. Start sliding scale insulin to avoid severe hyperglycemia and hyperosmolar coma associated with abiraterone.

E. Avoid foods with high potassium content.

9. Which of the following drugs used in the treatment of prostate cancer has a similar mechanism of action compared with leuprolide?

    A. Samarium-153
    B. Bicalutamide
    C. Degarelix
    D. Histrelin
    E. Docetaxel

10. A 65-year-old man who works in the local university as a professor of pharmacology is diagnosed with metastatic prostate cancer. He and his oncologist discuss treatment initiation with goserelin implant either monthly (3.6 mg subcutaneously every 28 days) or every 3 months (10.8 mg subcutaneously every 12 weeks). The patient is interested in knowing his plasma testosterone level in the first 4–5 weeks after initiation of the therapy and when he should expect to reach to the castration threshold level of <0.5 ng/mL plasma testosterone. Which of the following graphs accurately describes the pharmacology of goserelin with respect to plasma testosterone level?

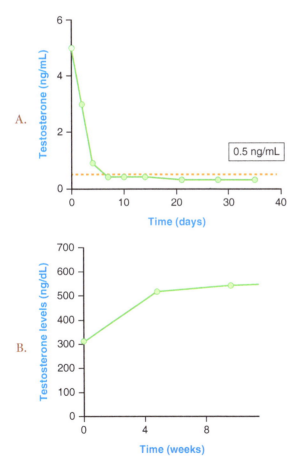

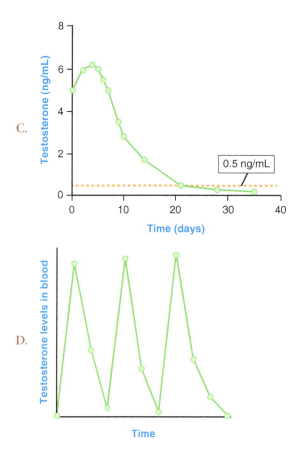

C.

D.

1. **C.** Degarelix is a GnRH antagonist that does not cause an initial release of LH, suppresses testosterone production, and avoids the androgen flare observed with GnRH agonists. Degarelix is useful when an immediate decrease in testosterone levels is desired.

2. **A.** Two large randomized clinical trials (LATITUDE and STAMPEDE trials) have demonstrated that the combination of ADT plus abiraterone significantly prolongs overall survival and secondary endpoints in patients with castration-sensitive prostate cancer. Two randomized trials (ENZAMET and TITAN trials) have shown benefit for either enzalutamide or apalutamide plus ADT over ADT alone for metastatic castration-sensitive (not resistant) prostate cancer. As it is explained in the Clinical Pearls section, continuous ADT is preferred compared with intermittent androgen deprivation (IAD). Baseline and periodic (every 2–3 years) measurement of bone density is recommended for men receiving ADT to detect and manage early osteoporosis. The recommended doses of supplemental vitamin D is 800 to 1,000 IU daily.

3. **C.** In three randomized trials (CHAARTED, STAMPEDE, and GETUG-AFU 15 trials), the combination of docetaxel plus ADT increased overall survival compared with ADT alone. High-risk or high-volume castration-sensitive metastatic prostate cancer should be treated with docetaxel plus ADT.

4. **C.** Approximately 15% to 20% of patients with prostate cancer may show a clinical or biochemical response after discontinuation of treatment with an antiandrogen. The majority of these responses are brief.

5. **A.** Nafarelin is a nasal spray (administered two or three times a day) GnRH agonist that is used in the treatment of endometriosis, uterine fibroids, and early puberty; in transgender hormone therapy; and in controlling ovarian stimulation in in vitro fertilization (IVF). Regulatory authorities have been evaluating whether GnRH agonists may increase the risk of diabetes and cardiovascular diseases (e.g., myocardial infarction, sudden cardiac death, stroke) in men receiving GnRH agonists (e.g., leuprolide acetate, goserelin acetate, triptorelin pamoate, histrelin acetate, nafarelin acetate) for the treatment of prostate cancer.

6. **B.** The clinical efficacy (including overall survival and progression-free survial) of enzalutamide was demonstrated in five randomized multicenter clinical trials, as explained in the FDA label of enzalutamide. Enzalutamide is metabolized by CYP2C8 and CYP3A4. The most common adverse reactions (≥10%) that occurred more frequently in the enzalutamide-treated patients were asthenia/fatigue, back pain, hot flushes, constipation, arthralgia, decreased appetite, diarrhea, and hypertension. Seizure occurred in <1% of patients after treatment with enzalutamide. Falls and fractures occurred in ~10% of patients treated with enzalutamide. No exposure-response relationship for the efficacy endpoint of overall survival was identified after once daily dosing of 160 mg enzalutamide. Additionally, no clinically meaningful exposure-response relationship for adverse events (e.g., fatigue, flushing, headache, or hypertension) was observed after exposure to 160 mg/day of enzalutamide.

7. **D.** Cabazitaxel is a microtubule inhibitor indicated in combination with prednisone for treatment of patients with metastatic castration-resistant prostate cancer (mCRPC) previously treated with a docetaxel-containing treatment regimen. In patients with mCRPC, overall survival (OS) was statistically significantly improved with cabazitaxel (median OS 15.1 months) versus mitoxantrone (median OS 12.7 months) after prior docetaxel treatment. Common adverse effects of cabazitaxel are neutropenia (including febrile neutropenia) and diarrhea.

8. **A.** Patients who are taking abiraterone should not eat food 2 hours before and 1 hour after taking the medication and the tablets must be swallowed whole with water. In patients who are taking abiraterone, severe hypoglycemia has been reported in patients with preexisting diabetes who are taking medications containing thiazolidinediones. Blood glucose in patients with diabetes should be monitored and antidiabetic agent dosages should be modified if clinically indicated. In the combined data from four placebo-controlled trials using prednisone 5 mg twice daily in combination with 1,000 mg abiraterone acetate daily, grades 3–4 hypokalemia were detected in 4% of patients on the abiraterone arm and 2% of patients on the placebo arm. In a randomized placebo-controlled, multicenter clinical trial (LATITUDE study), prednisone 5 mg daily in combination with 1,000 mg abiraterone acetate daily was used and grades 3–4 hypokalemia were reported in 10% of patients on the abiraterone group and 1%

of patients on the placebo group. In patients who are receiving abiraterone, increases in blood pressure, hypokalemia, or fluid retention should be monitored closely. In postmarketing reports, QT prolongation and torsades de pointes have been reported in patients who develop hypokalemia while taking abiraterone.

9. **D.** The currently available GnRH agonists (and the year of approval in the United States) include leuprolide (also called leuprorelin and Lupron; 1985), goserelin (also called Zoladex; 1989), histrelin (also called Supprelin and Vantas; 1991 and 2004), and triptorelin (also called Trelstar; 2000). Degarelix (also called Firmagon; 2008) is a GnRH antagonist.

10. **C.** Figure A depicts testosterone level over time under therapy with GnRH antagonists with no initial flare after treatment. Figure B represents testosterone time course under therapy with androgen receptor (AR) antagonists. Figure C illustrates testosterone level over time under therapy with GnRH agonist such as goserelin with initial flare, which is recommended to administer concomitant therapy with AR antagonists within the first 3 weeks. Figure D shows blood testosterone levels with bipolar androgen therapy (BAT) designed to work against castration-resistant prostate cancer by coadministering ADT and high doses of testosterone to rapidly achieve a supraphysiologic level of testosterone in the blood in order to hamper the ability of cancer cells to adapt.

SELECTED REFERENCES

Abida W, Patnaik A, Campbell D, et al. Rucaparib in men with metastatic castration-resistant prostate cancer harboring a BRCA1 or BRCA2 gene alteration. J Clin Oncol. 2020;38(32):3763–72. https://doi.org/10.1200/JCO.20.01035

Antonarakis ES, Lu C, Wang H, et al. AR-V7 and resistance to enzalutamide and abiraterone in prostate cancer. N Engl J Med. 2014;371(11):1028–38. https://doi.org/10.1056/NEJMoa1315815

Armstrong AJ, Azad AA, Iguchi T, et al. Improved survival with enzalutamide in patients with metastatic hormone-sensitive prostate cancer. J Clin Oncol. 2022;40(15):1616–22. https://doi.org/10.1200/JCO.22.00193

Auchus RJ. The backdoor pathway to dihydrotestosterone. Trends Endocrinol Metab. 2004;15(9):432–8. https://doi.org/10.1016/j.tem.2004.09.004

Beer TM, Armstrong AJ, Rathkopf DE, et al. Enzalutamide in metastatic prostate cancer before chemotherapy. N Engl J Med. 2014;371(5):424–33. https://doi.org/10.1056/NEJMoa1405095

Boddy JL, Fox SB, Han C, et al. The androgen receptor is significantly associated with vascular endothelial growth factor and hypoxia sensing via hypoxia-inducible factors HIF-1a, HIF-2a, and the prolyl hydroxylases in human prostate cancer. Clin Cancer Res. 2005;11(21):7658–63. https://doi.org/10.1158/1078-0432.CCR-05-0460

Burki T. Darolutamide for non-metastatic, castration-resistant prostate cancer. Lancet Oncol. 2019;20(3):e139. https://doi.org/10.1016/S1470-2045(19)30102-0

Chi KN, Agarwal N, Bjartell A, et al. Apalutamide for metastatic, castration-sensitive prostate cancer. N Engl J Med. 2019;381(1):13–24. https://doi.org/10.1056/NEJMoa1903307

Chi KN, Chowdhury S, Bjartell A, et al. Apalutamide in patients with metastatic castration-sensitive prostate cancer: Final survival analysis of the randomized, double-blind, phase III TITAN study. J Clin Oncol. 2021;39(20):2294–303. https://doi.org/10.1200/JCO.20.03488

Davis ID, Martin AJ, Stockler MR, et al. Enzalutamide with standard first-line therapy in metastatic prostate cancer. N Engl J Med. 2019;381(2):121–31. https://doi.org/10.1056/NEJMoa1903835

de Bono JS, Logothetis CJ, Molina A, et al. Abiraterone and increased survival in metastatic prostate cancer. N Engl J Med. 2011;364(21):1995–2005. https://doi.org/10.1056/NEJMoa1014618

Dehm SM, Tindall DJ. Regulation of androgen receptor signaling in prostate cancer. Expert Rev Anticancer Ther. 2005;5(1):63–74. https://doi.org/10.1586/14737140.5.1.63

Edwards J, Bartlett JM. The androgen receptor and signal-transduction pathways in hormone-refractory prostate cancer. Part 1: Modifications to the androgen receptor. BJU Int. 2005;95(9):1320–6. https://doi.org/10.1111/j.1464-410X.2005.05526.x

Evans RM. The steroid and thyroid hormone receptor superfamily. Science. 1988;240(4854):889–95. https://doi.org/10.1126/science.3283939

Fizazi K, Shore N, Tammela TL, et al. Darolutamide in nonmetastatic, castration-resistant prostate cancer. N Engl J Med. 2019;380(13):1235–46. https://doi.org/10.1056/NEJMoa1815671

Fizazi K, Tran N, Fein L, et al. Abiraterone plus prednisone in metastatic, castration-sensitive prostate cancer. N Engl J Med. 2017;377(4):352–60. https://doi.org/10.1056/NEJMoa1704174

Gillessen S, Attard G, Beer TM, et al. Management of patients with advanced prostate cancer: The report of the advanced prostate cancer consensus conference APCCC 2017. Eur Urol. 2018;73(2):178–211. https://doi.org/10.1016/j.eururo.2017.06.002

Gomella LG. Prostate cancer statistics: Anything you want them to be. Can J Urol. 2017;24(1):8603–4.

Huggins C, Hodges CV. Studies on prostatic cancer. I. The effect of castration, of estrogen and of androgen injection on serum phosphatases in metastatic carcinoma of the prostate. 1941. J Urol. 2002;167:948–51.

Hussain M, Fizazi K, Saad F, et al. Enzalutamide in men with nonmetastatic, castration-resistant prostate cancer. N Engl J Med. 2018;378(26):2465–74. https://doi.org/10.1056/NEJMoa1800536

Hussain M, Mateo J, Fizazi K, et al. Survival with olaparib in metastatic castration-resistant prostate cancer. N Engl J Med. 2020;383(24):2345–57. https://doi.org/10.1056/NEJMoa2022485

James ND, de Bono JS, Spears MR, et al. Abiraterone for prostate cancer not previously treated with hormone therapy. N Engl J Med. 2017;377(4):338–51. https://doi.org/10.1056/NEJMoa1702900

Labrie F. Blockade of testicular and adrenal androgens in prostate cancer treatment. Nat Rev Urol. 2011;8(2):73–85. https://doi.org/10.1038/nrurol.2010.231

Li Y, Chan SC, Brand LJ, et al. Androgen receptor splice variants mediate enzalutamide resistance in castration-resistant prostate cancer cell lines. Cancer Res. 2013;73(2):483–9. https://doi.org/10.1158/0008-5472.CAN-12-3630

Manning G, Whyte DB, Martinez R, et al. The protein kinase complement of the human genome. Science. 2002;298(5600):1912–34. https://doi.org/10.1126/science.1075762

Moul JW. Utility of LHRH antagonists for advanced prostate cancer. Can J Urol. 2014;21(2 Supp 1):22–7.

Parker C, Nilsson S, Heinrich D, et al. Alpha emitter radium-223 and survival in metastatic prostate cancer. N Engl J Med. 2013;369(3):213–23. https://doi.org/10.1056/NEJMoa1213755

Pratt WB, Toft DO. Steroid receptor interactions with heat shock protein and immunophilin chaperones. Endocr Rev. 1997;18(3):306–60. https://doi.org/10.1210/edrv.18.3.0303

Ryan CJ, Smith MR, de Bono JS, et al. Abiraterone in metastatic prostate cancer without previous chemotherapy. N Engl J Med. 2013;368(2):138–48. https://doi.org/10.1056/NEJMoa1209096

Ryan CJ, Smith MR, Fizazi K, et al. Abiraterone acetate plus prednisone versus placebo plus prednisone in chemotherapy-naive men with metastatic castration-resistant prostate cancer (COU-AA-302): Final overall survival analysis of a randomised, double-blind, placebo-controlled phase 3 study. Lancet Oncol. 2015;16(2):152–60. https://doi.org/10.1016/S1470-2045(14)71205-7

Sartor O, de Bono J, Chi KN, et al. Lutetium-177-PSMA-617 for metastatic castration-resistant prostate cancer. N Engl J Med. 2021;385(12):1091–103. https://doi.org/10.1056/NEJMoa2107322

Scher HI, Fizazi K, Saad F, et al. Increased survival with enzalutamide in prostate cancer after chemotherapy. N Engl J Med. 2012;367(13):1187–97. https://doi.org/10.1056/NEJMoa1207506

Shore ND, Saad F, Cookson MS, et al. Oral relugolix for androgen-deprivation therapy in advanced prostate cancer. N Engl J Med. 2020;382(23):2187–96. https://doi.org/10.1056/NEJMoa2004325

Smith MR, Hussain M, Saad F, et al. Darolutamide and survival in metastatic, hormone-sensitive prostate cancer. N Engl J Med. 2022;386(12):1132–42. https://doi.org/10.1056/NEJMoa2119115

Smith MR, Saad F, Chowdhury S, et al. Apalutamide treatment and metastasis-free survival in prostate cancer. N Engl J Med. 2018;378(15):1408–18. https://doi.org/10.1056/NEJMoa1715546

Smith MR, Shore N, Tammela TL, et al. Darolutamide and health-related quality of life in patients with non-metastatic castration-resistant prostate cancer: An analysis of the phase III ARAMIS trial. Eur J Cancer. 2021;154:138–46. https://doi.org/10.1016/j.ejca.2021.06.010

Sugawara T, Baumgart SJ, Nevedomskaya E, et al. Darolutamide is a potent androgen receptor antagonist with strong efficacy in prostate cancer models. Int J Cancer. 2019;145(5):1382–94. https://doi.org/10.1002/ijc.32242

Teutonico D, Montanari S, Ponchel G. Leuprolide acetate: Pharmaceutical use and delivery potentials. Expert Opin Drug Deliv. 2012;9(3):343–54. https://doi.org/10.1517/17425247.2012.662484

Tolis G, Ackman D, Stellos A, et al. Tumor growth inhibition in patients with prostatic carcinoma treated with luteinizing hormone-releasing hormone agonists. Proc Natl Acad Sci U S A. 1982;79(5):1658–62. https://doi.org/10.1073/pnas.79.5.1658

Tran C, Ouk S, Clegg NJ, et al. Development of a second-generation antiandrogen for treatment of advanced prostate cancer. Science. 2009;324(5928):787–90. https://doi.org/10.1126/science.1168175

Vasaitis TS, Bruno RD, Njar VC. CYP17 inhibitors for prostate cancer therapy. J Steroid Biochem Mol Biol. 2011;125(1–2):23–31. https://doi.org/10.1016/j.jsbmb.2010.11.005

CHAPTER 15

Multiple Myeloma as a Paradigm for Multi-Targeted Intervention

KATHRYN MAPLES ● **SAGAR LONIAL**

INTRODUCTION

Multiple myeloma (MM) is the second most common hematologic malignancy in the United States; it is characterized by uncontrolled plasma cell proliferation, osteolytic bone lesions, and immunodeficiency. Developing from two precursor states, including monoclonal gammopathy of undetermined significance (MGUS) and smoldering multiple myeloma (SMM), data estimated approximately 34,920 new cases of MM in 2021, with 12,410 deaths. Significant advancements in the treatment of MM have occurred over the last decade, with the U.S. Food and Drug Administration (FDA) approving 12 new agents during this period, which has led to deeper and more durable responses. Despite these improvements, this malignancy remains incurable, largely due to the development of drug resistance, and the need for novel treatment regimens remains critical. Selecting the optimal treatment regimen at diagnosis and at relapse remains a challenge as numerous monotherapy and combination therapies have gained approved and inclusion in national guidelines. Here, we review different classes of myeloma-directed therapy and important clinical considerations when selecting a multi-targeted intervention.

INITIAL THERAPY

The initial treatment decision largely depends upon the patient's eligibility for autologous stem cell transplant (ASCT), which is determined by the patient's age, comorbidities, and performance status. The standard approach for a transplant-eligible patient includes induction therapy with a three- or four-drug regimen for four to six cycles, followed by high-dose chemotherapy and ASCT, followed by consolidation and maintenance therapy. For transplant-ineligible patients, induction therapy may constitute a two- or three-drug regimen that lasts for 12 to 18 months followed by maintenance therapy. In recent years, it has become evident that disease characteristics, such as high-risk cytogenetics, should also be considered when selecting a frontline regimen and many centers are developing a risk-stratified approach to induction therapy. This modernized overall approach to induction therapy in patients with newly diagnosed MM is shown in **Figure 15.1**, and induction regimens consist

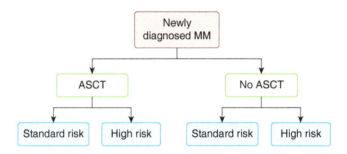

FIGURE 15.1 Novel approach to newly diagnosed treatment selection.
This diagram illustrates the movement toward a risk-stratified approach to induction therapy for MM. The regimen selected may differ in each of the four categories.

ASCT, autologous stem cell transplant; MM, multiple myeloma.

of immunomodulatory agents, proteasome inhibitors, and corticosteroids, with the recent addition of daratumumab.

IMMUNOMODULATORY AGENTS

Immunomodulatory drugs (IMiDs) have become a critical backbone in the treatment of MM over the last decade. The first-generation IMiD, thalidomide, was originally utilized not for MM, but rather for the treatment of hyperemesis gravidarum in the late 1950s. However, this ended with the eventual ban of thalidomide because it was found to cause phocomelia (birth with partial or complete absence of limbs) in thousands of babies. Years later, the anti-tumor necrosis factor (anti-TNF) and angiogenic properties of this drug were noted in leprosy patients followed by its discovery of antimyeloma activity. The exact mechanism of action (MOA) of the IMiDs was not always well understood but is thought to be multifactorial including direct cytotoxicity, antiangiogenic activity, increasing natural killer (NK) T cell activity, T cell modulating activity, and inhibition of proinflammatory cytokines, depicted in Figure 15.2. We have now learned that the IMiDs are largely believed to work by binding to cereblon, a subunit of ubiquitin ligase that eventually leads to ubiquitination and proteasomal degradation of essential transcription factors in plasma cell function and survival such as Ikaros and Aiolos (IKZF1 and IKZF3, respectively). Today, in addition to thalidomide, we now have the second- and third-generation IMiDs, lenalidomide (Revlimid) and pomalidomide (Pomalyst).

As a drug class, IMiDs cause an increased risk for embryo-fetal toxicity, venous thromboembolism (VTE), and a risk for secondary malignancies. Due to the embryo-fetal toxicity, all three IMiDs have a Risk Evaluation and Mitigation Strategy (REMS) program, which requires females of childbearing age to have a negative pregnancy test prior to each new prescription and both male and female patients must complete a survey acknowledging the risk associated with the therapy before the medication can be dispensed from the pharmacy. The VTE risk with IMiDs can be further increased in the setting of high-dose dexamethasone, and there are two scoring systems, the IMPEDE and the SAVED scores, that can assist with identifying an individual patient's risk for VTE. At a minimum, all patients on an IMiD need to be on aspirin

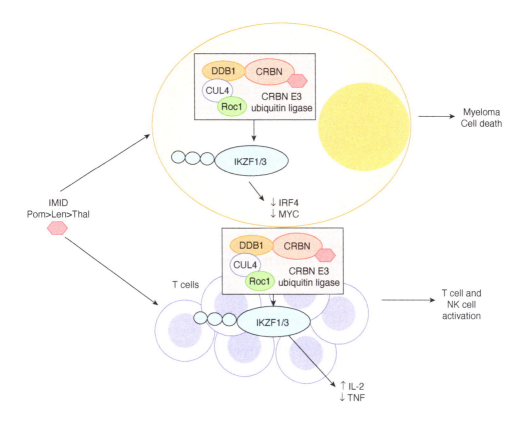

FIGURE 15.2 **Differential effects of IMiDs on myeloma cells as well as T cells and NK cells.**

The multifactorial mechanisms of action of the IMiDs. These agents with bind to cereblon, a subunit of ubiquitin ligase that eventually leads to ubiquitination, proteasomal degradatdon, T cell and NK activation and expansion, and MM cell death.

CRBN, cereblon; DDB1, damaged DNA binding protein 1; IKZF, Ikaros Zinc Finger family; IL, interleukin; IMiD, immunomodulatory drug; IRF4, interferon regulatory factor 4; NK, natural killer; Roc1, regulator of cullins 1; TNF, tumor necrosis factor.

prophylaxis, and the oral anticoagulants (e.g., apixaban and rivaroxaban) can be used at prophylaxis and treatment doses if indicated. The risk for developing a secondary malignancy is mostly documented with lenalidomide following high-dose melphalan, but practitioners may want to avoid the IMiD class in someone with a significant history of other malignancies.

Despite similarities in their structure (**Figure 15.3**) and the overlapping class effects, these three IMiDs do have some distinct properties and adverse effects. First, thalidomide and pomalidomide do not require dose adjustments in patients with impaired renal functions; however, 82% of lenalidomide is excreted as unchanged drug in the urine, which precipitates the need for dose adjustments in patients with impaired kidney functions. Thalidomide has significantly less myelosuppressive potential compared to lenalidomide and pomalidomide, which makes it an attractive option for a patient who has underlying cytopenias. Nevertheless, thalidomide is also associated with much higher rates of peripheral neuropathy and sedation and since these agents are often combined with bortezomib, the neuropathy associated with thalidomide can be limiting. Lenalidomide and pomalidomide commonly

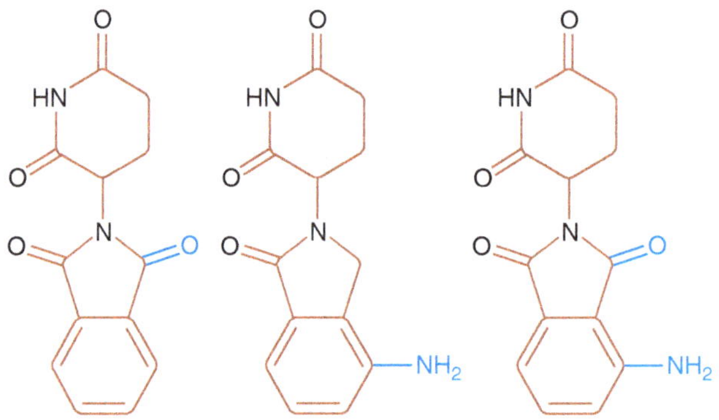

Thalidomide   Lenalidomide   Pomalidomide

FIGURE 15.3 Immunomodulatory drugs (IMiDs) molecular structure.
Three FDA-approved IMiDs are shown here. Despite the structural similarities and overlapping class effects, each agent has unique characteristics.

FDA, U.S. Food and Drug Administration.

cause myelosuppression and despite their inherent immunostimulatory properties, they do increase infection risk. Skin rash can occur with all three IMiDs but is most commonly seen with lenalidomide and may require a topical steroid cream if the rash is large and/or pruritic. Additionally, lenalidomide-induced diarrhea has been shown to be a result of bile acid malabsorption, so utilizing bile acid sequestrants such as colestipol or cholestyramine can significantly improve the diarrhea burden.

Although not widely used in the United States, thalidomide has indications for newly diagnosed and relapsed refractory MM (RRMM). Lenalidomide is the most common IMiD utilized in induction regimens, is critical in maintenance therapy, and also has indications for RRMM. Pomalidomide is currently only being utilized in the RRMM setting. Next-generation IMiDs, including iberdomide (CC-220) and mezigdomide (CC-92480), are currently under investigation and have activity in pomalidomide-refractory disease. Iberdomide and mezigdomide are oral agents that are structurally similar to the currently available IMiDs; however, these novel cereblon modulators (CELMoDs) bind to cereblon with higher affinity than lenalidomide or pomalidomide. Iberdomide in combination with dexamethasone proved to be an effective and safe regimen in heavily pretreated MM patients, which led to current investigations in a variety of different combinations for MM. Additionally, iberdomide is being investigated as monotherapy and in combination with dexamethasone for high-risk smoldering MM patients. Mezigdomide in combination with bortezomib and dexamethasone showed encouraging preliminary response rates including in patients with extramedullary disease. The complete adverse effect profile of these agents will be further answered in these ongoing trials.

PROTEASOME INHIBITORS

The multi-targeted intervention approach in MM is rooted in combining agents from different drug classes with unique mechanisms of action. The most commonly combined drugs

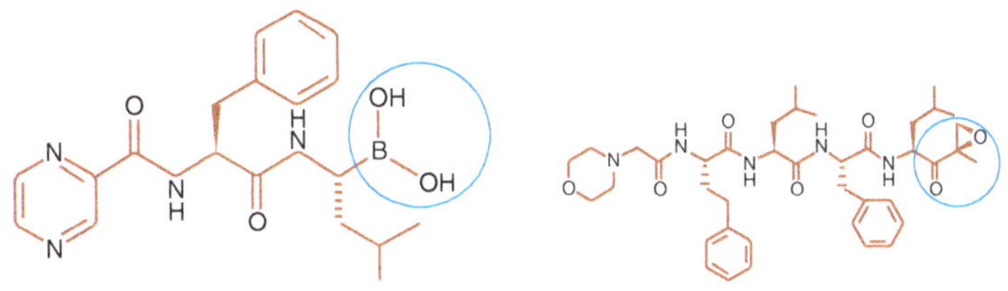

FIGURE 15.4 Proteasome inhibitor molecular structure.
Examples of boronic acid (left, bortezomib) and epoxyketone (right, carfilzomib) proteasome inhibitors. Circles indicate the boron (left) and epoxyketone (right) moieties.

for induction treatment include the IMiDs and proteasome inhibitors (PIs). Proteasomes are enzyme complexes within MM cells that are responsible for regulating protein homeostasis. Proteasome inhibitors will either reversibly or irreversibly inhibit the ubiquitin proteasome pathway, which leads to decreased protein degradation, activation of signaling cascades, cell-cycle arrest, and apoptosis. Clinically relevant PIs can be grouped into two major groups based on whether or not they carry a boron atom or epoxyketone moiety in their chemical structure (Figure 15.4). Boronic acid derivatives such as bortezomib (Velcade) and ixazomib (Ninlaro) inhibit the proteasome in a reversible manner, whereas the epoxyketone derivative carfilzomib (Kyprolis) demonstrates irreversible inhibition. As a drug class, all PIs increase the risk for herpes (zoster and simplex) reactivation, so all patients on a PI-containing regimen need to be on herpes simplex virus/varicella zoster virus (HSV/VZV) prophylaxis with an agent like acyclovir or valacyclovir for the entire duration of therapy and for at least 3 months after.

Bortezomib was the first-in-class PI to be approved in 2003 and it specifically blocks chymotrypsin-like activity at the 26S proteasome. The dose-limiting adverse effect of bortezomib is neuropathy, which most commonly presents as peripheral neuropathy (numbness, tingling, pins-and-needles sensation) in the hands and feet, but can also cause autonomic neuropathy. Bortezomib was originally administered as an intravenous (IV) infusion, but a subcutaneous (SC) formulation was later developed. When compared head-to-head, the efficacy of SC bortezomib was noninferior to IV, but the rates of peripheral neuropathy were significantly lower with SC. Therefore, SC bortezomib is the preferred route of administration in order to reduce the risk for neuropathy. If neuropathy develops, this can be managed through dose reductions as well as with neuropathic agents such as gabapentin, pregabalin, and duloxetine. Ixazomib is often referred to as "oral bortezomib" since it is also a boronic acid oral PI, but it blocks chymotrypsin-like activity of the beta 5 subunit of the 20S proteasome. Ixazomib has less neuropathy but more gastrointestinal (GI) toxicities like nausea, vomiting, and diarrhea. Ixazomib has to be taken on an empty stomach, 1 hour before a meal, so it can be helpful to premedicate with an antiemetic. The boronic acid PIs have unique drug-drug interactions for which patients need to be educated. High dose of vitamin C (>500 mg) and green tea interact with bortezomib and ixazomib and can reduce the efficacy of these agents, so patients should be advised to avoid these products for at least 12 hours before and after each dose of PI.

Carfilzomib is a potent, selective, and irreversible inhibitor of chymotrypsin-like activity of the 20S proteasome. While this second-generation PI does not have the neuropathy concerns, carfilzomib can cause cardiovascular toxicity including hypertension, new-onset or worsening heart failure, cardiomyopathy, and arrhythmias. Heart failure secondary to carfilzomib is usually reversible so it's important to have patients report symptoms of any new or worsening shortness of breath or edema. Compared to bortezomib, carfilzomib causes more myelosuppression and infusion reactions, which can be mitigated by premedication with dexamethasone. All three PIs can be utilized in both the newly diagnosed and relapsed/refractory setting depending on the specific patient and disease characteristics.

CORTICOSTEROIDS

Corticosteroids make up the third component of a "triplet" regimen for the treatment of MM and their role is multifactorial. First, plasma cells, similar to their lymphoid precursors, are highly susceptible to the lymphocytic properties of corticosteroids, resulting in direct cytotoxicity of myeloma cells by corticosteroids. Nuances do exist between the type and dose of steroids utilized. In older regimens, such as the classic all-oral MP (melphalan, prednisone) regimen, prednisone was the favored agent; however, in today's oncology practice, particularly in the United States, there is a preference for the more potent steroid dexamethasone. It is worth mentioning that historically, dexamethasone was dosed more aggressively, giving rise to the term "high-dose Dex." This practice changed as further clinical studies confirmed the noninferiority of "low-dose Dex," which is the dose of dexamethasone used in the majority of antimyeloma induction regimens today, although the term "low-dose" can be misleading since this still constitutes 40 mg per week of dexamethasone. The second role of dexamethasone in MM regimens is to provide synergy with other myeloma-directed therapies, such as the IMiDs, and PIs. Lastly, dexamethasone can serve as an antiemetic for regimens that have a higher incidence of nausea (e.g., ixazomib, cyclophosphamide, and selinexor containing regimens).

The most common acute adverse effects of steroids include insomnia, mood changes, poor glycemic control, blood pressure dysregulations, and fluid retention. Some of these adverse effects can cause significant distress for patients or their caregivers, so it's important to monitor for these occurrences and reduce the dose as needed. Further, due to the long-term side effects of steroids, including myopathy, weight gain, and osteoporosis, we can try to titrate the dexamethasone to the lowest effect dose or even completely discontinue if a patient's disease is stable. Dexamethasone is often a myeloma patient's best friend or biggest enemy but its role in MM-directed therapy is undeniable.

APPROACH TO RELAPSED REFRACTORY DISEASE

Several factors impact treatment selection for relapsed and refractory MM (RRMM) including patient age and comorbidities, cytogenetics, timing and aggressiveness of the relapse, and the response to frontline therapy. There is currently no universal standard on the optimal sequencing of available regimens but treatment can be broken down into early versus late relapse therapies. Table 15.1 lists impactful studies for early relapse regimens, and here we review the drug classes that can be introduced for early or late RRMM.

TABLE 15.1 Recent Advancements in Treatment for Early RRMM

REGIMEN	COMPARATOR	STUDY
DaraRd	Rd	POLLUX
DaraVd	Vd	CASTOR
DaraKd	Kd	CANDOR
DaraPd	Pd	APOLLO
IsaKd	Kd	IKEMA
IsaPd	Pd	ICARIA-MM
SVd	Vd	BOSTON
Venetoclax/Dex	N/a	Phase 1 and 2 studies in t(11;14 only)

Dara, daratumumab; Dex,dexamethasone; Isa, isatuximab; Kd, carfilzomib/dexamethasone; N/a, not applicable; Pd, pomalidomide/dexamethasone; Rd, lenalidomide/dexamethasone; RRMM, relapsed and refractory multiple myeloma; S, selinexor; Vd, bortezomib/dexamethasone.

MONOCLONAL ANTIBODIES

Anti-CD38 Monoclonal Antibodies

CD38 is a transmembrane glycoprotein expressed on lymphoid and myeloma cells that serves as a receptor for the transduction of activation signals and aids in the production of nucleotides that are involved in calcium signaling. CD38 is an ideal therapeutic target in MM because it is highly expressed on abnormal plasma cells, but has much lower expression on normal myeloid and lymphoid cells. Anti-CD38 antibodies induce cell death through multiple mechanisms (shown in Figure 15.5) that include antibody-dependent cell-mediated cytotoxicity, antibody-dependent cellular phagocytosis, complement-dependent cytotoxicity, induction of apoptosis, and modulation of CD38 enzyme activity. Monoclonal anitbodies are discussed extensively in Chapter 17.

Daratumumab (Darzalex) is a first-in-class human immunoglobulin G1 kappa (IgG1κ) CD38-directed monoclonal antibody (mAb) that was initially approved as a single agent in the treatment of RRMM in patients with three or more prior lines of therapy. Since this first indication, daratumumab has been approved in various combinations (with lenalidomide, pomalidomide, bortezomib, and carfilzomib) in both the newly diagnosed setting as well as for patients with at least one prior line of therapy. As reviewed in detail in Chapter 17, infusion-related reactions are a common side effect associated with mAbs. IV daratumumab is no exception, with all-grade infusion reactions reported to be 48% and the first-dose infusion can take approximately 8 to 10 hours to complete. In 2020, the novel subcutaneous formulation of daratumumab combined with hyaluronidase-fihj (Darzalex Faspro) was approved, which revolutionized the administration of daratumumab. Unlike other mAbs that have a SC formulation (e.g., rituximab), there is no need to give an initial dose of IV daratumumab.

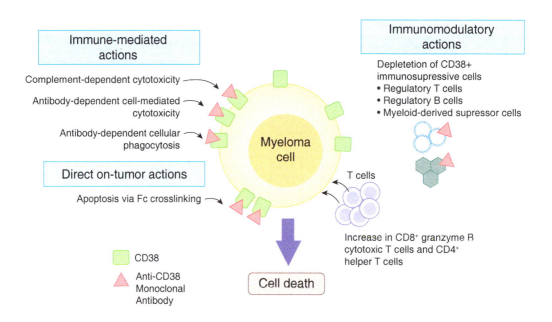

FIGURE 15.5 Anti-CD38 mechanism of action.
Mechanisms of action of anti-CD38 monoclonal antibodies (daratumumab and isatuximab) targeting surface CD38 antigen on multiple myeloma cells. Monoclonal antibodies against CD38 antigen can induce tumor cell killing via immune-mediated ac ions, direct cytotoxicity, and immunomodulatory actions.

It is safe to start therapy with the SC formulation, which has a 5-minute administration time, and the all-grade infusion reactions are significantly less at 13%. Due to the lower incidence of infusion reactions with daratumumab-hyaluronidase, recent data support eliminating premedications as soon as cycle 1, day 15, and postinfusion medications have also largely been eliminated in clinical practice. The National Comprehensive Cancer Network (NCCN) Guidelines state that for any regimen that includes daratumumab, either the IV or SC product can be utilized; however, it is important to note that IV daratumumab is a weight-based dose and SC daratumumab is a flat dose. Isatuximab-irfc (Sarclisa), the newest IgG kappa CD38 mAb, binds to a different epitope on the human cell surface antigen CD38. Isatuximab is available as an IV infusion that is weight-based and given weekly for cycle one and then biweekly thereafter. It has received FDA approval for the treatment of early relapse (one to three prior therapies) MM in combination with pomalidomide and dexamethasone (IsaPd) as well as in combination with carfilzomib and dexamethasone (IsaKd). There are limited data to support the use of switching from daratumumab to isatuximab, or vice versa, and it is believed that failure of one anti-CD38 mAb can be extrapolated to the other agent as well.

Upper respiratory tract infections are observed in approximately 20% of patients treated with an anti-CD38 based regimen, so it is recommend that all patients remain up to date on pneumococcal and influenza vaccines. Additionally, hepatitis B reactivation can occur during anti-CD38 therapy, so hepatitis B serologies should be checked prior to initiating therapy, and proper prophylaxis should be prescribed if indicated. Anti-CD38 mAbs have a few unique test interactions that have clinical significance for patients. First, both daratumumab and isatuximab can bind to CD38 on red blood cells, which may result in a positive indirect antiglobulin test (indirect Coombs test). The anti-CD38-mediated Coombs test positivity can persist for up to 6 months after the last dose. Lastly, anti-CD38 mAbs also can interfere with serologic testing by masking antibody detection to minor antigens in the patient's serum, so a blood type and screen must be drawn before administration.

Anti-SLAMF7 Monoclonal Antibody

Elotuzumab (Empliciti) is a humanized IgG1 mAb that directly targets SLAM family member 7 (SLAMF7), also known as cell-surface glycoprotein CD2 subset 1 (CS1). Elotuzumab allows for the selective destruction of MM cells with minimal effects on healthy tissues because the glycoprotein CS1 is expressed at low levels on most immune cells, including natural killer (NK) cells, while retaining high expression on MM cells. Of note, elotuzumab does not have any monotherapy activity in MM; however, it produces durable responses when combined with an IMiD. The dual MOA includes direct activation of NK cells and antibody-dependent cytotoxicity via the CD16 pathway as well as inhibiting the adhesion of MM cells to bone marrow stromal cells. Infusion reactions and infections, including opportunistic infections, are the most common side effects with elotuzumab. Premedications are required prior to each infusion and proper anti-infective prophylaxis should be given.

Because daratumumab, isatuximab, and elotuzumab are all IgG kappa antibodies, it is important to note that the presence of these antibodies may interfere with the serum protein electrophoresis (SPEP) and immunofixation assays that are used to monitor disease response. Patients treated with these mAbs may have iatrogenic bands observed on the SPEP and this should be carefully noted when determining the complete response and disease progression in patients with IgG kappa MM.

B CELL MATURATION ANTIGEN TARGET

B cell maturation antigen (BCMA), also known as tumor necrosis factor receptor superfamily member 17 (TNFRS17), is a type III transmembrane glycoprotein found universally on MM cells but rarely expressed on healthy naive and memory B cells. BCMA is required for the survival of malignant plasma cells and has become a favorable target for immune-based therapy. Further, BCMA on MM cells is associated with an immunosuppressive bone marrow microenvironment, and increased levels of soluble BCMA (sBCMA) are associated with disease progression and worse outcomes. Figure 15.6 illustrates the various mechanisms for targeting BCMA.

Antibody–Drug Conjugate

Belantamab mafodotin (Blenrep) is a first-in-class BCMA-directed monoclonal antibody–drug conjugate (ADC) that is approved for the treatment of patients with RRMM who have received at least four prior therapies, including a CD38 mAb, a PI, and an IMiD. The antibody component of belantamab mafodotin binds to BCMA and the entire molecule is then internalized by myeloma cells. Once internalized, the linker is cleaved, releasing a microtubule-disrupting agent called monomethyl auristatin F (MMAF), which causes destruction of the myeloma cells via cellular apoptosis, cell cycle arrest, and antibody-dependent cell-mediated

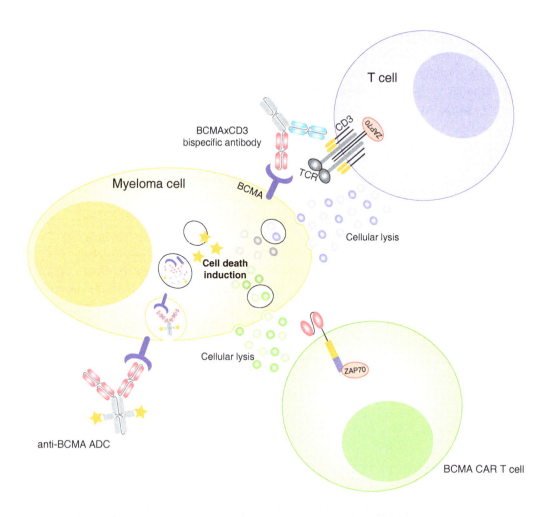

FIGURE 15.6 Three different mechanisms of action for BCMA-directed therapies. The BCMA is targeted via three different mechanism of action: antibody–drug conjugates (ADCs), bispecific antibodies, and chimeri antigen receptor (CAR) T cell therapy.

BCMA, B-cell maturation antigen; TCR, T cell receptor.

Source: Strassl I, Schreder M, Steiner N, et al., Cancers (Basel), 2021.

cytotoxicity. Prior to belantamab mafodotin, triple-class refractory MM patients had poor outcomes with a median overall survival of less than 1 year. Belantamab mafodotin offered a novel target and produced both deep and durable responses in heavily pretreated patients. The most common grade 3 or higher adverse effects with belantamab mafodotin are keratopathy (27%), thrombocytopenia (20%), and anemia (20%). Keratopathy refers to microcyst-like epithelial changes observed on the cornea of the eye and can present with or without symptoms such as blurry vision, dry eyes, or a decline in best corrected vision acuity (BCVA). A REMS program was established along with the approval of this medication to ensure completion of an ophthalmic examination before every dose. It's important to note that the corneal adverse reactions associated with belantamab mafodotin are a known side effect of MMAF, and the proposed mechanism of toxicity is related to the nonspecific uptake of belantamab mafodotin into the basal corneal epithelial cells. While the ocular toxicities are not permanent sequelae, it can take several weeks for symptoms to resolve to grade 1 or better. Dose reductions and dose delays are the primary management strategies for ocular toxicity, with a median time to reinitiation of treatment of 83 days (range, 28–146 days) after a dose hold. Patients should be instructed to apply 1 to 2 drops of preservative-free artificial tears in each eye at least four times daily starting with the first infusion and to avoid contact lenses. Corticosteroid eye drops are no longer being recommended because they did not demonstrate benefit in DREAMM-2. Additional BCMA-directed ADCs are currently under investigation, including HDP-101 and MEDI2228. Antibody-drug conjugates are also addressed in Chapter 17.

Chimeric Antigen Receptor T Cell Therapy

Chimeric antigen receptor (CAR) T cell therapy genetically modifies autologous T cells with a transgene encoding a CAR to identify and eliminate a tumor-associated antigen-expressing cells. CAR T cell therapy is discussed in Chapter 18. Anti-BCMA CAR T cells will bind to the BCMA-expressing cells, which then transmits a signal to promote T cell expansion, activation, target cell elimination, and persistence of the CAR T cells. Idecabtagene vicleucel (ide-cel; bb2121) is the first-in-class BCMA targeted CAR T cell therapy to be approved by the FDA for the treatment of RRMM after four prior lines therapies, including an anti-CD38 mAb, PI, and IMiD. Ciltacabtagene autoleucel (cilta-cel; LCAR-B38M, JNJ-4528) was the second CAR T cell therapy to be FDA approved for RRMM also after four prior lines of therapy. Cilta-cel is a dual epitope-binding CAR T cell construct directed against two distinct BCMA epitopes. The bi-epitope target improves the binding avidity and is unique to cilta-cel. Both ide-cel and cilta-cel produced deep and durable responses in patients with a median of six prior lines of therapy and allowed patients to have a break from chronic treatment because there is no recommended maintenance therapy following CAR T cells at this time. With the success of ide-cel and cilta-cel in heavily pretreated patients, these products are now currently being investigated in earlier lines of therapy in combination with traditional MM-directed agents such as IMiDs. There are also more than 10 additional BCMA-targeted CAR T cell products being investigated in clinical trials. While these CAR T cell constructs have similarities, there are differences in the costimulatory domains, the species used to generate the anti-BCMA single-chain variable fragment (scFv), the method of transduction (lentivirus vs. retrovirus), and the presence of additional safety domains. CAR T cell therapies are further discussed in Chapter 18 but the most common toxicities are cytokine release syndrome (CRS) and neurotoxicity. These products have a REMS program associated with them; however, differing from the antibody–drug conjugates that target BCMA, CAR T cell therapy is not an "off-the-shelf" product and requires approximately a 4-week manufacturing period, during which patients may require bridging therapy.

NOVEL MECHANISM OF ACTION AGENTS

XPO1 Inhibitors

Selinexor is a first-in-class, oral agent that reversibly inhibits nuclear export of tumor suppressor proteins, growth regulators, and mRNAs of oncogenic proteins by blocking exportin

1 (XPO1), which is overexpressed in myeloma. Inhibition of XPO1 results in accumulation of tumor suppressor proteins within the nucleus causing cell cycle arrest and apoptosis. Selinexor was initially approved in combination with dexamethasone for the treatment of late RRMM in patients previously treated with two PIs, two IMiDs, and a CD38 mAb. Selinexor demonstrated synergistic activity with PIs, even in those with PI-refractory disease. This led to the more recent approval of selinexor in combination with bortezomib and dexamethaonse for patients with one to three prior lines of therapy. Selinexor is currently being investigated in an ongoing trial in multiple combinations including with carfilzomib, with pomalidomide, and with daratumumab. The optimal dose of selinexor when combined with these different agents is yet to be determined, but a weekly dosing strategy has proved to be more tolerable than the original twice weekly dosing indication. The most common grade 3/4 adverse effects are anemia, thrombocytopenia, and fatigue. Utilizing a platelet stimulating factor, such as romiplostim or a thrombopoietin receptor agonist, can help mitigate the thrombocytopenia. Additionally, selinexor is associated with a moderate or high emetic potential. In the Phase 2 STORM trial, all-grade nausea and decreased appetite occurred in 72% and 56% of patients, respectively. It is recommended to use a dual antiemetic approach for selinexor-based regimens with a long-acting agent (e.g., olanzapine or rolapitant) and a breakthrough agent (e.g., ondansetron or prochlorperazine).

BCL-2 Inhibitors

As addressed in Chapter 9, BCL-2 is an antiapoptotic protein that is heterogeneously overexpressed on a subset of myeloma cells, specifically in those that have the 11;14 translocation (t(11;14)). Venetoclax is a selective, oral BCL-2 inhibitor that induces cell death in these MM cells and is recommended in combination with dexamethasone for early relapse disease in those with t(11;14). Venetoclax for MM has had some controversial moments following the results from the Phase 3 BELLINI trial in which venetoclax was combined with bortezomib and dexamethasone (VenVd) and compared to bortezomib and dexamethasone (Vd) alone. There was a higher incidence of death noted in the VenVd arm compared to Vd, so this raised questions regarding the safety of venetoclax for MM. However, the BELLINI trial did not exclude non-t(11;14) patients and only 13% of the population had t(11;14). In a subgroup analysis of only t(11;14) patients, both progression-free survival and overall survival favored VenVd. These updated BELLINI data, in addition to prior Phase 1 studies, highlight the importance of utilizing venetoclax only in the select group of MM patients with t(11;14). Venetoclax is currently under investigation in combination with daratumumab and carfilzomib and the dosing ranges from 400 to 800 mg daily, which is higher than the doses used in leukemia and lymphoma. Additionally, tumor lysis syndrome is very rare in MM; therefore, a dose ramp-up is not required. Due to the increase in pneumonia seen in the BELLINI study, it is recommended that patients receiving venetoclax be vaccinated against pneumonia per the Centers for Disease Control and Prevention Guidelines. The most common adverse effects with venetoclax-based therapy include nausea, diarrhea, and cytopenia. Patients may require growth factor while on this treatment to prevent dose holds and prolonged neutropenia.

ALKYLATORS

The role of alkylating agents in the treatment of MM has greatly evolved in the presence of the novel therapies already described. Alkylating agents and other cytotoxics are addressed in Chapter 5. Prior to the approval of lenalidomide and bortezomib, oral melphalan and prednisone were the mainstay of therapy. Nowadays, melphalan is largely only utilized as part of the high-dose conditioning chemotherapy regimen prior to ASCT, which causes expected side effects of myelosuppression, GI toxicity, and mucositis. While low-dose oral melphalan as part of the daratumumab, bortezomib, melphalan, and prednisone (Dara-VMP) regimen can still be considered for newly diagnosed, transplant-ineligible patients, recent data suggest that the triplet of daratumumab plus lenalidomide and dexamethasone is as good as triple- or quad-drug melphalan-based therapies.

The more common role for alkylating agents in the current era is in patients who have an aggressive or rapid progression. In this setting, there is often an urgent need for disease control and end-organ preservation. Cytotoxic chemotherapy combinations, such as DCEP (dexamethasone, cyclophosphamide, etoposide, and cisplatin) or VDT-PACE (bortezomib, dexamethasone, thalidomide, cisplatin, doxorubicin, cyclophosphamide, and etoposide), are administered as continuous infusions and provide rapid disease control. Synergy has also been noted when combining a PI with cytotoxic therapy, which has led to the utilization of bortezomib-DCEP (V-DCEP). Lastly, oral cyclophosphamide can be combined with a proteasome inhibitor and dexamethasone for newly diagnosed as well as RRMM in patients who have a contraindication to IMiDs.

PIPELINE AGENTS

Bispecific Antibodies

Bispecific antibodies (BiAbs), discussed further in Chapter 18, engage both CD3$^+$ T cells and a tumor-associated antigen (e.g., CD19, CD33, or BCMA), which lead to cancer cell death and T cell proliferation. Although no BiAbs are currently FDA approved for the treatment of MM, BiAbs targeting BCMA, GPRC5D, and FcRL5 are emerging as highly effective therapeutic options. Select BiAbs and preliminary results of ongoing studies are listed in Table 15.2. The first-generation BiAbs were relatively small proteins with short half-lives, which required an extended, continuous infusion administration that can be logistically challenging for patients. However, the new generation of BiAbs, including teclistamab and elranatamab, are given as weekly subcutaneous injections. Most BiAbs require step-up doses with 24-hour monitoring prior to reaching the full treatment dose due to CRS and neurotoxicity. While CRS is a common adverse event with BiAbs, neurotoxicity is much less common compared to CAR T cell therapy. Infections are a common complication with BiAbs and prophylactic measures should be implemented to reduce the risk for infection. Some of these measures may include intravenous immunoglobulin (IVIG) for patients with IgG levels less than 400 mg/dL, *Pneumocystis jirovecii* pneumonia (PJP) prophylaxis, and growth colony stimulating factor when neutropenic.

TABLE 15.2 Select Bispecific Antibodies (BiAbs): Dosing and CRS Results

AGENT	DOSING SCHEDULE	CRS ALL (GRADE 3+), %	SOURCE
BCMA/CD3 TARGET			
Elranatamab Phase 1, n=58	215–1,000 mcg/kg RP2D: 1 mg/kg or 76 mg SC weekly	87% (0)	Sebag et al., 2021
Pavurutamab Phase 1, n=75	5 mcg–12 mg IV QW	61% (7%)	Harrison et al., 2020
REGN5458 Phase 1, n=73	QW → Q2W; IV 3–400 mg	38% (0%)	Zonder et al., 2021
Teclistamab Phase 1/2, n=165	RP2D: 1.5 mg/kg SC weekly	71.5% (0.6%)	Moreau et al., 2021
FCRL5/CD3			
Cevostamab Phase 1/2, n=160	0.15–198 mg IV Q3W	81% (1%)	Trudel et al., 2021
GPRC5D/CD3			
Talquetamab Phase 1, n=102	405 mcg/kg SC QW (n=30) 800 mcg/kg SC Q2W (n=25)	72–77% (0–3%)	Krishnan et al., 2021

Note: These bispecific agents are currently under investigation for the treatment of multiple myeloma; data here include their target and preliminary safety information. Studies cited here are listed in the Selected References at the end of the chapter.

ASH, American Society of Hematology; BCMA, B-cell maturation antigen; CRS, cytokine release syndrome; IV, intravenous; QW, weekly; Q2W, every 2 weeks; Q3W, every 3 weeks; RP2D, recommended phase 2 dose; SC, subcutaneous.

BRAF/MEK Inhibitors

Mutation driven therapy allows for a customized treatment plan, and the BRAF V600E mutation is one that has been described in MM with a reported incidence of approximately 4% to 10%. Targeting the BRAF V600E mutation with BRAF inhibitors has produced positive results in solid tumor malignancies including metastatic melanoma, papillary thyroid cancer, and non-small cell lung cancer, and these agents are now being studied in MM as well. Vemurafenib and dabrafenib alone are being investigated as treatment options for MM patients who have a BRAF mutation. There are also ongoing trials combining a BRAF inhibitor with a MEK inhibitor (dabrafenib with trametinib or encorafenib with binimetinib) in attempts to subvert potential escape mechanisms and development of resistance. These combinations offer an all-oral drug therapy option with novel mechanisms of action and are an intriguing option for personalized medicine.

SUPPORTIVE CARE

One of the challenges in treating an MM patient is that symptom burden can arise from the disease itself (e.g., infections, bone destruction) as well as from the therapies that have just been described. It is critical to delineate what is contributing to symptom burden and is also important to provide supportive adjunctive treatment from the start.

Bone Disease

All newly diagnosed MM patients should receive a bone-modifying agent with bisphosphonates or denosumab. Zoledronic acid is preferred or pamidronate and denosumab are preferred in patients with renal disease. Patients should obtain a baseline dental exam and monitor for osteonecrosis of the jaw. If invasive dental work is needed, the bone-modifying agent should be held ideally for 2 months before and after the dental procedure. Radiation therapy and kyphoplasty can be adjunctive to systemic therapy if needed for pain relief from bone disease.

Infection

As previously described, MM patients on a PI-based or mAB-based regimen should be on HSV/VZV prophylaxis, and based upon the steroid dose, PJP prophylaxis may be indicated. Antibacterial and antifungal prophylaxis should be given to patients while neutropenic after ASCT or CAR T cell therapy. In addition to patients who received CAR T cells or a BiAb, IVIG is recommend for all MM patients who are experiencing recurrent infections and have an IgG less than 400 mg/dL Lastly starting two times or three times weekly growth factor can reduce the risk for infections and assist with maintaining the dose intensity of the MM-directed therapy for patients who require better disease control.

Renal Dysfunction

Patients may have renal dysfunction due to their disease, so it's important to avoid aggravating factors such as nonsteroidal anti-inflammatory drugs (NSAIDs) and reduce dosage for all medications (MM-directed therapy, supportive care, and medications for comorbidities) for renal impairment. Renal dysfunction is not a contraindication to ASCT and likely will improve if MM-directed therapy can be started quickly.

CHAPTER SUMMARY

Survival outcomes for MM have significantly improved over the last decade due to the approval of new drug therapies and the utilization of these agents as part of a multi-targeted approach. **Figure 15.7** summarizes the numerous drug classes and their mechanisms of action for targeting MM cells. Induction therapy has historically been based upon a patient's eligibility for ASCT, and we are now also starting to incorporate a risk-stratified approach with IMiDs, PIs, and corticosteroids being the mainstay for induction therapy. While there is no universally agreed-upon standard for the sequencing of therapies in

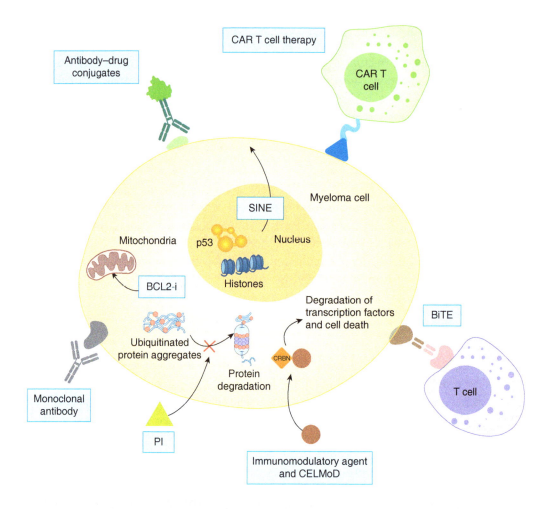

FIGURE 15.7 Summary of the mechanisms of action for all MM-directed therapies.
Various targets and–drug therapy mechanisms of action are critical to the multi-targeted approach to the management of MM.

BCL2, B-cell lymphoma 2; BiTE, bispecific T cell engager; CAR, chimeric antigen receptor; CELMoDs, cereblon E3 ligase modulating drugs; CRBN, cereblon; MM, multiple myeloma; PI, proteasome inhibitor.

the relapsed and refractory setting, it is important to select a regimen based upon the patient's disease biology, prior therapies, comorbidities, and lifestyle. Strategies for patients in second or later relapse include the following: (a) consider a clinical trial, or (b) select a combination regimen that is effective and appropriate based upon the above-mentioned factors. Monoclonal antibodies, BCMA-directed therapy, and drugs with novel mechanisms of action (e.g., selinexor and venetoclax) have proved to be successful in achieving deep and durable responses in patients who become refractory to IMiDs and PIs. Lastly, supportive care is critical to the success of treating an MM patient as adverse effects can arise from the disease itself as well as from the treatment. It is important to recognize that novel treatment options and new combinations of available therapies are at various stages of development and the treatment landscape for MM is evolving rapidly. We will likely continue to see more personalized approaches to MM-directed treatments as we continue to move in the direction of a cure.

CLINICAL PEARLS

- Triplets (and now quadruplets) are preferred over doublets when selecting a multi-targeted regimen for induction therapy, which most often combines an IMiD, PI, and corticosteroid.
- BCMA is an ideal target for MM-directed therapy and can be targeted with antibody-drug conjugates, CAR T cell therapy, and bispecific antibodies.
- Bone-modifying agents, VTE prophylaxis, and infection prophylaxis should be addressed for all MM patients.

MULTIPLE-CHOICE QUESTIONS

1. A 58-year-old professional guitar player is diagnosed with MM. He has no other co-morbidities but is fearful of developing peripheral neuropathy because it would end his career if he cannot play his guitar. Which proteasome inhibitor should be avoided for this induction therapy?

   A. Bortezomib
   B. Carfilzomib
   C. Ixazomib
   D. Oprozomib

2. A 67-year-old female is on lenalidomide maintenance after her autologous stem cell transplant and is complaining of significant diarrhea. She has tried and failed loperamide. Which of the following would be an appropriate drug to treat her lenalidomide-induced diarrhea?

   A. Ursodiol
   B. Colestipol
   C. Rifaximin
   D. Probiotic

3. Selinexor is considered to have moderate to high emetic potential. Which of the following antiemetic prophylaxis is most appropriate for a selinexor-based regimen?

   A. No prophylaxis required since selinexor is not an IV medication
   B. Dexamethasone alone
   C. Dexamethasone plus olanzapine
   D. 5-HT3 antagonist (e.g., ondansetron) plus a long-acting agent (e.g., olanzapine or rolapitant)

4. A 63-year-old female with RRMM has had two prior lines of therapy and is interested in an all-oral regimen. You would like to recommend venetoclax plus dexamethasone. Which cytogenetic abnormality must be present on her bone marrow biopsy for venetoclax to be appropriate?

    A. Del17p
    B. t(4:14)
    C. t(11;14)
    D. t(14;16)

5. Which of the following agents can interfere with the serum protein electrophoresis and immunofixation assays that are used to monitor disease response?

    A. Daratumumab
    B. Elotuzumab
    C. Isatuximab
    D. All of the above

6. Which of the following supportive care measures is not recommended for patients on belantamab mafodotin?

    A. Corticosteroid eye drops
    B. Preservative-free eye drops
    C. Avoiding contact lenses
    D. Premedications for infusion reactions

7. Which of the following therapies will require monitoring for cytokine release syndrome?

    A. Idecabtagene vicleucel
    B. Ciltacabtagene autoleucel
    C. Teclistamab
    D. All of the above

8. Which of the following class effects of the immunomodulatory agents (IMiDs) is the reasoning behind the REMS program?

    A. The venous thromboembolism risk
    B. The embryo-fetal risk
    C. The risk for secondary malignancies
    D. The risk for myelosuppression

9. A newly diagnosed MM patient with significant bone disease and renal failure requiring hemodialysis is starting induction therapy. Which of the following bone-modifying agents would be most appropriate to also start?

    A. Denosumab
    B. Pamidronate
    C. Zoledronic acid
    D. Bone modifying agents are only needed for relapsed disease.

10. Which of the following cannot be used as monotherapy to treatment MM?

A. Carfilzomib
B. Daratumumab
C. Elotuzumab
D. Pomalidomide

ANSWERS TO MULTIPLE-CHOICE QUESTIONS

1. **A.** Peripheral neuropathy is a dose-limiting side effect of bortezomib and should be avoided in patients who have significant underlying peripheral neuropathy or if developing peripheral neuropathy would be detrimental. Carfilzomib and ixazomib are both included in the national guidelines as options for frontline therapy.

2. **B.** Lenalidomide-induced diarrhea is secondary to bile acid malabsorption. So using a bile acid sequestrant, such as colestipol, is very effective at treating lenalidomide-induced diarrhea.

3. **D.** Dual-agent prophylaxis with a 5-HT3 antagonist and a long-acting antiemetic is recommended due to the high rates of nausea and vomiting seen with selinexor-based therapies.

4. **C.** BCL2 is heterogeneously overexpressed in those who have t(11;14). Venetoclax is a selective, oral BCL-2 inhibitor that induces cell death in these MM cells and is recommended in combination with dexamethasone for early relapse disease in those with t(11;14).

5. **D.** Daratumumab, isatuximab, and elotuzumab are all IgG kappa antibodies so the presence of these antibodies may interfere with the serum protein electrophoresis and immunofixation assays that are used to monitor disease response.

6. **A.** Corticosteroid eye drops were not shown to reduce the ocular toxicities in the DREAMM-2 study and are therefore not recommended. Patients are instructed to avoid contact lenses and use preservative-free artificial tears.

7. **D.** Both CAR T cell products and bispecific antibodies can cause cytokine release syndrome and patients should be monitored closely.

8. **B.** Thalidomide was removed from the market due to the embryo-fetal toxicities. Therefore, all of the IMiDs are now only available through the REMS program.

9. **A.** All newly diagnosed MM patients should receive a bone-modifying agent. Denosumab is the preferred agent for those with significant renal impairment.

10. **C.** Elotuzumab has no monotherapy activity against MM but induces responses when combined with IMiDs and dexamethasone.

SELECTED REFERENCES

Arnall JR, Maples KT, Harvey RD, Moore DC. Daratumumab for the treatment of multiple myeloma: A review of clinical applicability and operational considerations. Ann Pharmacother. 2022 Aug;56(8):927–40. https://doi.org/10.1177/10600280211058754

Berdeja JG, Madduri D, Usmani SZ, et al. Ciltacabtagene autoleucel, a B-cell maturation antigen-directed chimeric antigen receptor T cell therapy in patients with relapsed or refractory multiple myeloma (CARTITUDE-1): A phase 1b/2 open-label study. Lancet. 2021;398(10297):314–24. https://doi.org/10.1016/S0140-6736(21)00933-8

Chari A, Vogl DT, Gavriatopoulou M, et al. Oral selinexor-dexamethasone for triple-class refractory multiple myeloma. N Engl J Med. 2019 Aug 22;381(8):727–38. https://doi.org/10.1056/NEJMoa1903455

Collins SM, Bakan CE, Swartzel GD, et al. Elotuzumab directly enhances NK cell cytotoxicity against myeloma via CS1 ligation: Evidence for augmented NK cell function complementing ADCC. Cancer Immunol Immunother. 2013;62(12):1841–9. https://doi.org/10.1007/s00262-013-1493-8

Crawford LJ, Walker B, Irvine AE. Proteasome inhibitors in cancer therapy. J Cell Commun Signal. 2011 Jun;5(2):101–10. https://doi.org/10.1007/s12079-011-0121-7

de Weers M, Tai YT, van der Veer MS, et al. Daratumumab, a novel therapeutic human CD38 monoclonal antibody, induces killing of multiple myeloma and other hematological tumors. J Immunol. 2011;186(3):1840–8. https://doi.org/10.4049/jimmunol.1003032

Faiman B. Disease and symptom care: A focus on specific needs of patients with multiple myeloma. Clin J Oncol Nurs. 2017;21(Suppl 5):3–6. https://doi.org/10.1188/17.CJON.S5.3-6

Harrison SJ, Minnema MC, Lee HC, et al. A phase 1 first in human (FIH) study of AMG 701, an anti-B-cell maturation antigen (BCMA) half-life extended (HLE) BiTE (bispecific T-cell engager) molecule, in relapsed/refractory (RR) multiple myeloma (MM). Blood. 2020;136(Suppl 1):28. http://doi.org/10.1182/blood-2020-134063

Joseph NS, Kaufman JL, Dhodapkar MV, et al. Long-term follow-up results of lenalidomide, bortezomib, and dexamethasone induction therapy and risk-adapted maintenance approach in newly diagnosed multiple myeloma. J Clin Oncol. 2020 Jun 10;38(17):1928–37. https://doi.org/10.1200/JCO.19.02515

Krishnan AY, Minnema MC, Berdeja JG, et al. Updated phase 1 results from MonumenTAL-1: First-in-human study of talquetamab, a G protein-coupled receptor family C group 5 member D x CD3 bispecific antibody, in patients with relapsed/refractory multiple myeloma. Blood. 2021;138(Suppl 1):158. https://doi.org/10.1182/blood-2021-146868

Kumar S, Kaufman JL, Gasparetto C, et al. Efficacy of venetoclax as targeted therapy for relapsed/refractory t(11;14) multiple myeloma. Blood. 2017;130(22):2401–9. https://doi.org/10.1182/blood-2017-06-788786

Lonial S, Lee HC, Badros A, et al. Belantamab mafodotin for relapsed or refractory multiple myeloma (DREAMM-2): A two-arm, randomised, open-label, phase 2 study. Lancet Oncol. 2020 Feb;21(2):207–21. https://doi.org/10.1016/S1470-2045(19)30788-0

Maples KT, Johnson C, Lonial S. Antibody treatment in multiple myeloma. Clin Adv Hematol Oncol. 2021 Mar;19(3):166–74.

Maples KT, Joseph NS, Harvey RD. Current developments in the combination therapy of relapsed/refractory multiple myeloma. Expert Rev Anticancer Ther. 2020;20(12):1021–35. https://doi.org/10.1080/14737140.2020.1828071

Mateos MV, Nahi H, Legiec W, et al. Subcutaneous versus intravenous daratumumab in patients with relapsed or refractory multiple myeloma (COLUMBA): A multicentre, open-label, non-inferiority, randomised, phase 3 trial. Lancet Haematol. 2020 May;7(5):e370–80. https://doi.org/10.1016/S2352-3026(20)30070-3

Moreau P. How I treat myeloma with new agents. Blood. 2017;130(13):1507–13. https://doi.org/10.1182/blood-2017-05-743203

Moreau P, Kumar SK, San Miguel JS, et al. Treatment of relapsed and refractory multiple myeloma: Recommendations from the International Myeloma Working Group. Lancet Oncol. 2021;22(3):e105–18. https://doi.org/10.1016/S1470-2045(20)30756-7

Moreau P, Usmani SZ, Garfall AL, et al. Updated results from MajesTEC-1: phase 1/2 study of teclistamab, a B-cell maturation antigen x CD3 bispecific antibody, in relapsed/refractory multiple myeloma. Blood. 2021;138(Suppl 1):896. https://doi.org/10.1182/blood-2021-147915

Munshi NC, Anderson LD, Shah N, et al. Idecabtagene Vicleucel in relapsed and refractory multiple myeloma. N Engl J Med. 2021;384(8):705–16. https://doi.org/10.1056/NEJMoa2024850

National Comprehensive Cancer Network. Multiple myeloma. Version 5.2022 [cited October 2022]. Available from: https://www.nccn.org/professionals/physician_gls/pdf/myeloma.pdf

Nooka AK, Gleason C, Sargeant MO, et al. Managing infusion reactions to new monoclonal antibodies in multiple myeloma: Daratumumab and elotuzumab. J Oncol Pract. 2018;14(7):414–22. https://doi.org/10.1200/JOP.18.00143

Nooka AK, Lonial S. Mechanisms of action and novel IMiD-based compounds and combinations in multiple myeloma. Cancer J. 2019;25(1):19–31. https://doi.org/10.1097/PPO.0000000000000354

Palumbo A, Anderson K. Multiple myeloma. N Engl J Med. 2011;364(11):1046–60. https://doi.org/10.1056/NEJMra1011442

Raab MS, Giesen N, Scheid C, et al. Safety and preliminary efficacy results from a Phase II study evaluating combined BRAF and MEK inhibition in relapsed/refractory multiple myeloma (rrMM) patients with activating BRAF V600E mutations: The GMMG-Birma trial. Blood. 2020;136(Suppl 1):44–5. https://doi.org/10.1182/blood-2020-142600

Rajkumar SV, Dimopoulos MA, Palumbo A, et al. International Myeloma Working Group updated criteria for the diagnosis of multiple myeloma. Lancet Oncol. 2014;15(12):e538–48. https://doi.org/10.1016/S1470-2045(14)70442-5

Sebag M, Raje NS, Bahlis NJ, et al. Elranatamab (PF-06863135), a B-cell maturation antigen (BCMA) targeted CD3-engaging bispecific molecule, for patients with relapsed or refractory multiple myeloma: Results from magnetismm-1. Blood. 2021;138(Suppl 1):895. https://doi.org/10.1182/blood-2021-150519

Shah N, Chari A, Scott E, et al. B-cell maturation antigen (BCMA) in multiple myeloma: Rationale for targeting and current therapeutic approaches. Leukemia. 2020;34(4):985–1005. https://doi.org/10.1038/s41375-020-0734-z

Shah Z, Malik MN, Batool SS, et al. Bispecific T cell engager (BiTE) antibody based immunotherapy for treatment of relapsed refractory multiple myeloma (RRMM): A systematic review of preclinical and clinical trials. Blood. 2019;134(Suppl 1):5567. https://doi.org/10.1182/blood-2019-129652

Strassl I, Schreder M, Steiner N, et al. The agony of choice—where to place the wave of BCMA-targeted therapies in the multiple myeloma treatment puzzle in 2022 and beyond. Cancers (Basel). 2021;13(18):4701. https://doi.org/10.3390/cancers13184701

Trudel S, Cohen AD, Krishnan AY, et al. Cevostamab monotherapy continues to show clinically meaningful activity and manageable safety in patients with heavily pre-treated relapsed/refractory multiple myeloma: Updated results from an ongoing phase. Blood. 2021;138(Suppl 1):157. https://doi.org/10.1182/blood-2021-147983

Zonder JA, Richter J, Bumma N, et al. Early, deep, and durable responses, and low rates of cytokine release syndrome with REGN5458, a BCMAxCD3 bispecific monoclonal antibody, in a phase 1/2 first-in-human study in patients with relapsed/refractory multiple myeloma. Blood. 2021;138(Suppl 1):160. https://doi.org/10.1182/blood-2021-144921

PART V

Immune-Targeted Strategies

CHAPTER 16

Transplant-Related Agents: Focus on Graft-Versus-Host Disease Prevention and Treatment

VEDRAN RADOJCIC

Allogeneic hematopoietic stem cell transplantation (alloHSCT) remains the only curative procedure for a range of advanced hematologic malignancies and is increasingly used to treat noncancerous hematologic conditions (e.g., sickle cell disease) or inborn errors of metabolism. Advances in alloHSCT approaches and supportive care have significantly improved outcome of alloHSCT and led to a significant increase in transplant activity. Currently, ~40,000 alloHSCT procedures are performed worldwide each year, although fewer than 50% of patients with eligible disease ultimately undergo the procedure.

In patients with hematologic malignancies the key therapeutic benefit of alloHSCT is the immunotherapeutic antitumor effect (GVL, from graft-versus-leukemia/lymphoma) driven by the incoming new lymphohematopoietic system. The immunologic basis of GVL effect and its reliance on the antigenic disparity between the patient and alloHSCT donor have been well described. However, the same immunologic difference is responsible for occurrence of graft-versus-host disease (GVHD), where recipient (host) organs become a target of donor (graft) activated immune system.

GVHD affects more than 50% of transplanted patients and remains the major post-transplant complication and the limiting factor to broader use of alloHSCT in clinical practice. Occurrence and severity of GVHD are influenced by the range of factors beyond the immunologic mismatch and include aspects of transplant procedure (conditioning intensity and modality) and recipient and donor characteristics (such as age, gender mismatch, status of disease at transplantation). GVHD can present at any time after alloHSCT as acute or chronic disease (aGVHD and cGVHD, respectively), or as an overlap syndrome with features of both acute and chronic disease. Distinction between acute and chronic GVHD is based on underlying pathophysiologic mechanisms, affected organs, and ensuing clinical findings.

Effective GVHD prophylaxis is the major prerequisite for an overall success of alloHSCT since established GVHD, despite recent improvements, remains accompanied by high morbidity and mortality rates. Furthermore, escalated immunosuppression use during active GVHD treatment blunts the therapeutic GVL effect, while further contributing to GVHD morbidity through enhanced risk of opportunistic infections, accelerated cardiovascular disease, endocrinopathies, and secondary cancers. Thus, effective GVHD prevention and treatment remain areas of unmet need in alloHSCT.

BIOLOGY-DRIVEN INTERVENTIONS TO PREVENT AND TREAT GRAFT-VERSUS-HOST DISEASE

Recent advancements in understanding of GVHD pathophysiology, particularly those addressing disparate operational mechanisms in acute and chronic disease, have been instrumental for devising novel strategies of GVHD prevention and treatment.

aGVHD is characterized by the early post-transplant occurrence of injury to the skin, gastrointestinal, and liver epithelium mediated by activated donor T cells that play an essential effector role in the tissue destruction process. Both experimental models and clinical observations provide unequivocal evidence supporting the cascading and autocatalytic process of aGVHD pathophysiology (**Figure 16.1**), which includes (a) conditioning regimen-induced

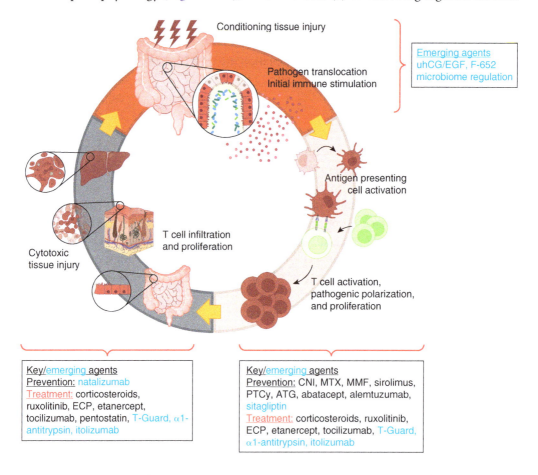

FIGURE 16.1 Key steps and mediators of acute GVHD pathophysiology.
Existing and emerging (blue typeface) agents targeting the disease processes are highlighted.

ATG, antithymocyte globulin; CNI, calcineurin inhibitor; ECP, extracorporeal photopheresis; EGF, epidermal growth factor; GVHD, graft-versus-host disease; MMF, mycophenolate mofetil; MTX, methotrexate; PTCy, post-transplant cyclophosphamide; uhCG, urinary human chorionic gonadotropin.

loss of gastrointestinal epithelium integrity with pathogen translocation and initial stimulation of innate and adaptive immune system, (b) T cell activation and pathogenic polarization through antigen presenting cells and increased proinflammatory cytokine and chemokine production, and (c) direct cellular damage to target organs and impaired tissue regeneration, which may be further worsened by GVHD therapy.

cGVHD, a generally delayed complication of alloHSCT, closely reflects range of human autoimmune conditions, such as scleroderma or systemic lupus erythematosus. It is characterized by dysregulated cellular and humoral responses leading to chronic inflammation, impaired tissue remodeling, and terminal fibroproliferative process leading to organ dysfunction. Current understanding of cGVHD recognizes three phases of disease development (Figure 16.2), with the first step closely reflecting processes seen in aGVHD. In the subsequent step, loss of immune tolerance due to damage to thymus and secondary lymphoid organs,

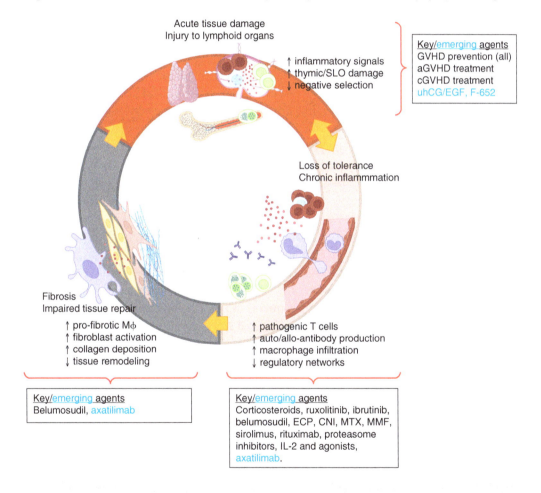

FIGURE 16.2 Key steps and mediators of chronic GVHD pathophysiology.
Existing and emerging (blue typeface) agents targeting the disease processes are highlighted.

aGVHD, acute GVHD; cGVHD, chronic GVHD; CNI, calcineurin inhibitor; ECP, extracorporeal photopheresis; EGF, epidermal growth factor; GVHD, graft-versus-host disease; IL-2, interleukin 2; MMF, mycophenolate mofetil; MTX, methotrexate; SLO, secondary lymphoid organs; uhCG, urinary human chorionic gonadotropin.

functional suppression and loss of regulatory T cells, expansion of pathogenic T helper 2 and 17 T cell subsets, and development of autoantibodies through impaired B cell regulation are essential to sustain chronic inflammation and tissue injury. Finally, skewed macrophage activation and polarization in response to tissue damage instructs fibroblast activation and collagen deposition, with the progressive deposition of extracellular matrix altering physical properties of the tissues, perpetuating the path of chronic inflammation and fibrosis.

While the self-sustaining activity of distinct immunopathologic processes seen in GVHD creates a significant challenge for management of acute and chronic disease forms, it has also allowed for an increased investigation and identification of key molecular nodes that may serve as therapeutic targets. Following sections will provide an overview of biology-driven strategies for prevention and treatment of GVHD, highlight clinical pharmacology of agents that represent the cornerstone of current GVHD management, and provide insight into the future directions in the field.

AGENTS FOR PREVENTION OF GVHD

While pathophysiology of acute and chronic GVHD recognizes contribution of multiple immune cell subsets to the disease, alloreactive T cells represent the core GVHD effectors and suppression of their activity is the cornerstone of GVHD prophylaxis (Figure 16.3). Summary of agent properties is provided in the Table 16.1.

Calcineurin inhibitors (CNIs) cyclosporine A (CsA) and tacrolimus represent the backbone of most GVHD prevention regimens and have been used continuously for almost five decades. Combination with an antimetabolite (methotrexate) remains the most used GVHD prevention regimen to date. None of the GVHD prevention agents have to date unequivocally demonstrated improved transplant outcomes that would prompt CNI-based regimen displacement from conventional transplant practice. CsA and tacrolimus share comparable clinical properties and are used interchangeably.

Antimetabolites methotrexate (MTX) and mycophenolate mofetil (MMF) are commonly used in conjunction with a CNI for GVHD prevention and remain an option for corticosteroid (CS)-refractory GVHD treatment. MTX is more commonly used with the myeloablative (MAC) and MMF with the reduced intensity (RIC) and nonmyeloablative (NMA) conditioning regimens. MMF is generally given for ~1 month for matched subling donor (MSD) and ~3 months for matched unrelated donor (MUD) transplants.

Post-transplant cyclophosphamide (PTCy) has emerged as one of the most consequential advances in GVHD prevention. It has ushered in the era of haploidentical alloHSCT and allowed transplant access to many patients without a suitable matched donor. PTCy selectively targets rapidly proliferating alloreactive effector T cells, while sparing regulatory (Tregs) and memory T cells to promote development of immune tolerance. Additional immunosuppressive agents (CNIs and/or MMF) are commonly added to the PTCy backbone but are usually tapered/discontinued on an accelerated schedule when compared to CNI-based regimens. Enhanced GVHD prevention benefits are more prominent with the use of bone marrow over the peripheral blood stem cell source.

Antithymocyte globulin (ATG) is an animal-sourced polyclonal immune globulin that has been used as a GVHD prophylaxis agent due to its ability to induce in vivo T cell depletion. This effect is based on complement-mediated and activation-induced cell death. Two formulations of ATG exist based on their animal origin, with rabbit ATG preferred over the horse ATG due to its higher efficacy and greater product consistency.

Abatacept, a humanized cytotoxic T lymphocyte–associated antigen 4 (CTLA4) and immunoglobulin G1 (IgG1) fusion protein, is the first drug approved by the U.S. Food and Drug Administration (FDA) for aGVHD prophylaxis. Abatacept approval was based on the results of a Phase 2 study where improvement in aGVHD was seen in mismatched unrelated donor (MMUD; grade III–IV) and MUD (grade II–IV) setting, without impact on cGVHD.

Sirolimus inhibits mammalian target of rapamycin (mTOR), which disrupts phosphatidylinositol 3-kinase (PI3K)-Akt signaling and blocks T cell activation, proliferation, and differentiation, while preserving Tregs. The main benefit of sirolimus is aGVHD reduction but it is not widely used because of the risk of hepatic sinusoidal obstruction syndrome (SOS; more common with use of busulfan-based MAC regimens or MUD/MMUD grafts).

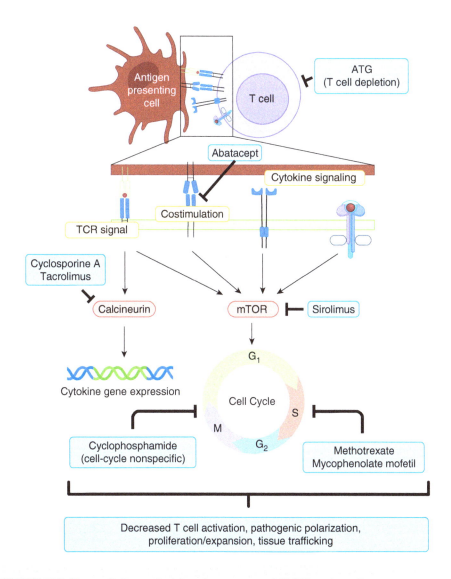

FIGURE 16.3 Key cellular and molecular targets of GVHD prevention.

GVHD, graft-versus-host disease; mTOR, mammalian target of rapamycin.

TABLE 16.1 Properties of Agents Used for Prevention of GVHD

AGENT	MECHANISM OF ACTION	METABOLISM / PHARMACOKINETICS / INTERACTIONS	DOSING / DURATION
CNI (CsA, tacrolimus)	Inhibition of signaling downstream of TCR → ↓ Cytokine expression (IL-2) ↓ T cell proliferation, function, survival CsA: inhibits cyclophilin Tacrolimus: inhibits FK binding proteins	Cytochrome P450 metabolism ↑ levels with CYP inhibitors Impacted by genetic polymorphisms (CYP, P-gp) Excreted in bile	IV (early peritransplant) PO
Antimetabolites (MTX, MMF)	Inhibition of purine and DNA synthesis → ↓ T cell proliferation, function, survival MTX: added inhibition of T cell activation and migration MMF: added effect on B cells	MTX: • eliminated in urine unchanged • ↑ levels with multiple drugs (NSAIDs; PPIs) • ↓ clearance with fluid collections (e.g., ascites) MMF: • metabolized in liver to an active metabolite • inactivated by glucuronidation; excreted in urine	MTX: IV (days +1, +3, +6, +11) together with a CNI SQ for chronic GVHD MMF: IV or PO (1–3 months)
Cyclophosphamide (PTCy)	Blockade of DNA synthesis → ↓ T effectors (number/function) ↑ Treg:effector T cell ratio Treg / hematopoietic stem cells → ↑ ALDH expression → protects from PTCy effects	Metabolized in liver (CYP) to active metabolites CYP inducers potentiate efficacy and toxicity Eliminated in urine or via ALDH inactivation Acrolein metabolite behind hemorrhagic cystitis	IV dosing on day +3 and +4

(continued)

TABLE 16.1 Properties of Agents Used for Prevention of GVHD (*continued*)

AGENT	MECHANISM OF ACTION	METABOLISM / PHARMACOKINETICS / INTERACTIONS	DOSING / DURATION
Antithymocyte globulin (ATG)	↓ Effector T cells (depletion) Broad immunomodulatory effects (B cells, NK cells, DCs)	Poorly characterized	IV in the early peritransplant period (different dosing regimens) Prophylactic antihistamines, acetaminophen, and cortico-steroids are used
Abatacept	Costimulatory blockade (CD80/86:CD28 engagement) → ↓ T cell activation	Clearance ↑ with: ● body weight increase ● MUD over MMUD setting	IV on days -1, +5, +14, +28
Sirolimus	Inhibition of mTOR (downstream of TCR/CD28/IL2 receptor) → ↓ T cell proliferation, function → Treg sparing	Metabolized in the intestine and liver (CYP) ↑ levels with CYP inhibitors	IV (early peritransplant) PO

AGENT	MONITORING	TOXICITIES
CNI (CsA, tacrolimus)	Trough level (collected immediately prior to the next dose) correlates with efficacy and toxicity Target levels may differ based on timing after alloHSCT (↑ if closer to day 0) Leach into plastic → do not collect from lumens used to infuse	Renal toxicity Neurotoxicity (PRES, neuropathy) Hypertension Metabolic/endocrine changes (hypomagnesemia) Thrombotic microangiopathy (TMA) Mechanisms: ● Endothelial damage ● Vasoconstriction ● Neuronal calcineurin inhibition

(continued)

TABLE 16.1 Properties of Agents Used for Prevention of GVHD (*continued*)

AGENT	MONITORING	TOXICITIES
Antimetabolites (MTX, MMF)	MTX: level may be monitored in patient at risk for toxicities to guide leucovorin rescue	MTX: ● Renal toxicity (tubular precipitation; risk ↓with alkalinization (pH≥ 8) ● Hepatic toxicity ● Mucositis ● Myelosuppression MMF: ● Myelosuppression (<MTX) ● GI toxicity (nausea, diarrhea)
Cyclophosphamide (PTCy)	N/A	Myelosuppression (delayed engraftment) Hemorrhagic cystitis can be >20% ● Prevention with mesna, IV fluids, and forced diuresis Possible cardiac toxicity ↑ CMV reactivation
Antithymocyte globulin (ATG)	N/A	Acute infusion reaction, anaphylaxis, serum sickness, and cytokine release syndrome ↑ EBV reactivation / PTLD
Abatacept	N/A	No additional toxicities over CNI/MTX alone seen in the Phase 2 randomized controlled trial
Sirolimus	Trough level	Hypertension, edema, dyslipidemias (hypertriglyceridemia), headaches, mucositis TMA Hepatic SOS
AGENT	USE	COMMENT
CNI (CsA, tacrolimus)	GVHD prevention Acute and chronic GVHD treatment	PRES and TMA require immediate agent discontinuation
Antimetabolites (MTX, MMF)	GVHD prevention GVHD treatment: → aGVHD: MMF → cGVHD: MMF, MTX	If MTX is omitted due to toxicity for one or more doses → replacement with MMF

(*continued*)

TABLE 16.1 Properties of Agents Used for Prevention of GVHD (continued)

AGENT	USE	COMMENT
Cyclophosphamide (PTCy)	GVHD prevention ↓ Severe aGVHD / cGVHD ↑ Efficacy in: • Haploidentical alloHSCT • MMUD alloHSCT	Highly active in preventing GVHD in patients exposed to immune checkpoint blockade
Antithymocyte globulin (ATG)	GVHD prevention → ↓ severe aGVHD/cGVHD Acute GVHD treatment	Pooled analyses highlight ↑ relapse risk No OS improvement
Abatacept	GVHD prevention Chronic GVHD treatment	FDA approval based on Phase 2 study assessing two cohorts: 1. CNI/MTX with abatacept vs. placebo in the MUD setting (randomized, double-blinded) 2. CNI/MTX with abatacept in MMUD setting, compared with historical control subjects No impact on cGVHD prevention
Sirolimus	GVHD prevention → ↓ aGVHD Acute and chronic GVHD treatment	↑ Disease control, overall, and disease-free survival in patients with lymphoma after RIC alloHSCT Hepatic SOS more common with busulfan-based MAC or MUD/MMUD grafts

aGVHD, acute GVHD; ALDH, aldehyde dehydrogenase; alloHSCT, allogeneic hematopoietic stem cell transplantation; cGVHD, chronic GVHD; CMV, cytomegalovirus; CNI, calcineurin inhibitor; CsA, cyclosporine A; CYP, cytochrome P450; DCs, dendritic cells; EBV, Epstein-Barr virus; FDA, U.S. Food and Drug Administration; GI, gastrointestinal; GVHD, graft-versus-host disease; IL-2, interleukin 2; IV, intravenous; MAC, myeloablative conditioning; MMF, mycophenolate mofetil; MMUD, mismatched unrelated donor; mTOR, mammalian target of rapamycin; MTX, methotrexate; MUD, matched unrelated donor; N/A, not applicable; NK, natural killer; NSAIDs, nonsteroidal anti-inflammatory drugs; OS, overall survival; P-gp, P-glycoprotein; PO, oral; PPIs, proton pump inhibitors; PRES, posterior reversible encephalopathy syndrome; PTCy, post-transplant cyclophosphamide; PTLD, post-transplant lymphoproliferative disorder; RIC, reduced-intensity conditioning; SOS, sinusoidal obstruction syndrome; SQ, subcutaneous; TCR, T cell receptor.

AGENTS FOR TREATMENT OF GVHD

Once GVHD occurs, the disease characteristics (acute vs. chronic) and its severity guide the treatment interventions. While mild acute (grade I) or chronic GVHD may be controlled with use of topical or organ-specific therapies only (not discussed in this chapter), moderate/severe disease (grade ≥II for acute; three or more organs involved, and/or symptom score ≥2 for chronic GVHD] warrants use of systemic therapy. While the initial step in this process may include optimization of previously used GVHD prophylaxis regimen (e.g., restart or increase of a previously tapered CNI), additional therapy goal is to control the underlying immune dysregulation that drives tissue destruction (aGVHD) or complex autoimmunity-like disease and fibrosis (cGVHD), since alloreactive T cells are the key effectors of acute and chronic GVHD, treatments center on suppression of critical pathways mediating T cell responses.

SYSTEMIC CORTICOSTEROIDS

Systemic corticosteroids (CS) are the mainstay of frontline acute and chronic GVHD treatment. No agents to date have demonstrated the ability to improve benefits of CS when added to initial therapy.

This is likely due to CS activity and potent regulation of immune responses that impact complex GVHD pathophysiology cascade. CS bind to the intracellular glucocorticoid receptor and regulate expression of range of genes critical for function immune system. The key anti-inflammatory effects are seen in inhibited synthesis of almost all proinflammatory cytokines, promoted expression of regulatory cytokines (e.g., interleukin 10 [IL-10]), and decreased vascular permeability and leukocyte migration to the site of inflammation.

The broad activity of CS also explains the toxicities seen with prolonged exposure, which significantly contribute to GVHD morbidity and may enhance mortality risk. CS toxicities may include opportunistic infections, musculoskeletal toxicities (avascular necrosis, osteoporosis, myopathy, and growth retardation in children), endocrine changes (glucose intolerance or diabetes, hypothalamic-pituitary-adrenal axis suppression and adrenal insufficiency), cardiovascular disease, cataracts, and neuropsychiatric changes. Risk of opportunistic infections, already increased in alloHSCT, warrants use of infection prophylaxis (including reimmunizations) and intensive monitoring (including for cytomegalovirus and Epstein-Barr virus).

The initial CS dose used in aGVHD (2 mg/kg/day of methylprednisolone) is generally higher than that in cGVHD (1 mg/kg/day of prednisone). Use of low CS doses in aGVHD result in more common need for secondary immunosuppression, whereas high CS doses increase complication rates. Higher CS doses have not been beneficial in cGVHD. CS taper and discontinuation are based on disease response and toxicities and occur over a prolonged period (several months), with goal of maintaining the minimal dose required for sustained symptom control. Taper and discontinuation approaches are driven by consensus, clinician experience, and/or institutional preferences, since high-quality evidence is lacking.

Many studies have evaluated the addition of alternate agents to frontline steroids in both acute and chronic GVHD with an overall lack of high-quality data supporting benefit or demonstrating abject failure of such an approach. Nonabsorbable CS (e.g., beclomethasone dipropionate or budesonide) may be added to patients with grade II aGVHD as they reduce systemic CS exposure and may improve response and survival.

Resistance to CS is common and may impact ≥50% of all patients. A unified definition of CS resistance is lacking; however, if appropriate CS exposure is accompanied by overt disease progression (by day 5 for acute, or by day 15 for chronic GVHD) or lack of response (by day 7 for acute or 4–6 weeks for chronic GVHD) second-line therapies should be considered. Inability to taper CS is often considered as an additional manifestation of CS resistance due to the impact of long-term CS use on patient morbidity and mortality.

TREATMENT OF CORTICOSTEROID-RESISTANT GRAFT-VERSUS-HOST DISEASE

Enhanced understanding of GVHD biology and improved disease classification systems have accelerated drug development in both acute and chronic GVHD. This has been accompanied by first FDA approvals for treatment of CS-resistant acute and chronic GVHD, with three new drug agents approved across these indications.

Ruxolitinib

Ruxolitinib, a selective inhibitor of Janus kinase (JAK)1 and JAK2, is the only agent approved by the FDA for treatment of both acute and chronic GVHD in patients 12 years or older after failure of the initial therapy.

JAK-signal transducers and activators of transcription (STAT) pathway mediates signaling transduction downstream of proinflammatory cytokine receptors. Ruxolitinib binding inhibits JAK-STAT signaling and modulates adaptive and innate immune responses critical in acute and chronic GVHD. This includes decreased generation of pathogenic CD4 helper T cells (Th), B cells, and reduced cytokine production.

Ruxolitinib is primarily metabolized by the CYP3A4 enzyme, with up to 50% of metabolites active. Concomitant use with strong CYP3A4 inhibitors warrants close monitoring and dose reduction, as does renal (drug is excreted in urine) and hepatic dysfunction. Key adverse event (AE) in alloHSCT population, based on the mechanism of action, is myelosuppression (anemia and thrombocytopenia are most common and related to JAK signaling role in mediating erythropoietin and thrombopoietin effects), which requires dose modifications. While heightened infectious risk has been described with JAK inhibitors when used outside the alloHSCT setting, published studies have shown that ruxolitinib safety profile is not significantly different from that seen in patients with CS-refractory acute and chronic GVHD treated with best available therapy (BAT).

Ruxolitinib is given orally, with target doses in acute and chronic GVHD lower than those in myelofibrosis. Gradual taper is recommended if response is achieved and sustained to allow CS discontinuation, with re-treatment advised if disease exacerbations occur during taper. While systemic inflammatory response with ruxolitinib withdrawal is documented in patients with myelofibrosis, there is insufficient data to suggest existence of the same in the setting of GVHD treatment.

Efficacy of ruxolitinib in acute and chronic GVHD after failure of CS use was clearly demonstrated in two large randomized controlled trials that compared ruxolitinib with BAT. In aGVHD, superior overall and durable responses were seen with ruxolitinib, which translated in improved median, but not 18-month overall, survival. In cGVHD, ruxolitinib led to superior overall and sustained responses and decreased the need for new therapy initiation but did not significantly impact the ability to reduce concomitant immunosuppression use. Based on these results, findings from a separate meta-analysis, and safety evidence from an expanded access program, ruxolitinib represents a bona fide choice for eligible patients for treatment of acute and chronic GVHD after failure of CS therapy.

EXTRACORPOREAL PHOTOPHERESIS

While not considered a pharmacologic intervention, extracorporeal photopheresis (ECP) remains among the most used treatment modalities for CS-refractory acute and chronic GVHD. Since its initial use in early 1990s, ECP has been administered to thousands of patients. During ECP, apheresis-collected peripheral blood mononuclear cells are incubated with 8-methoxypsoralen, then exposed to ultraviolet irradiation before reinfusion into the patient.

Despite its frequent use in GVHD, ECP mechanism of action remains poorly defined. Described effects include enhanced effector T cell apoptosis, increase in Tregs and regulatory dendritic cells, and reduction in pathogenic B cells.

ECP induces high response rates in acute and chronic GVHD, which are comparable to those seen with currently approved agents. ECP has demonstrated remarkable safety and is often considered a preferred modality in patients with significant infectious complications or at a very high risk of underlying disease relapse. Its major limitation remains the logistical challenge, where need for frequent and prolonged treatments confines its use to highly specialized care centers.

Ibrutinib

Ibrutinib is the first agent approved by the FDA for use in CS-refractory cGVHD. Ibrutinib inhibition of Bruton tyrosine and IL-2 inducible T cell kinase and suppression of pathologic B and T cell responses are reported as the mechanism of action behind cGVHD control.

Common ibrutinib AEs in patients with cGVHD are similar to those seen in other ibrutinib indications, including bleeding and bruising, thrombocytopenia, stomatitis, and diarrhea.

FDA approval was based on the results of an open-label single-arm Phase 1b/2 study that evaluated ibrutinib use in 42 adult patients who received three or fewer prior treatment lines for CS-refractory cGVHD. cGVHD responses were noted in two thirds of patients, with improvements seen in multiple organs accompanied by reduction in CS use in majority of patients. Subsequent study of ibrutinib use in a pediatric cGVHD population replicated adult findings, prompting the addition of cGVHD in pediatric patients ≥1 year of age to ibrutinib label. Study requirement for presence of highly inflammatory cGVHD manifestations at baseline, conflicting real-world experience, and lack of larger follow-up studies confirming the reported benefits limit full appraisal of ibrutinib role in treatment of cGVHD.

Belumosudil

Belumosudil is the first approved agent that targets Rho-associated coiled-coil–containing protein kinase 2 (ROCK2). ROCK2 inhibition promotes Treg homeostasis while reducing IL-17–producing CD4 and follicular helper T cells that promote cGVHD cascade.

Belumosudil was approved based on the results of an open-label Phase 2 study that randomized a total of 132 patients who received at least two prior treatment lines for cGVHD to one of two dosing arms (200 mg orally once vs. twice daily). Reported safety and efficacy outcomes were similar between both cohorts, with an overall cGVHD response seen in 76% of patients and was accompanied reduction of CS use in 65% and patient-reported symptomatic improvement in 70% of cases.

FDA approved the once daily dosing regimen, with twice daily dosing indicated with concurrent strong CYP3A inducer or a proton pump inhibitor use. AEs reported to date are consistent with those commonly seen in cGVHD patients (including fatigue, nausea, diarrhea). Liver function test abnormalities requiring dose modification were uncommon.

OTHER TREATMENTS AND NEW DIRECTIONS

The majority of agents used for GVHD prevention and treatment of established acute and chronic disease have not been approved by regulatory authorities and are used off-label, including CNIs. Many added agents have been evaluated over the years using emerging biology insights and borrowing from other therapeutic indications (usually autoimmunity) where pathophysiology parallels were identified. Challenges in applying the lessons learned to current day practice remain significant and are driven by the mixed quality of prior findings and refined understanding of GVHD. This is particularly true in cGVHD, where heterogeneity of disease classification and lack of agreed objective response metrics before the 2014 National Institutes of Health cGVHD consensus development project prohibits direct comparison to contemporary studies.

While numerous agents have been tested in GVHD over decades, a limited number remains in continued use and is highlighted in Table 16.2. The evidence supporting their benefit is limited; thus, their utilization continues to be based on consensus recommendations, provider experience, institutional practices, and general availability.

Over the past decade, significant progress has been made in prevention and treatment of GVHD, which is seen in the considerable decrease in overall rate of severe acute GVHD, and

TABLE 16.2 List of Additional Agents Used in the Management of Acute and Chronic GVHD After Corticosteroid Failure

AGENT	MECHANISM OF ACTION	INDICATION	COMMENT
Etanercept	Cytokine signaling inhibition (TNF-α)	aGVHD	Response more common with GI GVHD Increased risk of infection and relapse
Tocilizumab	Cytokine signaling inhibition (IL-6)	aGVHD	Evaluated primarily in intestinal GVHD No significant benefit when used as GVHD prevention agent
Alemtuzumab	T cell depletion	aGVHD	High rates of viral, invasive fungal, and bacterial infections
IL-2	Enhanced Treg balance	cGVHD	High early response rates; major AE a flu-like illness
Rituximab	B cell depletion	cGVHD	High response in skin and oral cGVHD (similar to ibrutinib)

(continued)

TABLE 16.2 List of Additional Agents Used in the Management of Acute and Chronic GVHD After Corticosteroid Failure (*continued*)

AGENT	MECHANISM OF ACTION	INDICATION	COMMENT
Proteasome inhibitors (bortezomib/ ixazomib)	B cell depletion	cGVHD	Evaluated in prevention and treatment of cGVHD; overall ixazomib response ~50%
Imatinib	Antifibrotic effects	cGVHD	~30% response rate in sclerotic cGVHD

AE, adverse event; aGVHD, acute GVHD; cGVHD, chronic GVHD; GI, gastrointestinal; GVHD, graft-versus-host disease; IL-6, interleukin 6; TNF-α, tumor necrosis factor alpha.

improved outcomes for acute and chronic GVHD patients. While improvements in supportive care may partly explain this, better understanding of GVHD biology and an expanded therapeutic armamentarium have played an important role as well. Table 16.3 highlights the emerging pharmacologic agents (nonpharmacologic modalities, including microbiome modulation and mesenchymal stem cell therapies are not included) for prevention and treatment of GVHD. Since GVHD is initiated and sustained through ongoing tissue injury, strategies targeting enhanced tissue repair may offer a great promise for future advances in GVHD management.

TABLE 16.3 Emerging Future Agents for Pharmacologic GVHD Prevention and Treatment

AGENT	TARGETED PROCESS	INDICATION
Sitagliptin	Costimulation blockade	GVHD prevention
T-Guard (CD3/ CD7-immunotoxin)	T cell depletion	aGVHD treatment
α1-Antitrypsin	Treg homeostasis Cytokine signaling	aGVHD treatment
Itolizumab	T cell trafficking	aGVHD treatment
Natalizumab		aGVHD treatment
Urinary-derived human chorionic gonadotropin	Tissue repair	aGVHD treatment
F-652 (human IL-22)		aGVHD treatment
Axatilimab	Fibrosis Inflammation	cGVHD treatment

aGVHD, acute GVHD; cGVHD, chronic GVHD; GVHD, graft-versus-host disease; IL-22, interleukin 22.

CHAPTER SUMMARY

GVHD is the major cause of morbidity and death after alloHSCT and strategies that enhance immune tolerance without diminishing anticancer benefits are essential for transplant success. This chapter provides a brief introduction to GVHD pathophysiology and reviews standard and emerging biology-driven interventions for GVHD prevention and treatment. High-yield concepts are shared on mechanism of action, pharmacokinetics, toxicity, and efficacy of key agents used to manipulate immune system after alloHSCT.

CLINICAL PEARLS

- In conventional matched sibling and unrelated donor alloHSCT, no superior alternative to CNI/antimetabolite combination has been identified to date.
- When measuring therapeutic CNI levels, ensure sample is not collected through the catheter lumen previously used for CNI infusion. CNI permeate the plastic and will leach into the sample, leading to falsely high troughs.
- PTCy has dramatically changed access to the alloHSCT by enabling use of haploidentical and mismatched unrelated donors without compromising safety and antitumor efficacy. PTCy use is characterized particularly by reduction in cGVHD.
- Corticosteroids remain the mainstay of upfront acute and chronic GVHD management despite significant long-term toxicities and high rate of treatment failure. Addition of secondary agents to frontline therapy has shown no measurable benefit to date.
- Improved understanding of GVHD biology has since 2017 been accompanied by five new agent approvals for GVHD prevention (abatacept) and treatment (ruxolitinib, acute and chronic; belumosudil, ibrutinib, chronic). Ruxolitinib superiority to alternative agents when used as a second-line therapy in acute and chronic GVHD has been demonstrated in randomized controlled trials.
- Novel strategies for GVHD prevention and treatment increasingly target tissue regeneration as the unresolved tissue damage continues to provide feed forward signals for sustained acute and chronic GVHD.

MULTIPLE-CHOICE QUESTIONS

1. Which of the following AEs is the least likely to be associated with use of CNI after alloHSCT?

    A. Hypomagnesemia
    B. Hypertension
    C. Atrial fibrillation
    D. Neurotoxicity
    E. Renal toxicity

2. A 62-year-old patient undergoing MUD alloHSCT with tacrolimus/MTX GVHD prophylaxis develops severe mucositis on day +9 that prevents oral intake and requires parenteral use of analgesics. Which of the following may have made this potential toxicity of MTX worse?

   A. Use of famotidine for acid reflux
   B. Addition of leucovorin after MTX on day +1, +3, and +6
   C. Use of morphine for analgesia
   D. Prior history of abnormal liver chemistry abnormalities with use of fluconazole
   E. Presence of pleural effusion

3. A 48-year-old patient has undergone haploidentical alloHSCT and received PTCy on day +3 and +4 and continues with tacrolimus/MMF prophylaxis. On day +16, patient developed bloody urine, and diagnosis of hemorrhagic cystitis is made. Which of the following may have predisposed to this known cyclophosphamide toxicity?

   A. Vigorous intravenous fluid repletion around the time of PTCy administration
   B. Use of mesna until the day +4
   C. Forced diuresis around the time of PTCy administration.
   D. Use of steroids for transient cytokine release syndrome on day +5.

4. Which of the following is true regarding PTCy use for GVHD prevention?

   A. Its benefit is limited to severe acute GVHD prevention.
   B. PTCy is more effective in preventing GVHD in MMUD transplantation than abatacept.
   C. Delayed engraftment is uncommon with PTCy use, when compared to conventional CNI-based prophylaxis.
   D. PTCy significantly reduces antitumor benefits of alloHSCT, but this is offset by improved nonrelapse mortalit risk.
   E. PTCy reduces both acute and chronic GVHD.

5. Which of the following agents has not been approved by the FDA for use in treatment of acute or chronic GVHD?

   A. Abatacept
   B. Ruxolitinib
   C. Ibrutinib
   D. Belumosudil

6. Which of the following agents used for GVHD prevention and treatment is associated with increased risk of sinusoidal obstruction syndrome after busulfan-based MAC alloHSCT?

   A. Abatacept
   B. MMF
   C. Sirolimus
   D. CsA
   E. ATG

7.   Which of the following is true regarding agents used for prevention or treatment of GVHD?

   A.   ATG reliably reduces acute and chronic GVHD through isolated depletion of T cells.
   B.   MTX and MMF are most often combined with CNI for prevention of GVHD, with choice of either agent largely driven by the conditioning regimen use (MAC for MTX vs. RIC for MMF).
   C.   Mechanism of action of PTCy rests on expansion of Tregs, while effects on other immune cells that contribute to GVHD are negligible.
   D.   Belumosudil blockade of ROCK2 was the basis of its benefit seen in the randomized Phase 3 clinical trial that led to the FDA approval.
   E.   CNI-based regimens are superior to other GVHD control strategies across all the transplant platforms; and remain the most commonly used prevention modality in alloHSCT.

8.   Which of the following is true regarding ruxolitinib use in GVHD management?

   A.   Its use in cGVHD improves overall survival.
   B.   Its use in cGVHD significantly improves CS discontinuation.
   C.   Systemic inflammatory syndrome is an uncommon AE of ruxolitinib taper in GVHD.
   D.   Thrombocytopenia with ruxolitinib is an unexpected AE in GVHD patients.

9.   Which of the following correctly pairs the agent used in GVHD management with its mechanism of action?

   A.   Abatacept directly causes T cell depletion.
   B.   Tacrolimus binds to cyclophilin to inhibit calcineurin.
   C.   Ibrutinib blocks Bruton tyrosine and IL-2 inducible T cell kinase.
   D.   MTX and MMF inhibit uracil synthesis and DNA transcription.
   E.   Ruxolitinib selectively inhibits JAK1 and JAK3.

10. Transplant-associated thrombotic microangiopathy (TMA) is a rare, but serious complication seen after alloHSCT. TMA may be related to drugs used for GVHD prevention. Which of the following statements regarding TMA is correct?

   A.   TMA is the most common cause of thrombocytopenia seen with ruxolitinib use.
   B.   If TMA is found to be related to agents used for GVHD management, because of the competing GVHD risk, therapy should not be changed.
   C.   TMA association with sirolimus has not been described.
   D.   Both CsA and tacrolimus can cause TMA.
   E.   Addition of abatacept to CNI/MTX regimens has been associated with a significant increase in TMA reporting.

ANSWERS TO MULTIPLE-CHOICE QUESTIONS

1. **C.** Other answers describe common AEs associated with CNI use. In addition, rare, but potentially life-threatening complications may include posterior reversible leukoencephalopathy and transplant-associated microangiopathy, which warrant prompt agent discontinuation.

2. **E.** Presence of third-space fluids leads to MTX accumulation and prolonged elimination, potentiating its toxic AEs. MTX levels may also be increased with concomitant use of proton-pump inhibitors (famotidine is a histamine-2 receptor antagonist) or nonsteroidal anti-inflammatory drugs (not opioids), whereas leucovorin addition would enhance MTX clearance. Resolved prior liver injury does not impact current MTX pharmacokinetics.

3. **B.** Mesna inactivates cyclophosphamide metabolite acrolein and provides uroprotective benefits when high-dose cyclophosphamide is used. Mesna half-life is shorter than that of cyclophosphamide, thus its use throughout the PTCy course is needed for its continued bladder presence and benefit. While CYP3A4 inducers and select azoles (fluconazole and itraconazole) may increase cyclophosphamide levels and promote toxic effects, such effects have not been described for prednisone.

4. **E.** PTCy reduces both acute and chronic GVHD, with significant cGVHD reduction reported across all reported transplant platforms. There is no data directly comparing efficacy of PTCy and abatacept in MMUD alloHSCT. When compared to CNI-based allografting, delayed engraftment is more common with PTCy. Effect of PTCy on relapse is not well defined, but GVL activity after PTCy-based alloHSCT appears largely unaffected.

5. **A.** Abatacept is approved only for GVHD prevention. Ruxolitinib is approved for treatment of both acute and chronic GVHD after failure of one or more lines of therapy. Ibrutinib and belumosudil are approved for treatment of cGVHD.

6. **C.** Sirolimus. Increased risk of sinusoidal obstruction syndrome with use of sirolimus after busulfan-based MAC conditioning and MUD/MMUD grafts was shown in select studies. For other listed agents, such association was not demonstrated.

7. **B.** While choice of an antimetabolite when combined with a CNI may be driven by institutional preference or experience, conditioning intensity is the most common reason for selecting MTX (for MAC) versus MMF (for RIC). ATG reliably reduces cGVHD, whereas mixed aGVHD effects (reduction vs. no effect) have been reported in key studies. While Treg sparing is a part of the mechanism of action of PTCy, it also affects alloreactive T cells (reduced numbers and/or function) and other lymphohematopoietic cells that may contribute to GVHD. While belumosudil inhibits ROCK2 and by doing so modulates immune system to generate cGVHD benefit, its approval was based on the results of a randomized open-label Phase 2 trial. CNI-based prevention remains the most common immunosuppression backbone after alloHSCT, there is no evidence supporting their superiority in all alloHSCT platforms. PTCy-based regimens appear more effective in haploidentical alloHSCT, but direct comparison is lacking.

8. **C.** Systemic inflammatory syndrome has been described in myelofibrosis, but evidence for its occurrence in GVHD patients treated with ruxolitinib is limited. Use of ruxolitinib does not improve survival nor does it significantly impact CS discontinuation in cGVHD. Thrombocytopenia is an expected AE based on ruxolitinib mechanism of action, which involves blockade of JAK signaling necessary for the thrombopoietin activity on megakaryocytes.

9. **C.** Ibrutinib blocks both Bruton tyrosine and IL-2 inducible T cell kinase to inhibit B and T cell pathology in cGVHD. Abatacept blocks costimulation and T cell activation, but does not directly deplete T cells, which is seen with ATG, alemtuzumab, and to an extent PTCy. Tacrolimus binds to FK binding protein to inhibit calcineurin; cyclophilin is a target for CsA. MTX and MMF are antimetabolites that block purine (uracil is a pyrimidine) and DNA synthesis (not transcription) to inhibit T cell proliferation. Ruxolitinib is a selective inhibitor of JAK1 and JAK2, not JAK3.

10. **D.** TMA has been described with sirolimus and both CNIs currently in use without significant difference in its incidence with use of CsA or tacrolimus. Ruxolitinib caused myelosuppression is the most common cause of thrombocytopenia, which improves with dose reduction or drug holding. If TMA is identified and an immunosuppressive agent is considered the cause, the same should be discontinued and alternative immunosuppression considered. Abatacept addition to CNI/MTX-based prophylaxis did not lead to an increase in AE reporting, when compared to CNI/MTX alone.

SELECTED REFERENCES

Abu-Dalle I, Reljic T, Nishihori T, et al. Extracorporeal photopheresis in steroid-refractory acute or chronic graft-versus-host disease: Results of a systematic review of prospective studies. Biol Blood Marrow Transplant. 2014 Nov;20(11):1677–86. https://doi.org/10.1016/j.bbmt.2014.05.017

Carpenter PA, Kang HJ, Yoo KH, et al. Ibrutinib treatment of pediatric chronic graft-versus-host disease: Primary results from the phase 1/2 iMAGINE study. Transplant Cell Ther. 2022 Nov;28(11):771.e1–e10. https://doi.org/10.1016/j.jtct.2022.08.021

Chin KK, Kim HT, Inyang EA, et al. Ibrutinib in steroid-refractory chronic graft-versus-host disease, a single-center experience. Transplant Cell Ther. 2021;27(12):990.e1–e7. https://doi.org/10.1016/j.jtct.2021.08.017

Cooke KR, Luznik L, Sarantopoulos S, et al. The biology of chronic graft-versus-host disease: A task force report from the National Institutes of Health consensus development project on criteria for clinical trials in chronic graft-versus-host disease. Biol Blood Marrow Transplant. 2017 Feb;23(2):211–34. https://doi.org/10.1016/j.bbmt.2016.09.023

Cutler CS, Lee SJ, Arai S, et al. Belumosudil for chronic graft-versus-host disease (cGVHD) after 2 or more prior lines of therapy: The Rockstar study. Blood. 2021;138(22):2278–89. https://doi.org/10.1182/blood.2021012021

Flowers ME, Martin PJ. How we treat chronic graft-versus-host disease. Blood. 2015 Jan 22;125(4):606–15. https://doi.org/10.1182/blood-2014-08-551994

Hui L, Qi L, Guoyu H, et al. Ruxolitinib for treatment of steroid-refractory graft-versus-host disease in adults: A systematic review and meta-analysis. Expert Rev Hematol. 2020 May;13(5):565–75. https://doi.org/10.1080/17474086.2020.1738214

Jagasia MH, Greinix HT, Arora M, et al. National Institutes of Health consensus development project on criteria for clinical trials in chronic graft-versus-host disease: I. The 2014 Diagnosis and Staging

Working Group report. Biol Blood Marrow Transplant. 2015 Mar;21(3):389–401.e1. https://doi.org/10.1016/j.bbmt.2014.12.001

Miklos D, Cutler CS, Arora M, et al. Ibrutinib for chronic graft-versus-host disease after failure of prior therapy. Blood. 2017;130(21):2243–50. https://doi.org/10.1182/blood-2017-07-793786

Niederwieser D, Baldomero H, Bazuaye N, et al. One and a half million hematopoietic stem cell transplants: Continuous and differential improvement in worldwide access with the use of non-identical family donors. Haematologica. 2022;107(5):1045–53. https://doi.org/10.3324/haematol.2021.279189

Schroeder MA, Hari PN, Blithe A, et al. Safety analysis of patients who received ruxolitinib for steroid-refractory acute or chronic graft-versus-host disease in an expanded access program. Bone Marrow Transplant. 2022;57(6):975–81. https://doi.org/10.1038/s41409-022-01673-y

Zeiser R, Blazar BR. Acute graft-versus-host disease—Biologic process, prevention, and therapy. N Engl J Med. 2017 Nov 30;377(22):2167–79. https://doi.org/10.1056/NEJMra1609337

Zeiser R, Blazar BR. Pathophysiology of chronic graft-versus-host disease and therapeutic targets. N Engl J Med. 2017 Dec 28;377(26):2565–79. https://doi.org/10.1056/NEJMra1703472

Zeiser R, Polverelli N, Ram R, et al. Ruxolitinib for glucocorticoid-refractory chronic graft-versus-host disease. N Engl J Med. 2021;385(3):228–38. https://doi.org/10.1056/NEJMoa2033122

Zeiser R, Von Bubnoff N, Butler J, et al. Ruxolitinib for glucocorticoid-refractory acute graft-versus-host disease. N Engl J Med. 2020;382(19):1800–10. https://doi.org/10.1056/NEJMoa1917635

CHAPTER 17

Monoclonal Antibodies Including Antibody–Drug Conjugates, Immunoconjugates, and Cytokine-Directed Agents

ALISON DUFFY • CIERA BERNHARDI

INTRODUCTION

This chapter illustrates the key features of monoclonal antibodies and cytokine therapy. For monoclonal antibodies, both naked and conjugated types are described as well as common targets, classifications, common oncologic uses, structure, and mechanism of action. Understanding the cancer pharmacology of these agents informs the reader of the common class-wide and target-specific side effects, as well as how to prevent, monitor, and manage these toxicities. Similarly, the chapter also provides an overview of cytokine therapy efficacy and toxicity, and describes mechanism of action. It compares and contrasts the toxicities seen with interferon and high-dose interleukin therapy and describes their management. Although these cytokine-directed agents may have a restricted place in therapy, they paved the way for more recent immunotherapy drug approvals (Tables 17.1 and 17.2 and Figures 17.1–17.3).

Naked monoclonal antibodies are antibodies with no additional elements; these antibodies contribute to killing cancer cells alone and only by immunologic mechanisms. Conjugated monoclonal antibodies are structurally combined with chemotherapy or a radioactive compound and, in theory, kill the cancer cells in traditional manner albeit with much more selectivity.

TABLE 17.1 Monoclonal Antibody Class and Target Overview

TARGET	TYPE	DRUG	CLASSIFICATION	COMMON ONCOLOGIC USES
BCMA	Conjugate	Belantamab* mafodotin[†]	Humanized	Multiple myeloma
CCR4	Naked	Mogamulizumab	Humanized	Mycosis fungoides
CD19	Conjugate	Loncastuximab tesirine	Chimeric	NHL
CD19	Naked	Tafasitamab*	Humanized	NHL
CD20	Naked	Obinutuzumab	Humanized	CLL, NHL
CD20	Naked	Ofatumumab	Human	CLL
CD20	Naked	Rituximab	Chimeric	NHL, ALL, CLL
CD20	Radioisotope	Ibritumomab tiuxetan Y-90	Murine	NHL
CD22	Conjugate	Inotuzumab ozogamicin	Humanized	ALL
CD22	Conjugate	Moxetumomab pasudotox	Mouse	Hairy cell leukemia
CD30	Conjugate	Brentuximab vedotin	Chimeric	Hodgkin lymphoma, CTCL
CD33	Conjugate	Gemtuzumab ozogamicin	Humanized	AML
CD38	Naked	Daratumumab	Human	Multiple myeloma
CD38	Naked	Isatuximab	Chimeric	Multiple myeloma
CD52	Naked	Alemtuzumab	Humanized	CLL, T-PLL
CD79b	Conjugate	Polatuzumab vedotin	Humanized	NHL
EGFR	Naked	Cetuximab	Chimeric	Head and neck, colorectal, NSCLC
EGFR	Naked	Necitumumab	Human	NSCLC

(continued)

TABLE 17.1 Monoclonal Antibody Class and Target Overview (*continued*)

TARGET	TYPE	DRUG	CLASSIFICATION	COMMON ONCOLOGIC USES
EGFR	Naked	**Panitumumab**	Human	Colorectal
EGFR/ cMET	Naked, bispecific	**Amivantamab***	Human	NSCLC
GD2	Naked	**Dinutuximab**	Chimeric	Neuroblastoma
GD2	Naked	**Naxitamab***	Humanized	Neuroblastoma
HER2	Conjugate	**Ado-trastuzumab emtansine**	Humanized	Breast
HER2	Conjugate	**Trastuzumab deruxtecan**	Humanized	Breast
HER2	Naked	**Margetuximab**	Chimeric	Breast
HER2	Naked	**Pertuzumab**	Humanized	Breast
HER2	Naked	**Trastuzumab**	Humanized	Breast, gastric
Nectin-4	Conjugate	**Enfortumab vedotin**	Human	Urothelial
SLAMF7	Naked	**Elotuzumab**	Humanized	Multiple myeloma
Tissue factor	Conjugate	**Tisotumab vedotin**	Human	Cervical
Trop-2	Conjugate	**Sacituzumab govitecan**	Humanized	Breast
VEGF	Naked	**Bevacizumab**	Humanized	Colorectal, NSCLC, RCC, cervical, glioblastoma
VEGF	Naked	**Ramucirumab**	Human	Gastric, colorectal, NSCLC

*Does not follow typical nomenclature rules for monoclonal antibodies (described in Figure 17.1).
†In November 2022, the manufacturer and the sponsor of belantamab mafodotin-blmf announced that it has initiated the process for withdrawal of the U.S. marketing authorization for the agent. This decision was made after the request of the U.S. Food and Drug Administration (FDA), which was based on the previously announced outcome of the DREAMM-3, a Phase III confirmatory trial, which did not meet the requirements of the FDA Accelerated Approval regulations. Belantamab mafodotin-blmf, a monotherapy treatment, was used for treatment of adult patients with relapsed or refractory multiple myeloma who have received at least four prior therapies including an anti-CD38 monoclonal antibody, a proteasome inhibitor, and an immunomodulatory agent.

MONOCLONAL ANTIBODY STRUCTURE

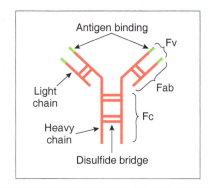

CLASSIFICATION

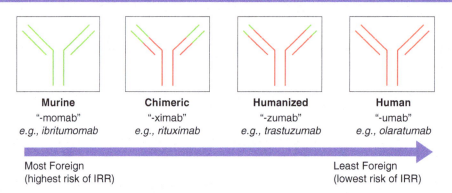

FIGURE 17.1 Monoclonal antibody structure and classification.
Naked monoclonal antibodies (Mabs) are modified immunoglubulin G (IgG) antibodies directed at tumor-specific markers to enhance the activity of the body's own immune system against the malignant cell. Similar to human IgG, Mabs generally consist of two identical heavy chains and two identical light chains. These chains are connected by multiple disulfide bridges. The integrity of these disulfide bridges is critical in maintaining stability and therapeutic effect of the Mab.

The fragment crystallizable (Fc) region is identical to human IgG and allows for coordination with the innate immune system. The active antibody fragment (Fv) region is contained within the fragment antigen-binding (Fab) region, and is the manufactured variation that is directed at the respective targeted tumor marker. Typically, monoclonal antibodies have two identical Fv regions (as they are typically made of the same heavy chains and light chains as mentioned previously). An exception is amivantamab, a bispecific Mab that has two different Fv regions: one that binds epidermal growth factor receptor (EGFR), one that binds cMET. This is different from a bispecific T cell engager (BiTE) Mab (e.g., blinatumomab), as amivantamab targets two separate tumor antigens and maintains an Fc region.

Mabs are classified based on the ratio of human-derived versus murine-derived components. The nomenclature of monoclonal antibodies is partially derived from its classification. For example, chimeric Mabs end in the suffix "-ximab" such as rituximab. Those that consist of more murine-derived components have a higher risk of infusion-related reaction (IRR) due to the degree of foreignness.

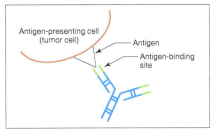

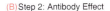

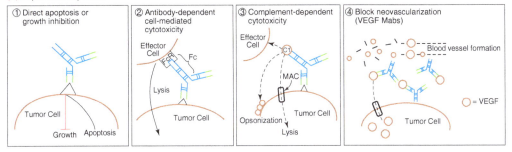

FIGURE 17.2 Naked monoclonal antibody mechanism of action.

Monoclonal antibodies (Mabs) exert their activity in a two-step process.

(A) Antibody recognition of the antigen occurs when the antigen-binding site of the Mab (Fv region) binds to the antigen on the antigen-presenting cell (tumor cell).

(B) Antibody effect predominantly occurs via one of four primary mechanisms, although many Mabs exert their activity via multiple mechanisms.

(1) Direct apoptosis or growth inhibition occurs when the antigen-binding site of the Mab binds to the antigen on the tumor cell, causing inhibition or activation of an intracellular process that promotes tumor growth or tumor death, respectively.

(2) Antibody-dependent cell-mediated cytotoxicity (ADCC) occurs when the Fc region of the Mab binds to the Fc receptor (FcR) on effector cells such as natural killer cells, resulting in a release of inflammatory and cytotoxic proteins that ultimately result in cell death.

(3) Complement-dependent cytotoxicity (CDC) is activated by the binding of complement component 1 (C1) to the Fc region of the Mab to initiate the classical complement pathway. The downstream effects of the complement cascade result in opsonization of the tumor cell surface, effector cell recruitment, and the formation of the membrane attack complex (MAC). The MAC forms pores in the surface of the tumor cell and results in cell lysis. Notably, both CDC and ADCC require a functioning innate immune system; therefore, activity via these mechanisms may be diminished in an immunocompromised patient.

(4) Block neovascularization is a mechanism specific to Mabs targeting vascular endothelial growth factor (VEGF). Tumor cells deprived of adequate blood supply may secrete VEGF to stimulate angiogenesis. This restores adequate perfusion to the tumor to allow for continued tumor growth. VEGF-targeted Mabs sequester VEGF, inhibiting its ability to promote angiogenesis.

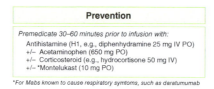

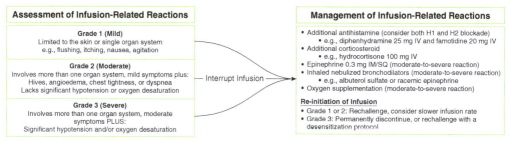

FIGURE 17.3 Prevention and management of infusion-related reactions due to monoclonal antibodies.

Infusion-related reactions (IRRs) are a possible reaction to all Mabs; however, they are more common with murine or chimeric Mabs. Prevention, identification, and management of such reactions are described in this figure.

Premedication selection is based on drug, infusion rate, and past toxicities. The reader is referred to the package insert for each Mab for guidance on specific agent selection. IRRs are usually a result of proinflammatory cytokines (TNF-α and IL-6) that are released upon binding of the Mab to its target. Predominantly these reactions occur acutely during the first infusion or just after completion of the infusion, and are frequently low grade. Rechallenging of the Mab is often feasible in these cytokine-mediated reactions.

It is possible that some infusion-related reactions are true allergies and are IgE-mediated rather than cytokine-mediated. IgE-mediated reactions usually occur at the second (or later) infusion, as initial sensitization must occur before an immune reaction can be mounted.

The exception is cetuximab, which frequently has an IgE-mediated reaction upon the first infusion due to a natural preexposure to an oligosaccharide, galactose-α-1,3-galactose, that is common to some geographical areas such as the southeast portion of the United States. IgE-mediated reactions are prohibitive in any further use of that Mab without a desensitization protocol.

EGFR, epidermal growth factor receptor; GD2, ganglioside typically on neuroectoderm-derived cells; HER2, human epidermal growth factor receptor 2; IgE, immunoglobulin E; IL-6, interleukin 6; IM, intramuscular; IV, intravenous; Mabs, monoclonal antibodies; PO, by mouth; SQ, subcutaneous; TNF-α, tumor necrosis factor alpha; VEGF, vascular endothelial growth factor.

TABLE 17.2 Select Target-Specific Toxicities and Management

Common toxicities of each Mab are related to the anatomic distribution of the corresponding receptor on nontumor cells.

EGFR and HER2 are related receptors and are both highly expressed on epithelial cells including that of the skin and gastrointestinal tract. Agents targeting either EGFR or HER2 therefore have a high prevalence of rash, diarrhea, and other related toxicities.

VEGF receptors are prevalent on vasculature endothelial cells that, when stimulated by VEGF, release nitric oxide to cause vasodilation and ultimately lower blood pressure. When VEGF is sequestered by a VEGF-inhibiting Mab, vasoconstriction occurs causing hypertension.

GD2 expression in peripheral pain fibers results in profound pain for patients when receiving GD2-directed therapy, necessitating inpatient admission and the use of patient-controlled analgesia.

TARGET	TOXICITY (INCIDENCE)	TOXICITY PREVENTION	TOXICITY MANAGEMENT
EGFR	Papulopustular rash (77%–96%)	<ul><li>Moisturizer cream</li><li>Sunscreen</li></ul> Can consider: <ul><li>Topical steroid (low potency)</li><li>Doxycycline</li></ul>	<ul><li>Topical steroid treatment<ul><li>○ Face: low potency</li><li>○ Body: high potency</li></ul></li><li>Systemic treatment (grade 3 or 4 only):<ul><li>○ Corticosteroids</li><li>○ Tetracyclines</li></ul></li></ul> *Consider dose reduction or discontinuation for grade 3 or 4*
	Diarrhea (16%–72%)	<ul><li>Adequate hydration</li></ul>	<ul><li>Loperamide</li><li>Fluid and electrolyte repletion as needed</li></ul>
	Stomatitis (7%–32%)	<ul><li>Adequate oral hygiene</li><li>Consider sodium bicarbonate mouth rinse after each meal</li></ul>	<ul><li>Pain management with topical and/or systemic analgesics</li></ul>

(continued)

TABLE 17.2 Select Target-Specific Toxicities and Management (*continued*)

TARGET	TOXICITY (INCIDENCE)	TOXICITY PREVENTION	TOXICITY MANAGEMENT
HER2	Diarrhea (7%–67%)	● Adequate hydration	● Loperamide ● Fluid and electrolyte repletion as needed

	Rash (4%–34%)	● Moisturizer cream
		● Sunscreen
			● Topical steroid treatment:
			  ○ Face: low potency
			  ○ Body: high potency
			● Systemic treatment (grade 3 or 4 only):
			  ○ Corticosteroids
			  ○ Tetracyclines

	Decreased LVEF (4%–22%)	● Separate from administration schedule of anthracyclines	● Manage as per current guidelines for HF ● Hold therapy for at least 4 weeks; may consider rechallenging if LVEF resolves
VEGF	HTN (12%–34%)	N/A	● Manage as per current guidelines for HTN, preference for ACEi or ARB therapy ● Avoid nifedipine, which has been associated with increased VEGF secretion
	Proteinuria/nephrotic syndrome (4%–36%)	● Optimize HTN management	● Grade 1: no intervention needed ● Grade 2: hold therapy until resolves, reinitiate at reduced dose ● Grade >3 or nephrotic syndrome: discontinue permanently
	Thrombosis (2%–15%)	● VTE prophylaxis is not routinely recommended, unless other indications exist	● Hold therapy while anticoagulation is initiated and stabilized ● Permanently discontinue for arterial thrombosis or grade 4 venous thrombosis
	Bleeding (up to 40%)	● Optimize HTN management	● Discontinue permanently for grade 3 or 4
	Wound dehiscence (1%–15%)	N/A	● Discontinue permanently
	Gastrointestinal perforation (<1%–3%)	N/A	● Discontinue permanently

(continued)

TABLE 17.2 Select Target-Specific Toxicities and Management (*continued*)

TARGET	TOXICITY (INCIDENCE)	TOXICITY PREVENTION	TOXICITY MANAGEMENT
GD2	Neuropathic pain (52% severe, 85% all grade)	• Dinutuximab: morphine 50 mcg/kg IV once, then 20–50 mcg/kg/hour CIVI with PCA • Naxitamab: administer 12-day course of gabapentin starting 5 days prior to first dose each cycle	If inadequately controlled: • Consider additional opioids/lidocaine 2 mg/kg IV once, then 1 mg/kg/hour
	Capillary leak syndrome (23%) Hypotension (18%)	• 0.9% NaCl bolus—10 mL/kg	• Interrupt infusion; upon resolution, resume infusion at 50% previous rate
	Infection or sepsis (18%)	N/A	• Discontinue until resolution; continue to next cycle, even if previous cycle incomplete
	Neurologic eye disorders (2%)	N/A	• No visual impairment: decrease dose by 50% • Visual impairment: permanently discontinue

Note: Black box warnings are denoted with a bold outline.

ACEi, angiotensin conversion enzyme inhibitor; ARB, angiotensin receptor blocker; CIVI, continuous intravenous infusion; EGFR, epidermal growth factor receptor; GD2, ganglioside typically on neuro-ectoderm-derived cells; HER2, human epidermal growth factor receptor 2; HF, heart failure; HTN, hypertension; IV, intravenous; LVEF, left ventricular ejection fraction; N/A, not applicable; NaCl, sodium chloride; PCA, patient-controlled analgesia; VEGF, vascular endothelial growth factor; VTE, venous thromboembolism.

MONOCLONAL ANTIBODIES IN COMBINATION WITH OTHER CHEMOTHERAPEUTICS

In modern oncology clinical practice, Mabs are often combined with conventional cytotoxic chemotherapeutic agents, with targeted therapies, with other immunotherapy, or with radiation therapy to improve clinical outcomes both in frontline setting as well as in the relapsed or refractory conditions. Some of the common examples of "chemoimmunotherapy" for treatment of different oncologic conditions include:

• **Rituximab**: (a) in combination with cyclophosphamide, doxorubicin, vincristine, and prednisone (CHOP) or other anthracycline-based chemotherapy regimens or in combination with cyclophosphamide, vincristine, and prednisone (CVP) chemotherapy for untreated diffuse large B cell, CD20[+] non-Hodgkin lymphoma (NHL), Burkitt lymphoma, Burkitt-like lymphoma, or mature B cell acute leukemia; (b) in combination with fludarabine and cyclophosphamide for patients with previously untreated and previously treated CD20⁺ chronic lymphocytic leukemia (CLL); (c) in combination with hyper-CVAD/HiDAC-HDMTX (hyperfractionated cyclophosphamide, vincristine, doxorubicin, dexamethasome/high-dose methotrexate–high-dose cytarbine) for treatment of CD20⁺ B cell acute lymphoblastic leukemia (B-ALL)

- ***Rituximab biosimilars (Riabni [rituximab-arrx], Ruxience [rituximab-pvvr], Truxima [rituximab-abbs])***: in general are used as monotherapy or in combination with conventional chemotherapy with similar indications as rituximab

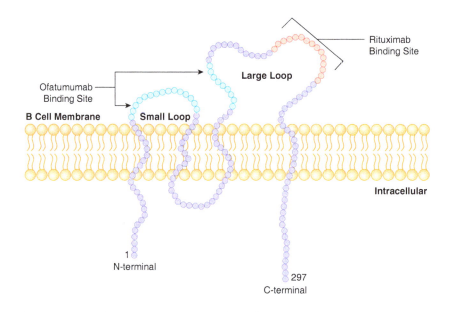

FIGURE 17.4 The structure of CD20 and different binding sites of different anti-CD20 monoclonal antibodies.

- ***Tafasitamab-cxix***: in combination with lenalidomide for the treatment of adult patients with relapsed or refractory diffuse large B cell lymphoma who are not eligible for autologous stem cell transplant
- ***Cetuximab***
  ○ Head and neck cancer: locally or regionally advanced squamous cell carcinoma in combination with radiation therapy (initial dose: 400 mg/m² administered as a 2-hour intravenous [IV] infusion 1 week prior to initiating a course of radiation therapy; subsequent doses: 250 mg/m² administered as a 1-hour infusion every week for the duration of radiation therapy). Cetuximab administration should be completed 1 hour prior to radiation therapy.
  ○ Colorectal cancer (*KRAS* wild-type, *EGFR*-expressing, metastatic disease): (a) in combination with FOLFIRI for first-line treatment, (b) in combination with irinotecan in patients who are refractory to irinotecan-based chemotherapy, (c) in combination with encorafenib, for the treatment of adult patients with metastatic colorectal cancer with a BRAF V600E mutation

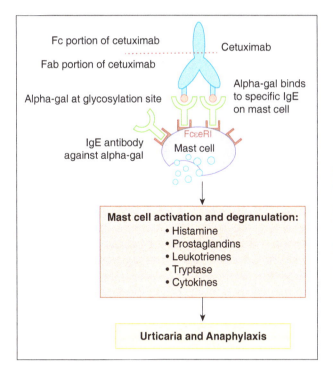

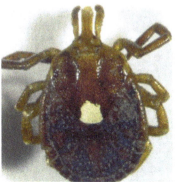

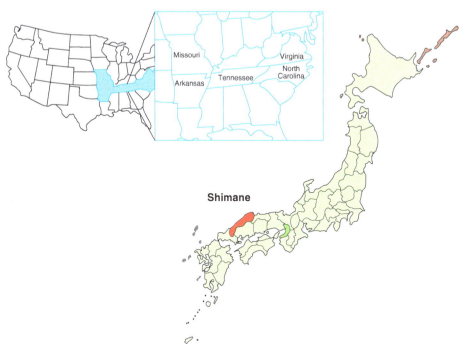

FIGURE 17.5 Cetuximab- and red meat–induced anaphylaxis in the southern United States, where tick-mediated Rocky Mountain spotted fever is common.

(continued)

FIGURE 17.5 Cetuximab- and red meat–induced anaphylaxis in the southern United States, where tick-mediated Rocky Mountain spotted fever is common. (*continued*) Immunoglobulin E (IgE) antibodies against cetuximab are present prior to therapy in a majority of patients who develop allergic reactions during cetuximab administration. The antibodies are specific for galactose-α-1,3-galactose (alpha-gal), which is present on the Fab portion of the cetuximab heavy chain.

Patients with IgE antibodies against galactose-α-1,3-galactose often experience delayed anaphylaxis after eating red meat with the abundant expression of the galactose-α-1,3-galactose epitope in the tissues of non-primate mammals.

IgE antibodies to galactose-α-1,3-galactose are produced in response to tick bites; as it is known that anti-galactose-α-1,3-galactose IgE antibodies reacted with proteins of *Amblyomma americanum*, a tick common in the southeastern United States. Hence, anti-galactose-α-1,3-galactose IgE antibodies formed by recurrent tick bites is associated with the development of anaphylaxis, both during cetuximab infusion and after consuming red meat.

High incidences of both cetuximab- and red meat–induced anaphylaxis have been reported in the southern United States, where tick-mediated Rocky Mountain spotted fever is common as well as in Japan, in eastern Shimane region, where tick-mediated Japanese spotted fever is common.

- *Panitumumab*: in combination with FOLFOX for first-line treatment of wild-type RAS (defined as wild-type in both KRAS and NRAS) metastatic colorectal cancer
- *Necitumumab*: in combination with gemcitabine and cisplatin, for first-line treatment of patients with metastatic squamous non-small cell lung cancer. It is not indicated for treatment of nonsquamous non-small cell lung cancer.
- *Trastuzumab*: (a) in combination with eribulin and pertuzumab for HER2$^+$ advanced or metastatic breast cancer, (b) in combination with docetaxel and carboplatin as neoadjuvant therapy for HER2$^+$ breast cancer, (c) doxorubicin plus cyclophosphamide followed by paclitaxel with trastuzumab followed by extended trastuzumab as adjuvant therapy for HER2$^+$ breast cancer
- *Pertuzumab*: (a) in combination with trastuzumab and docetaxel for treatment of patients with HER2$^+$ metastatic breast cancer who have not received prior anti-HER2 therapy or chemotherapy for metastatic disease; (b) in combination with trastuzumab and chemotherapy as neoadjuvant treatment of patients with HER2$^+$, locally advanced, inflammatory, or early-stage breast cancer as part of a complete treatment regimen for early breast cancer; (c) in combination with trastuzumab and chemotherapy as adjuvant treatment of patients with HER2$^+$ early breast cancer at high risk of recurrence
- *Brentuximab vedotin*: (a) in combination with doxorubicin, vinblastine, and dacarbazine for previously untreated stage III or IV classical Hodgkin lymphoma; (b) in combination with doxorubicin, vincristine, etoposide, prednisone, and cyclophosphamide for pediatric patients 2 years and older with previously untreated high-risk classical Hodgkin lymphoma; (c) as monotherapy for adult patients with classical Hodgkin lymphoma at high risk of relapse or progression as post-autologous hematopoietic stem cell transplantation (auto-HSCT) consolidation; (d) for adult patients with classical Hodgkin

lymphoma after failure of auto-HSCT or after failure of at least two prior multiagent chemotherapy regimens in patients who are not auto-HSCT candidates; (e) for adult patients with systemic anaplastic large cell lymphoma after failure of at least one prior multiagent chemotherapy regimen; (f) in combination with cyclophosphamide, doxorubicin, and prednisone for adult patients with previously untreated systemic anaplastic large cell lymphoma or other CD30-expressing peripheral T cell lymphomas (PTCL), including angioimmunoblastic T cell lymphoma and PTCL not otherwise specified; (g) as monotherapy for adult patients with primary cutaneous anaplastic large cell lymphoma or CD30-expressing mycosis fungoides (MF) who have received prior systemic therapy

- *Gemtuzumab ozogamicin*: in combination with an anthracycline (e.g., daunorubicin or idarubicin) and cytarabine [e.g., 7+3] for treatment of newly diagnosed $CD33^+$ acute myeloid leukemia in adults and pediatric patients 1 month and older

- *Daratumumab* (see also Chapter 15): (a) in combination with bortezomib, melphalan, and prednisone in newly diagnosed patients with multiple myeloma (MM) who are ineligible for auto-HSCT; (b) in combination with lenalidomide and dexamethasone in newly diagnosed patients with MM who are ineligible for auto-HSCT and in patients with relapsed or refractory multiple myeloma (RRMM) who have received a least one prior therapy; (c) in combination with bortezomib, thalidomide, and dexamethasone in newly diagnosed patients with MM who are eligible for auto-HSCT; (d) in combination with bortezomib and dexamethasone in patients with RRMM who have received at least one prior therapy; (e) in combination with carfilzomib and dexamethasone in patients with RRMM who have received one to three prior lines of therapy; (f) in combination with pomalidomide and dexamethasone in patients with RRMM who have received at least two prior therapies including lenalidomide and a proteasome inhibitor; (g) as single agent in patients with RRMM who have received at least three prior lines of therapy including a proteasome inhibitor and an immunomodulatory agent or who are double-refractory to a proteasome inhibitor and an immunomodulatory agent

- *Polatuzumab vedotin*: in combination with bendamustine and rituximab or a rituximab biosimilar for the treatment of adult patients with relapsed or refractory diffuse large B cell lymphoma after at least two prior therapies

- *Bevacizumab*: (a) in combination with IV 5-fluorouracil-based chemotherapy for first or second-line treatment of metastatic colorectal cancer, (b) in combination with fluoropyrimidine+irinotecan- or fluoropyrimidine+oxaliplatin-based chemotherapy for second-line treatment in patients with metastatic colorectal cancer who have progressed on a first-line bevacizumab or bevacizumab biosimilar-containing regimen, (c) in combination with carboplatin and paclitaxel for first-line treatment of patients with unresectable, locally advanced, recurrent or metastatic nonsquamous non-small cell lung cancer, (d) in combination with interferon-α for metastatic renal cell carcinoma, (e) in combination with paclitaxel and cisplatin, or paclitaxel and topotecan for persistent, recurrent, or metastatic cervical cancer, (f) in combination with carboplatin and paclitaxel, followed by bevacizumab as monotherapy for stage III or IV epithelial ovarian, fallopian tube, or primary peritoneal cancer following initial surgical resection, (g) in combination with paclitaxel, pegylated liposomal doxorubicin, or topotecan for platinum-resistant recurrent epithelial ovarian, fallopian tube, or primary peritoneal cancer who received no more than two prior chemotherapy regimens, (h) in combination with carboplatin and paclitaxel or carboplatin and gemcitabine, followed by bevacizumab as monotherapy for platinum-sensitive recurrent epithelial ovarian, fallopian tube, or primary peritoneal cancer, (i) in combination with atezolizumab for the treatment of patients with unresectable or metastatic hepatocellular carcinoma (HCC) who have not received prior systemic therapy, (j) as monotherapy for recurrent glioblastoma in adults. Of note, bevacizumab is not indicated for adjuvant treatment of colon cancer.

ANTIBODY–DRUG CONJUGATES

Conjugates of antibodies with drugs and isotopes have also been shown to be effective in the treatment of cancer and have the intent of increasing the therapeutic index of the drug or isotope by delivering the cytoxic "warhead" or "payload" directly to the tumor cell or tumor microenvironment (Figure 17.6).

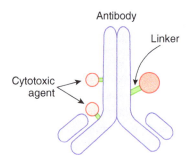

FIGURE 17.6 Elements of an antibody–drug conjugate (ADC).
The ADC is a three-component system including a potent cytotoxic anticancer agent linked via a biodegradable linker to an antibody. The antibody binds to specific markers (antigens or receptors) at the surface of the cancer cell. The cytotoxic agent or "warhead" is designed to kill the target cells when internalized and released. There are three main categories of cytotoxic agents for commercially available ADCs: microtubule inhibitors, DNA-damaging agents, and most recently, protein synthesis inhibitors. The linker attaches the cytotoxic agent to the antibody. Newer linker systems are stable in circulation and are able to release the cytotoxic agent inside the target cells.

TABLE 17.3 Available Antibody–Drug Conjugates

CYTOTOXIC AGENT	DRUG	DOSE-LIMITING TOXICITIES	CLINICAL PEARLS
Microtubule Inhibitors			
DM-1	**Ado-trastuzumab emtansine**	**Hepatotoxicity, embryo-fetal toxicity**, thrombocytopenia, **cardiotoxicity**, pulmonary toxicity (interstitial lung disease/pneumonitis), peripheral neuropathy	**Not interchangeable with conventional trastuzumab**
Monomethyl auristatin E (MMAE)	**Enfortumab vedotin**	Hyperglycemia, peripheral neuropathy, ocular disorders, skin reactions, infusion site extravasations, embryo-fetal toxicity	Clinically relevant drug interactions with CYP3A4 strong inhibitors and inducers; consider artificial tears prophylactically
MMAE	**Tisotumab vedotin**	**Ocular disorders**, hemorrhage, pneumonitis, peripheral neuropathy, embryo-fetal toxicity	Eye drop pre-medications and eye care requirements
MMAE	**Polatuzumab vedotin**	Peripheral neuropathy, infusion-related reactions, myelosuppression, opportunistic infections, progressive multifocal leukoencephalopathy (PML), tumor lysis syndrome, hepatotoxicity, embryo-fetal toxicity	Antipyretic and antihistamine premedications
MMAE	**Brentuximab vedotin**	Peripheral neuropathy, myelosuppression, hepatotoxicity, renal impairment, **JC virus and PML**	Clinically relevant drug interactions with CYP3A4 strong inhibitors and inducers
MMAF	**Belantamab mafodotin**	**Ocular changes,** infusion reactions, embryo-fetal toxicity, thrombocytopenia	Available through restriction program, BLENREP REMS, eye exams required
DNA Damaging Agents			
DXd (Topoisomerase inhibitor)	**Trastuzumab deruxtecan**	Cardiotoxicity, **pulmonary toxicity (interstitial lung disease/pneumonitis), embryo-fetal toxicity,** neutropenia	**Not interchangeable with conventional trastuzumab**

(continued)

TABLE 17.3 Available Antibody–Drug Conjugates (continued)

CYTOTOXIC AGENT	DRUG	DOSE-LIMITING TOXICITIES	CLINICAL PEARLS
SN-38 (Topoisomerase inhibitor)	**Sacituzumab govitecan**	**Severe neutropenia and diarrhea,** nausea/vomiting, embryo-fetal toxicity, hypersensitivity	Infusion reaction and antiemetic pre-medications, diarrhea treatment and pharmacogenomic considerations (UGT1A1 activity) similar to irinotecan
SG3199 (alkylating agent)	**Loncastuximab tesirine**	Effusions/edema, myelosuppression, infections, cutaneous reactions, embryo-fetal toxicity	Steroid premedication
Calicheamicin (DNA minor groove inhibitor)	**Inotuzumab ozogamicin**	**Hepatotoxicity** [including **veno-occlusive disease (VOD)** also called **sinusoidal obstruction syndrome (SOS)**], myelosuppression	Premedicate with antihistamine, antipyretic, corti-costeroid, consider cytoreductive therapy
Calicheamicin (DNA distruption)	**Gemtuzumab ozogamicin**	**Hepatotoxicity [VOD/SOS],** myelosuppression, **hemorrhage**	Premedicate with antihistamine, antipyretic, corticosteroid, consider cytoreductive therapy
Protein Synthesis Inhibitors			
PE38 (*Pseudomonas* exotoxin-protein synthesis inhibitor)	**Moxetumomab pasudotox**	**Capillary leak syndrome (CLS), hemolytic uremic syndrome (HUS),** renal toxicity, infusion-related reactions, electrolyte abnormalities	Avoid if creatinine clearance <29 mL/min; premedicate with antipyretic, antihistamine, H2 receptor antagonist, hydration, thrombo-prophylaxis with low-dose aspirin (day 1–8/cycle), consider post-infusion medications; see package insert for monitoring for toxicities (similar to high-dose interleukin)

Bold text indicates a black box warning; similar to naked monoclonal antibodies, all agents have a risk of infusion reactions with varying likelihood based on monoclonal antibody classification (nomenclature).

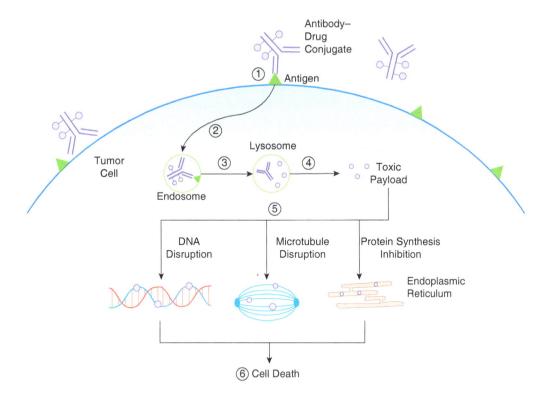

FIGURE 17.7 **Antibody–drug conjugate mechanism of action.**

Antibody–drug conjugates (ADCs) follow a six-step pathway to exert their toxic effect on the tumor cell. In describing these six steps, an example antibody–drug conjugate, ado-trastuzumab emtansine, is used. Ado-trastuzumab emtansine, also referred to as ado-trastuzumab, is an antibody–drug conjugate that shows valuable activity in patients with breast cancer who have developed resistance to the "naked" antibody. This antibody–drug conjugate is made up of trastuzumab and the highly potent microtubule targeted agent DM1 (derived from maytansine isolated from an Ethiopian plant, *Maytenus ovatus*), linked together by a nonreducible thioether linker (SMCC, referred to as MCC in conjugated form). This molecule T-MCC-DM1 is referred to more commonly as T-DM1.

Step 1: Antibody–drug conjugate recognizes and binds to its antigen target: T-DM1 binds to the HER2 protein on the extracellular domain of breast cancer cells and begins to exert its antitumor effects.

Step 2: Antibody–drug conjugate internalization: The HER2–T-DM1 complex undergoes internalization via an endosome.

Step 3: Fusion with lysosome: This internalized complex is then fused with a lysosome, followed by proteolytic degradation of the linker to release DM-1.

Step 4: Toxic payload release: DM-1-containing catabolites are released. The primary active metabolite, lysine-SMCC-DM1, does not cross the plasma membrane readily and thus should not impact neighboring cells.

Step 5: Cytotoxic effect of the antibody–drug conjugate's payload: DM-1-containing catabolites work similarly to vinca alkaloids by binding to tubulin, preventing microtubule polymerization, promoting depolymerization, and

(continued)

FIGURE 17.7 Antibody–drug conjugate mechanism of action. (*continued*) suppressing microtubule dynamic instability. The in vitro activity of maytansine is dramatic; it is 100 times more potent than the vinca alkaloids. Upon exposure to T-DM1, cells with HER2 overexpression, regardless of trastuzumab sensitivity and resistance, undergo apoptosis and mitotic disruptions, leaving normal cell lines unharmed.

To note, Step 5 is similar for other microtubule disruptors such as brentuximab vedotin and belantamab mafodotin. Alternate cytotoxic effects include DNA disruption (as is the case for gemtuzumab ozogamicin, for example) and protein synthesis inhibition via action through the endoplasmic reticulum (as is the case for moxetumomab pasudotox).

Step 6: Tumor cell death: Of note, in addition to the steps described here, T-DM1 retains other trastuzumab mechanism of actions, such as FCγ receptor-mediated engagement of immune effector cells that leads to antibody-dependent cellular cytotoxicity and HER3/PI3K/AKT signaling pathway disturbance.

RADIOIMMUNOCONJUGATES

- A radioimmunoconjugate targeting CD20 available for use in treatment of lymphoma is ibritumomab tiuxetan (Zevalin) using yttrium-90; Figure 17.6). This agent may be especially helpful in bulky tumors or those that are poorly vascularized.
- For both dosimetry/imaging and therapeutic effect, rituximab is given prior to ibritumomab tiuxetan. Lutetium Lu-177 dotatate (Lutathera) is a radiolabeled somatostatin analog for neuroendocrine tumors.
  - Somatostatin analogs (octreotide) should be discontinued for at least 4 weeks (long-acting formulations) or 24 hours (short-acting formulations) prior to each dose.
  - Antiemetic premedications followed by an IV amino acid solution (for nephroprotection) should be given prior to, during, and 3 hours following lutetium Lu-177 dotatate administration.

Toxicities of radioimmunoconjugates, which may limit their use, include:
  - Myelosuppression (thrombocytopenia), infusion reaction, hypersensitivity reaction, mucocutaneous reaction, secondary malignancy, infertility, embryo-fetal toxicity
  - Minimize radiation exposure during and after treatment consistent with institutional good radiation safety practices and patient management procedures.

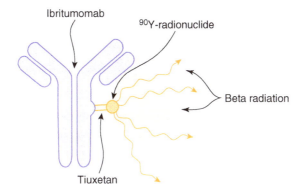

FIGURE 17.8 **Components of ^{90}Y-ibritumomab tiuxetan.**
Ibritumomab is a murine IgG1-kappa monoclonal antibody conjugated with
a linker-chelator tiuxetan. When bound to the radionuclide indium (In)-111 or
yttrium (Y)-90, this agent delivers a potentially cytotoxic dose of high beta
energy (maximum energy of 2.3 MeV with a half-life of 64 hours) and has a path
length of 5 to 10 mm, which improves its ability to kill bulky, poorly vascularized
tumors.

Through a "crossfire effect," neighboring malignant cells that do not bind
antibody are targeted with radiation emitted from bound cells.

Stem cells do not have the CD20 antigen and are therefore allowed to
regenerate after treatment.

In addition, the antibody itself may trigger cell death via antibody-dependent
cell-mediated cytotoxicity (ADCC), complement-dependent cytotoxicity (CDC),
and apoptosis.

BISPECIFIC ANTIBODIES

Bispecific monoclonal antibodies are artificial proteins that can simultaneously bind to two
different types of antigens/epitopes on the same antigen designed to recruit and activate immune cells against specific targets on cancer cells.

The BiTEs (bispecific T cell engagers) are connected by a linker molecule, which delineates the flexibility of the construct and antigen-binding kinetics in conjunction with the specific antigens. DARTs have a analogous structure to BiTEs but include a disulfide linker for additional stability. BiKEs and trispecific killer cell engagers (TriKEs) comprise two (BiKE) or three (TriKE) variable antigen regions; they activate NK cells either by binding to interleukin 16 (IL-16) or containing an IL-15 linker.

In addition to blinatumomab (Figure 17.9), the other clinically used bispecific antibodies include amivantamab (Table 17.1), which targets epidermal growth factor (EGF) and MET receptors, for adult patients with locally advanced or metastatic non-small cell lung cancer (NSCLC) with EGFR exon 20 insertion mutations; emicizumab, which targets clotting factors IXa and X and is used in the treatment of hemophilia A; and catumaxomab, which was used for the treatment of malignant ascites in people with epithelial cell adhesion molecule (EpCAM)–positive cancer (withdrawn from the market due to commercial reasons).

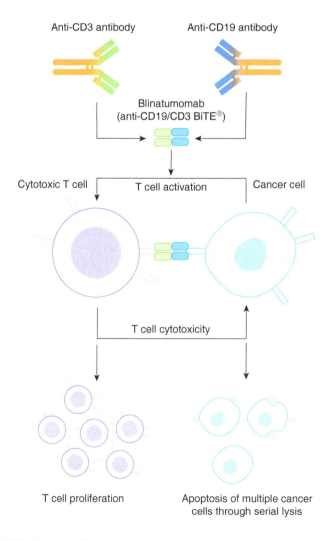

FIGURE 17.9 Blinatumomab.

(continued)

FIGURE 17.9 Blinatumomab. (*continued*)
Blinatumomab (Blincyto) is a anti-CD19-CD3 bi-specific T cell engager (BiTE). The mechanism of action of blinatumomab involves the patient's own cytotoxic T ce ls to att ck CD19[+] B cells; after connection of endogenous T cells via CD3 by blinatumomab to a CD19-expressing B cell, the activated T cells kill the B cells and proliferate, creating more killer T cells.

Blinatumomab is FDA (U.S. Food and Drug Administration) approved for (1) treatment of relapsed or refractory CD19[+] B cell precursor acute lymphoblastic leukemia (ALL), and (2) treatment of CD19[+] B-ALL in first or second complete remission (CR) with minimal residual disease (MRD) ≥0.1%. Of note, the confirmatory study (ECOG-ACRIN E1910 Randomized Phase III National Cooperative Clinical Trials Network Trial) investigated consolidation therapy with blinatumomab in newly diagnosed adult patients with B-ALL in MRD-negative remission demonstrated an improvement in overall survival.

Cytokine release syndrome (CRS) and neurologic toxicities, which may be severe, life-threatening, or fatal, occurred in patients receiving blinatumomab.

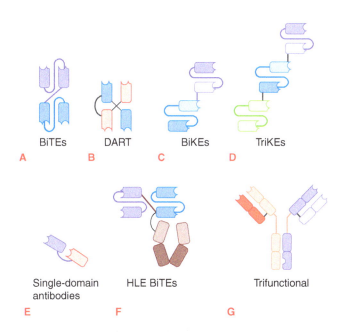

FIGURE 17.10 Bispecific antibodies can be manufactured in several structural formats.
(A) BiTEs (bispecific T cell engagers), (B) DARTs (dual affinity retargeting antibodies), (C) BiKEs (bispecific NK-cell engagers), (D) TriKEs (trispecific NK-cell engagers), (E) single-domain antibodies with only one variable chain per target, (F) HLE BiTEs (half-life extended bispecific T cell engagers) are BiTEs with an Fc portion that increases its half-life. (G) Trifunctional antibodies conserved their Fc domain to be able to bind to cells expressing Fc receptors.

CYTOKINE THERAPY

There are more than 70 separate proteins and glycoproteins with biologic effects in humans including interferon (IFN)-alpha, -beta, -gamma; interleukin (IL) 1 through 29 (so far); the tumor necrosis factor (TNF) family, and the chemokine family. Only pegylated interferon alpha and high-dose IL-2 are in use in oncology practice, although they are used infrequently (Figure 17.12).

- Interferon
  - About 20 different genes encode IFN-α and their biologic effects are indistinguishable. IFN induces the expression of many genes, inhibits protein synthesis, and exerts a number of different effects on diverse cellular processes.
  - Interferon is not curative for any tumor but can induce partial responses in follicular lymphoma, hairy cell leukemia, chronic myeloid leukemia, polycythemia vera (and essential thrombocythemia), melanoma, and Kaposi sarcoma. IFN-α products may cause or exacerbate lethal or life-threatening neuropsychiatric, autoimmune, ischemic, and infectious disorders.
  - Ropeginterferon alfa-2b-njft (Besremi) is an interferon alfa-2b that is approved for the treatment of adults with polycythemia vera. Recommended starting dose is 100 mcg by subcutaneous injection every 2 weeks (50 mcg if receiving hydroxyurea), and the dose is increased by 50 mcg every 2 weeks (up to a maximum of 500 mcg) until hematologic parameters are stabilized.
  - IFN-α and IL-2 are associated with substantial toxicity in relation to the neurologic, cutaneous, musculoskeletal, gastrointestinal, cardiovascular, renal, hepatic, and hematologic systems. Patients should be closely monitored; those with persistent severe or worsening signs and symptoms of conditions shown in Figure 17.11 should be withdrawn from therapy. Some toxicities are reversible.

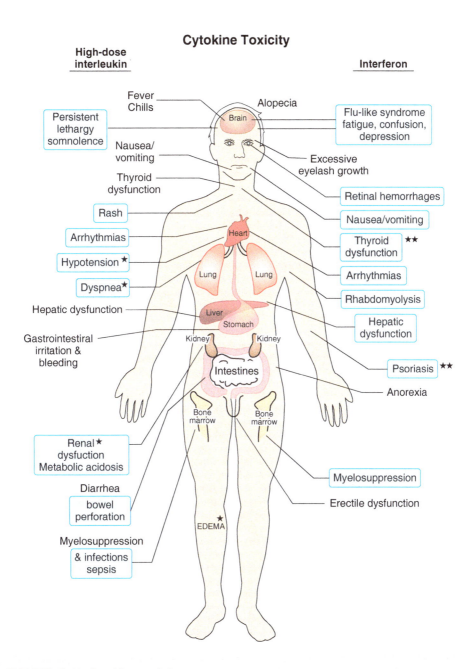

FIGURE 17.11 Cytokine toxicity.
The left side of the picture describes toxicity seen with high-dose interleukin 2 (IL-2) therapy. The right side of the picture describes toxicity seen with high-dose interferon therapy. *Indicates a component of capillary leak syndrome (hypotension, dyspnea, renal dysfunction, labeled on the left). **Indicates that this-could be an autoimmune reaction (psoriasis and thyroid dysfunction, labeled on the right). A box indicates a contraindication to therapy or a reason to withhold therapy until a resolution in toxicity. For IL-2, doses are held. For interferon, doses are reduced or treatment is discontinued.

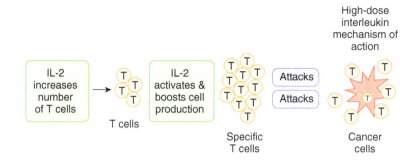

FIGURE 17.12 Mechanism of action for high-dose interleukin (IL).

- Interleukin-2 (IL-2) (aldesleukin)
  - High-dose IL-2 has been used in the adjuvant setting in stage II melanoma, multiple myeloma, and follicular lymphoma, with uncertain effects on survival.
  - IL-2 exerts its antitumor effects indirectly through augmentation of immune function. Its biologic activity is to promote the growth and activity of T cells and NK cells.
  - Historically, IL-2 was one of the few treatments for adults with metastatic solid tumors that could produce complete responses (CRs) that were often durable for decades without further treatment.
  - IL-2 should be restricted to those with normal cardiac and pulmonary function. It should be administered in a hospital setting; an intensive care facility and specialists skilled in cardiopulmonary or intensive care medicine must be available.
  - IL-2 is associated with capillary leak syndrome (CLS) characterized by a loss of vascular tone and extravasation of plasma proteins and fluid into the extravascular space. See Figure 17.11 and Table 17.4 for more information on identifying and managing toxicities. In terms of holding therapy based on toxicities, most toxicities reverse completely within 3 to 6 days.

TABLE 17.4 Management of Cytokine Therapy Toxicities

	TOXICITY	PRE-MEDICATION	PHARMACOLOGIC MANAGEMENT
Central nervous system	Delusions, visual hallucinations		Lorazepam, haloperidol
	Depression	Antidepressants (if high risk)	
	Fatigue		Hydration
Endocrine	Hypothyroidism		Levothyroxine

(continued)

TABLE 17.4 Management of Cytokine Therapy Toxicities (*continued*)

	TOXICITY	PRE-MEDICATION	PHARMACOLOGIC MANAGEMENT
Cardio-pulmonary, renal and metabolic	Hypotension/oliguria/rising serum creatinine		Fluids, vasopressors
	Cardiotoxicity		Consider rate-controlling agent
	Metabolic acidosis		Sodium bicarbonate
	Dyspnea and peripheral edema		Diuretics
	Fevers/chills/muscle aches	Acetaminophen ± NSAID (e.g., indomethacin)	Meperidine (rigors/chills)
	Flu-like symptoms		Hydration, analgesics, antiemetics, bedtime administration
Gastrointestinal	Nausea/vomiting	Serotonin and/or dopamine antagonist **Do not use steroid**	Serotonin and/or dopamine antagonist
	Epigastric pain	H2-receptor antagonist	
	Diarrhea		Antimotility agents (e.g., loperamide)
	Anorexia		High-protein supplements, multivitamins
	Hepatotoxicity		Avoid alcohol consumption
Dermatologic	Skin rash, pruritus		Emollients (nonsteroid-containing) and antihistamines
	Psoriasis		Pharmacologic or phototherapy

Note: Nonpharmacologic interventions may also be successful.

NSAID, nonsteroidal anti-inflammatory drug.

CHAPTER SUMMARY

Monoclonal antibodies and cytokine-directed therapies derive both their efficacy and their toxicities from the specific targets they affect. Additionally, hypersensitivity reactions are a common toxicity with all of these agents, and the frequency by which it occurs is directly correlated with the extent of foreign sequence used to formulate the drug. The addition of a cytotoxic agent to form a conjugate with monoclonal antibodies maintains the specificity of the drug to target the tumor cell, while simultaneously increasing the cytotoxic properties of the drug. Although the use of cytokine-directed therapies is limited, clinicians should be aware of the severe toxicity profiles of these agents so that appropriate management can occur preemptively and promptly. Understanding the mechanism and toxicity profile of cytokine-directed therapy is pivotal to understanding the mechanisms of action and toxicity of more current immunotherapy options used routinely in practice.

CLINICAL PEARLS

- Anti-EGFR antibodies can induce papulopustular rash, which can be managed with tetracyclines and steroids. Depending on the severity of the rash, topical or systemic corticosteroids or tetracyclines should be used for management as well as dose interruptions, reductions, and discontinuations for grade 3 or 4 rashes.
- Anti-HER2$^+$ antibodies decrease left ventricular ejection fraction (LVEF) that most likely is reversible. Trastuzumab should be held if 16% or more absolute decrease in EF from pretreatment value occurs or if baseline EF is below the limit of normal and there is a 10% or more absolute decrease in EF from pretreatment values. Trastuzumab can be resumed if within 4 to 8 weeks EF returns to normal limits and the absolute decrease from baseline is less than or equal to 15%. Permanently discontinue trastuzumab if there have been more than 8 weeks of EF decline or if there are more than three episodes of cardiomyopathy.
- VEGF receptors are prevalent on vasculature endothelial cells that, when stimulated by VEGF, release nitric oxide to cause vasodilation and ultimately lower blood pressure. When VEGF is sequestered by VEGF-inhibiting monoclonal antibodies, vasoconstriction occurs causing hypertension. However, nifedipine should be avoided as it has been associated with increased VEGF secretion. The anti-VEGF monoclonal antibody bevacizumab, used for ovarian, breast, colorectal, and lung cancers, can be associated with tumor necrosis (e.g., intestinal perforation, pulmonary hemorrhage), anaerobic liver abscess (*Bacteroides fragilis*), and *Fusarium* nasal septal infections.
- Progressive multifocal leukoencephalopathy (PML) can occur as a complication of therapy with alemtuzumab (anti-CD52, used for chronic lymphocytic leukemia and multiple sclerosis), rituximab (anti-CD20, used for B cell chronic lymphocytic leukemia, non-Hodgkin lymphomas, autoimmune disorders including rheumatoid arthritis, myasthenia gravis, and idiopathic thrombocytopenic purpura), brentuximab (anti-CD30, Hodgkin lymphoma, and anaplastic large cell lymphoma), and natalizumab (anti-α4-integrin, used for multiple sclerosis, Crohn disease).

1. A 45-year-old woman is referred to an oncologist by her primary care physician for an enlarging right supraclavicular mass currently 7 cm and a 2.5 cm left inguinal node. PET/CT shows a 5-cm retroperitoneal mass with standardized uptake value (SUV) of 10.5 in addition to the other two lesions with SUVs of 11 and 8. The bone marrow biopsy is negative. Complete blood count, lactic dehydrogenase, and blood chemistries are unremarkable. Excisional biopsy of the supraclavicular node confirms the diagnosis of diffuse large B cell lymphoma (DLBCL). What is the most appropriate treatment option for this patient?

    A. R-CHOP for six cycles
    B. Dose-adjusted EPOCH-R for six cycles
    C. R-hyper-CVAD alternating with HDMTX-HiDAC followed by auto-HSCT
    D. Ibrutinib

2. A 59-year-old woman with newly diagnosed ER/PR⁻, HER2⁺ breast cancer requests consultation about the use of pertuzumab and/or lapatinib for treatment of her disease. Which of the following statements is true?

    A. Lapatinib and pertuzumab are recommended as single agents for adjuvant therapy of patients with HER2⁺ breast cancer.
    B. Pertuzumab can be used for adjuvant treatment of breast cancer instead of trastuzumab.
    C. Pertuzumab can be used in combination with trastuzumab and chemotherapy as neoadjuvant treatment of patients with HER2⁺, locally advanced, inflammatory, or early-stage breast cancer (either >2 cm in diameter or node-positive) as part of a complete treatment regimen for early breast cancer.
    D. Pertuzumab is not indicated for treatment of metastatic breast cancer.

3. A 43-year-old man presents with history of anaplastic large T cell lymphoma. He was treated initially with six cycles of CHOP and remained in complete remission for 2 years. He subsequently relapsed and was treated with ICE (ifosfamide, carboplatin, and etoposide) chemotherapy followed by auto-HSCT and remained in remission for another 3 years. He currently has cervical lymphadenopathy with fever and weight loss. Biopsy reveals anaplastic large T cell lymphoma with t(2;5) by FISH (fluorescence in situ hybridization). Which of the following treatments is most appropriate now?

    A. Romidepsin
    B. Pralatrexate
    C. Ibrutinib plus venetoclax followed by allo-HSCT
    D. Brentuximab vedotin

4. Which of the following are possible components of antibody–drug conjugates?

   A. Microtubule inhibitor (e.g., calicheamicin)
   B. Cytotoxic agent (e.g., monomethyl auristatin E)
   C. Radioisotope (e.g., yttrium-90)
   D. Bispecific T cell engager

5. Which of the following statements is TRUE regarding high-dose IL-2 therapy?

   A. It should be given to a patient with normal pulmonary and cardiac function.
   B. It can be administered in an outpatient cancer center facility, similar to other immunotherapy agents.
   C. Patients should be monitored for depression, delusions, and visual hallucinations.
   D. If patients experience dyspnea, arrhythmia, or somnolence, doses should be escalated to optimize dose intensity as toxicities are reversible.

6. A 45-year-old man presents with 2 months history of fatigue, drenching night sweats, and 15 kg weight loss with recently progressive shortness of breath. PET/CT reveals a 22-cm mediastinal mass with SUV of 75. Biopsy confirms the diagnosis of primary mediastinal B cell lymphoma. What is the recommended management for this patient with curative intent?

   A. R-CHOP for six cycles
   B. Dose-adjusted EPOCH-R for six cycles
   C. R-hyper-CVAD alternating with HDMTX-HiDAC followed by auto-HSCT
   D. Debulking radiation followed by four to six cycles of R-CHOP followed by auto-HSCT

7. A 58-year-old man presents with KRAS mutant colon cancer with a single confirmed metastatic lesion in the right liver lobe measuring approximately 4.5 cm. What is the best next step in his management?

   A. FOLFOX + bevacizumab until disease progression or serious adverse events
   B. Neoadjuvant FOLFOX + cetuximab, followed by resection of the liver metastasis and primary colon tumor with en bloc resection of regional lymph node
   C. FOLFOX followed by maintenance cetuximab
   D. Synchronus resection of liver metastasis and primary colon tumor with en bloc resection of regional lymph node followed by adjuvant FOLFOX

8. Which of the following statements is TRUE regarding monoclonal antibody infusion-related reaction prevention and management?

   A. Standard premedications may include acetaminophen, hydrocortisone, and diphenhydramine.
   B. The reaction risk is related to lifetime cumulative dose; reactions occur several hours after infusion completion.
   C. Patients from the southeastern United States who experience life-threatening, IgE-mediated reactions to cetuximab after the first infusion can be rechallenged at the same infusion rate.
   D. For infusion-related reactions of any severity grade, the monoclonal antibody should be permanently discontinued.

9. A medical oncologist is requested to have a peer-to-peer discussion with an insurance company representative about ramucirumab, a VEGF receptor antagonist. The insurance representative is referencing U.S. Food and Drug Administration (FDA) approval for the drug coverage. Which one of the following indications is not approved by the FDA to use remucirumab?

    A. In combination with everolimus for treatment of renal cell cancer (RCC)
    B. As a single agent or in combination with paclitaxel, for treatment of advanced gastric or gastroesophageal junction adenocarcinoma
    C. In combination with docetaxel, for treatment of metastatic NSCLC with disease progression on or after platinum-based chemotherapy
    D. In combination with FOLFIRI, for the treatment of metastatic colorectal cancer with disease progression on or after prior therapy with bevacizumab, oxaliplatin, and a fluoropyrimidine

10. Which of the following are TRUE regarding structure, classification, and mechanism of action of monoclonal antibodies?

    A. Based on the ratio of human-derived versus murine-derived components, chimeric monoclonal antibodies are less foreign than humanized monoclonal antibodie.
    B. The fragment antigen-binding region on the naked monoclonal antibodies is targeted to tumor-specific marker.
    C. Monoclonal antibody effects may occur via antibody-dependent cell-mediated cytotoxicity and complement-dependent cytotoxicit.
    D. All of the above
    E. B and C only

ANSWERS TO MULTIPLE-CHOICE QUESTIONS

1. **A.** R-CHOP (rituximab [Rituxan], cyclophosphamide [Cytoxan], doxorubicin [Adriamycin], vincristine [Oncovin], and prednisone) is the most widely used therapeutic standard for DLBCL for nearly 20 years, with the addition of rituximab to the CHOP backbone in the 2000s significantly improving survival after several years and attempts of unsuccessful efforts to intensify CHOP with additional chemotherapeutics. This is based on meaningful improvement in outcomes (survival, quality of life) based on well-designed well-conducted Phase 3 clinical trials. The R-CHOP regimen is usually given in 21-day cycles (once every 21 days) for six cycles. In some cases 14-day cycles may be used, and occasionally for limited stage disease (stage I or II) three or four cycles may be used followed by radiation therapy.

2. **C.** Pertuzumab is a HER2/neu receptor antagonist indicated for (a) use in combination with trastuzumab and docetaxel for treatment of patients with HER2$^+$ metastatic breast cancer who have not received prior anti-HER2 therapy or chemotherapy for metastatic disease; (b) use in combination with trastuzumab and chemotherapy as neoadjuvant treatment of patients with HER2$^+$, locally advanced, inflammatory, or early-stage breast cancer (either >2 cm in diameter or

node-positive) as part of a complete treatment regimen for early breast cancer; and (c) use in combination with trastuzumab and chemotherapy as adjuvant treatment of patients with HER2$^+$ early breast cancer at high risk of recurrence.

3. **D.** Brentuximab vedotin (Adcetris) is approved for treatment of adult patients with systemic anaplastic large cell lymphoma (sALCL) after failure of at least one prior multiagent chemotherapy regimen. The recommended dosage as single agent for adult patients is 1.8 mg/kg up to a maximum of 180 mg every 3 weeks.

4. **B.** Choice A is incorrect; while microtubule inhibitors are an example of a cytotoxic agent that is a component of an antibody–drug conjugate, examples include DM-1 and monomethyl auristatin E (MMAE) not calicheamicin, a DNA-disrupting agent. Choice B is correct; this is an example of a cytotoxic, microtubule inhibitor. C is incorrect; radioisotopes are not a component of an antibody–drug conjugate but of a radioimmunoconjugate. D is incorrect; this is a unique type of monoclonal antibody that is not an antibody–drug conjugate. The first-in-class bispecific T cell engager is called blinatumomab.

5. **A.** IL-2 should be restricted to those with normal cardiac and pulmonary function. B is inccorect; it should be administered in a hospital setting; an ICU and specialists skilled in cardiopulmonary or intensive care medicine must be available. C is incorrect; these toxicities are related to interferon. D is incorrect; these are either contraindications to therapy or a reason to withhold therapy, until there is a resolution in toxicity. For IL-2, doses are held. In terms of holding therapy based on toxicities, most toxicities reverse completely within 3 to 6 days.

6. **B.** The efficacy of *infusional* dose-adjusted etoposide, doxorubicin, and cyclophosphamide with vincristine, prednisone, and rituximab (DA-EPOCH-R) and filgrastim without radiotherapy was studied in a single-arm, Phase 2, prospective study of 51 patients with untreated primary mediastinal B cell lymphoma. The event-free survival rate was 93%, and the overall survival rate was 97% (a median of 5 years of follow-up). This study, although nonrandomized, avoided the need for radiotherapy in patients with primary mediastinal B cell lymphoma. The use of R-CHOP and radiotherapy in patients with primary mediastinal B cell lymphoma in the Mabthera International Trial Group resulted in an event-free survival rate of 78% at 34 months among 44 patients of whom 73% received radiotherapy.

   The efficacy of DA-EPOCH-R compared with R-CHOP (both for six cycles) as frontline therapy for 491 eligible patients (74% with stage III or IV disease) with DL-BCL was assessed in the Phase III Intergroup Trial Alliance/CALGB 50303. The primary objective was progression-free survival (PFS); secondary objectives included response rate, overall survival (OS), and safety. At a median follow-up of 5 years, neither PFS was statistically different between the arms (hazard ratio .93; 95% CI 0.68 to 1.27; p = .65) nor was OS different (hazard ratio 1.09; 95% CI 0.75 to 1.59; p = .64). Grade 3 and 4 adverse events were more common in the DA-EPOCH-R arm than the R-CHOP arm, including infection (16.9% vs. 10.7%, respectively), febrile neutropenia (35.0% vs. 17.7%, respectively), mucositis (8.4% vs. 2.1%, respectively), and neuropathy (18.6% vs. 3.3%, respectively; p <.001). This study confirmed that the more intensive, infusional DA-EPOCH-R was more toxic and did not improve PFS or OS compared with R-CHOP.

7. **D.** Bevacizumab is not indicated for adjuvant treatment of colon cancer. The bevacizumab-Avastin adjuvant (AVANT) study did not show an improvement of disease-free survival (DFS) with the addition of bevacizumab to oxaliplatin-based chemotherapy in stage III colon cancer. Cetuximab is not indicated for treatment of Ras-mutant colorectal cancer or when the results of the Ras mutation tests are unknown.

8. **A.** These are standard premedications that may be used, depending on the agent, reaction history, time since last infusion, and infusion number. B is incorrect; predominantly these reactions occur acutely during the first infusion or just after completion of the infusion, and are frequently low grade. C is incorrect; cetuximab frequently has an IgE-mediated reaction upon the first infusion due to a natural preexposure to an oligosaccharide, galactose-α-1,3-galactose, that is common to some geographical areas such as the southeast portion of the United States. IgE-mediated reactions are prohibitive in any further use of that monoclonal antibody without a desensitization protocol. D is incorrect; rechallenging of the monoclonal antibody is often feasible as these are typically cytokine-mediated reactions and typically low grade in nature. Rechallenging should not occur if a patient experiences a grade 4, anaphylactic reaction.

9. **A.** Ramucirumab is not approved for treatment of RCC. In addition to B, C, and D indications, ramucirumab is approved as monotherapy, for the treatment of hepatocellular carcinoma in patients who have an alpha fetoprotein of ≥400 ng/mL and have been treated with sorafenib.

10. **E.** Choice A is incorrect; chimeric monoclonal antibodies are more foreign. B is correct; the Fab region is the manufactured variation that is directed at the respective targeted tumor marker. C is correct; in addition to these mechanisms, two additional mechanisms include direct apoptosis or growth inhibition and blocking neovascularization (by VEGF monoclonal antibody inhibitors).

SELECTED REFERENCES

Appleby L, Morrissey S, Bellmunt J, Rosenberg J. Management of treatment-related toxicity with targeted therapies for renal cell carcinoma: Evidence-based practice and best practices. Hematol Oncol Clin North Am. 2011;25(4):893–915. https://doi.org/10.1016/j.hoc.2011.05.004

Barroso-Sousa R, Santana IA, Testa L, et al. Biological therapies in breast cancer: Common toxicities and management strategies. Breast. 2013;22(6):1009–18. https://doi.org/10.1016/j.breast.2013.09.009

Bartlett NL, Wilson WH, Jung SH, et al. Dose-adjusted EPOCH-R compared with R-CHOP as frontline therapy for diffuse large B-cell lymphoma: Clinical outcomes of the phase III intergroup trial Alliance/CALGB 50303. J Clin Oncol. 2019;37(21):1790–9. https://doi.org/10.1200/JCO.18.01994

Diamantis N, Banerji U. Antibody-drug conjugates—An emerging class of cancer treatment. Br J Cancer. 2016;114(4):362–7. https://doi.org/10.1038/bjc.2015.435

Dunleavy K, Pittaluga S, Maeda LS, et al. Dose-adjusted EPOCH-rituximab therapy in primary mediastinal B-cell lymphoma. N Engl J Med. 2013;368(15):1408–16. https://doi.org/10.1056/NEJMoa1214561

Dutcher JP, Schwartzentruber DJ, Kaufman HL, et al. High dose interleukin-2-expert consensus on best management practices—2014. J Immunother Cancer. 2014;2(1):26. https://doi.org/10.1186/s40425-014-0026-0

Hauschild A, Gogas H, Tarhini A, et al. Practical guidelines for the management of interferon-α2b side effects in patients receiving adjuvant treatment for melanoma expert opinion. Cancer. 2008;112(5):982–94. https://doi.org/10.1002/cncr.23251

Hofheinz RD, Segaert S, Safont MJ, et al. Management of adverse events during treatment of gastrointestinal cancers with epidermal growth factor inhibitors. Crit Rev Oncol Hematol. 2017;114:102–13. https://doi.org/10.1016/j.critrevonc.2017.03.032

Jerjian TV, Glode AE, Thompson LA, O'Bryant CL. Antibody-drug conjugates: A clinical pharmacy perspective on an emerging cancer therapy. Pharmacotherapy. 2016;36(1):99–116. https://doi.org/10.1002/phar.1687

Khongorzul P, Ling CJ, Khan FU, et al. Antibody-drug conjugates: A comprehensive review. Mol Cancer Res. 2020;18(1):3–19. https://doi.org/10.1158/1541-7786.MCR-19-0582

Lacouture ME, Anadkat MJ, Bensadoun RJ, et al. Clinical practice guidelines for the prevention and treatment of EGFR inhibitor-associated dermatologic toxicities. Support Care Cancer. 2011;19(8):1079–95. https://doi.org/10.1007/s00520-011-1197-6

McGinty L, Kolesar J. Dinutuximab for maintenance therapy in pediatric neuroblastoma. Am J Health Syst Pharm. 2017;74(8):563–7. https://doi.org/10.2146/ajhp160228

Newsome BW, Ernstoff MS. The clinical pharmacology of therapeutic monoclonal antibodies in the treatment of malignancy; have the magic bullets arrived? Br J Clin Pharmacol. 2008;66(1):6–19. https://doi.org/10.1111/j.1365-2125.2008.03187.x

Peddi PF, Hurvitz SA. Trastuzumab emtansine: The first targeted chemotherapy for treatment of breast cancer. Future Oncol. 2013;9(3):319–26. https://doi.org/10.2217/fon.13.7

Picard M, Galvao VR. Current knowledge and management of hypersensitivity reactions to monoclonal antibodies. J Allergy Clin Immunol Pract. 2017;5(3):600–9. https://doi.org/10.1016/j.jaip.2016.12.001

Schwartz RN, Stover L, Dutcher JP. Managing toxicities of high-dose interleukin-2. Oncology (Williston Park). 2002;16(11 Suppl 13):11–20.

CHAPTER 18

Immunotherapeutics: Immune Checkpoint Inhibitors, Vaccines, Bispecifics, and Engineered T Cells

MARK YARCHOAN • **ELIZABETH JAFFEE**

INTRODUCTION

Over the past decade, novel immunotherapeutics have become firmly established as a major pillar of cancer therapy. Here we review the ways in which cancers learn to evade the immune system by coopting specific pathways that incude immune tolerance. Cancer immunotherapies aim to reverse tumor immune evasion, leading to durable immune-mediated tumor regression. Immune checkpoint inhibitors, including monoclonal antibodies targeting the programmed cell death protein 1 (PD-1) pathway, are cancer immunotherapies that reverse immune exhaustion in T cells. These therapies are widely used in clinical practice and have demonstrated improved survival for patients with many different forms of cancer. Bispecific T cell engaging antibodies, chimeric antigen receptor (CAR) T cells, and therapeutic cancer vaccines are cancer immunotherapies that activate the immune system against specific tumor antigens. The mechanism of action, present status, and future potential of these therapeutic modalities in the care of patients with cancer is reviewed here.

Tumorigenesis occurs as a multistep process through which normal cells acquire sequential mutations that favor uncontrolled tumor growth (Figure 18.1). Some early cancers and precancers are recognized and eliminated by the adaptive or the innate immune system. In some cases, transformed cells can coopt immunosuppressive pathways to avoid immune destruction and develop into established cancers. By the time cancers are clinically detected, they have often developed a myriad of different ways to evade immune destruction; some of the pathways they utilize are shown here. Tumor cells produce chemokines and cytokines that recruit immunosuppressive cell types to the tumor immune microenvironment (TiME), such as myeloid-derived suppressor cells (MDSCs), tumor-associated macrophages (TAMs), and T regulatory cells (Tregs). Tumors also directly avoid immune cell destruction by upregulating ligands for T cell inhibition (e.g., PD-L1), and through metabolic reprogramming to deplete the tumor microenvironment of factors required for T cell activation. The immunosuppressive signals from tumor cells and other immunosuppressive cell types that are recruited to the TiME impair the antitumor immune response and induce immune tolerance. The remaining T cells in the TiME are often dysfunctional as a result of anergy, exhaustion, or senescence. Finally, some tumors create a stroma that acts as a physical barrier shielding tumor cells from immune elimination. Many cancer immunotherapies attempt to normalize aberrant tumor-immune crosstalk by targeting specific pathways shown here. For example, monoclonal antibodies against PD-1 (on T cells) or its ligand PD-L1 (on tumor cells) that are used in the standard treatment of many tumor types can unleash powerful antitumor immunity in some patients. However, only a minority of patients who receive PD-1/PD-L1 inhibitors respond to these agents, and although immune responses can be durable, cure is rare. It is likely that other pathways will need to be targeted concurrently to overcome the potently immunosuppressive TiME of most established tumors, and many pathways shown here are being explored in combination with anti-PD-1 or anti-PD-L1 therapies in clinical trials.

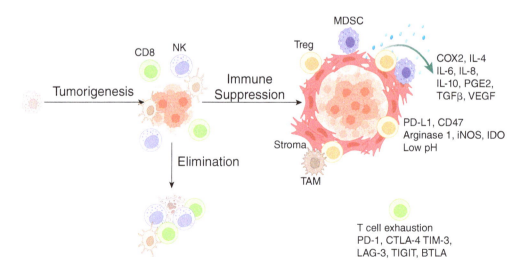

FIGURE 18.1 Tumors orchestrate a complex signaling network to evade immune destruction.

BTLA, B and T cell lymphocyte attenuator; CD8, cluster of differentiation 8; COX2, cyclooxygenase 2; CTLA-4, cytotoxic T lymphocyte-associated protein 4; IDO, indoleamine 2,3-dioxygenase; IL, interleukin; iNOS, inducible nitric oxide synthase; LAG-3, lymphocyte-activation gene 3; MDSC, myeloid-derived suppressor cell; NK, natural killer; PD-1, programmed cell death protein 1; PD-L1, programmed death ligand 1; PGE2, prostaglandin E2; TAM, tumor-associated macrophage; TGF, tranforming growth factor; TIGIT, T cell immunoglobulin and ITIM domain; TIM-3, T cell immunoglobulin and mucin domain–containing molecule 3; Treg, T regulatory cell; VEGF, vascular endothelial growth factor.

Tumor neoantigens are derived from genomic alterations within the tumor DNA, including but not limited to single-nucleotide variants (SNVs), insertions and deletions (indel), gene fusions, and frameshift mutations. Viral proteins are another type of tumor antigen that can be recognized by CD8 T cells. Some tumors can evade the immune system by upregulating the immunosuppressive ligand PD-L1. PD-L1 on tumor cells binds to PD-1 receptors on T cells, thereby inactivating the T cells. Antibodies against PD-1 or PD-L1 block the inhibitory interaction of the PD-1 receptor with PD-L1, which restores the antitumor activity of effector T cells. In some cancer types, the probability of benefit from anti-PD-1 therapies is related to the amount of PD-L1 expression on tumor cells, and PD-L1 expression is approved as a companion diagnostic test for use of PD-1 inhibitors in some cancers. However, PD-L1 expression is an imperfect biomarker due to issues pertaining to dynamic expression and heterogeneity of expression in the tumor microenvironment, a lack of assay standardization across PD-L1 platforms, and discrepancies related to assay interpretation. PD-L1 is also found on antigen presenting cells (APCs) where it can also drive T cells that recognize tumor antigens into an inactive state.

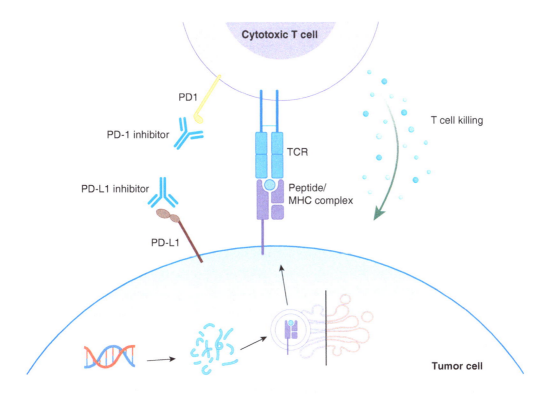

FIGURE 18.2 When functioning normally, cytotoxic T cells can recognize and destroy tumor cells through the identification of aberrant proteins (neoantigens) that are presented on the surface of tumors in the context of the major histocompatibility complex (MHC).

PD-1, programmed cell death protein 1; PD-L1, programmed death ligand 1; TCR, T cell receptor.

Anti-PD-1 and anti-PD-L1 immunotherapies demonstrate clinical activity in a wide range of different cancer types, while other cancers have not responded to these agents. One factor that contributes to the efficacy of anti-PD-1 immunotherapy in some cancer types is the tumor mutational burden (TMB). Each mutation in the tumor genome has the potential to create an abnormal protein (neoantigen) that can be recognized by the immune system. Tumors with a high TMB may appear more "foreign" to the immune system and are therefore more likely to induce a robust antitumor immune response in the setting of an immune checkpoint inhibitor (Figure 18.3). Several tumor types that respond exceptionally well to anti-PD-1 immunotherapy arise in the setting of specific mutagens (ultraviolet light in the case of melanoma and cutaneous squamous cell cancers, cigarette smoking in the case of lung cancer) and consequently have high TMB. In addition, cancers with DNA mismatch repair deficiency (MMRd) have a high TMB resulting from DNA copy errors and also have a high response rate to PD-1 immunotherapy. The PD-1 inhibitor pembrolizumab is approved for any cancer with MMRd or a high tumor mutation (>10 mutations/megabase). The U.S. Food and Drug Administration (FDA) approval of pembrolizumab in 2017 for patients with MMRd cancer was the first time that the agency ever approved a cancer drug to be used in a "tissue-agnostic" manner (based only on a biomarker test, regardless of tumor type). Cancers of the kidney, liver, esophagus, and ovary have a moderate mutational burden while leukemias and pediatric tumors show the lowest levels of TMB. A higher tumor mutational burden is also associated with a higher response rate to PD-1 immunotherapy within certain tumor types. Some tumors respond better to PD-1/PD-L1 inhibition than would be anticipated from the TMB. For example, Merkel cell carcinomas (MCCs) that are associated with the Merkel cell polyomavirus (MCPyV) have a modest TMB but a high response rate to PD-1 inhibition. In these tumors, a strong immune response against viral antigens on tumor cells may enhance PD-1 responsiveness. Therefore, both neoantigen quantity and quality may affect responses to cancer immunotherapies.

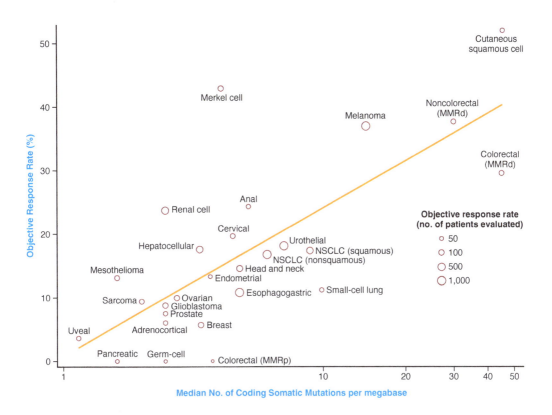

FIGURE 18.3 **Impact of tumor mutational burden on efficacy of anti-PD-1 immunotherapy.**

MMRd, mismatch repair deficiency; MMRp, mismatch repair proficiency; NSCLC, non-small cell lung cancer; PD-1, programmed cell death protein 1.

Source: Yarchoan M, Hopkins A, Jaffee EM., N Engl J Med, 2017.

Approved immune checkpoint inhibitors restore antitumor immunity by blocking inhibitor ligands on T cells, tumor cells, and/or APCs. Molecules targeted by currently approved immune checkpoint inhibitors are PD-1 (or its ligand, PD-L1), cytotoxic T-lymphocyte-associated protein 4 (CTLA-4), and lymphocyte-activation gene 3 (LAG-3). There is a burgeoning interest in developing other novel immune checkpoint inhibitors that can activate antitumor immunity alone or act synergistically with other immune checkpoint inhibitors to improve response rates. Figure 18.4 highlights several key emerging inhibitory and stimulatory immune checkpoint-modulating antibodies that are being tested both as single agents and in combination with anti-PD-1 in both preclinical and clinical settings. Upregulation of additional inhibitory immune checkpoints has been shown to contribute to resistance to anti-PD-1/PD-L1 therapy. Thus, combination inhibitory checkpoint blockade has emerged as one strategy of overcoming resistance as well as amplifying the immune response. Several promising inhibitory immune checkpoints, namely T cell immunoglobulin and mucin domain–containing molecule 3 (TIM-3), T cell immunoreceptor with immunoglobulin and ITIM domains (TIGIT), and V domain–containing Ig suppressor of T cell activation (VISTA), have been shown to augment antitumor immunity in preclinical studies and have demonstrated varying degrees of success in clinical trials. Likewise, combining inhibitory checkpoint blockade with activation of stimulatory pathways can produce a stronger antitumor immune response than anti-PD-1/PD-L1 or CTLA-4 blockade alone. Agonist antibodies against stimulatory immune checkpoint molecules such as T cell antigen 4-1BB homolog (4-1BB), CD40, and inducible T cell costimulator (ICOS) have demonstrated strong antitumor activity in preclinical studies, while their clinical efficacy remains to be further explored in the clinic.

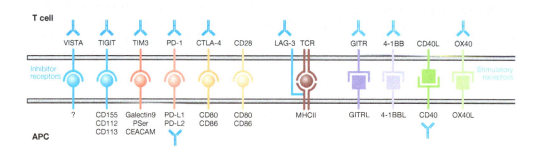

FIGURE 18.4 Cellular targets for immune checkpoint inhibitors.

APC, antigen-presenting cell; CEACAM, carcinoembryonic antigen-related cell adhesion molecule 1; CTLA-4, cytotoxic T lymphocyte-associated protein 4; GITR, glucocorticoid-induced tumor necrosis factor receptor; GITRL, GITR ligand; LAG-3, lymphocyte-activation gene 3; MHC, major histocompatibility complex; PD-1, programmed cell death protein 1; TCR, T cell receptor; TIGIT, T-cell immunoglobulin and ITIM domain; TIM3, T cell immunoglobulin and mucin domain–containing molecule 3; VISTA, V domain–containing Ig suppressor of T cell activation.

Source: Popovic A, Jaffee EM, Zaidi N., J Clin Invest, 2018.

Immune-related adverse effects (irAEs) from checkpoint inhibitors can be serious or life threatening, and limit the use of immune checkpoint inhibitors in patients with cancer. The frequency of irAEs is higher among patients treated with two immune checkpoint inhibitors (e.g., PD-1 inhibitor in combination with CTLA-4 inhibitor) versus PD-1 monotherapy. For example, severe treatment-related adverse events were noted in 16% of patients receiving PD-1 inhibitor monotherapy and 55% of patients receiving a PD-1 inhibitor plus a CTLA-4 inhibitor for melanoma. Some examples of common irAEs are shown in the Figure 18.5, but immune checkpoint inhibitors can impact any organ system. Myocarditis is an infrequent irAE from immune checkpoint inhibitor therapy, but has the highest fatality rate of the reported irAEs. Treatment of irAEs generally involves administration of steroids. Other immunosuppressive agents including but not limited to tumor necrosis factor-alpha inhibitors or mycophenylate mofetil are sometimes used in the management of severe or steroid-refractory cases.

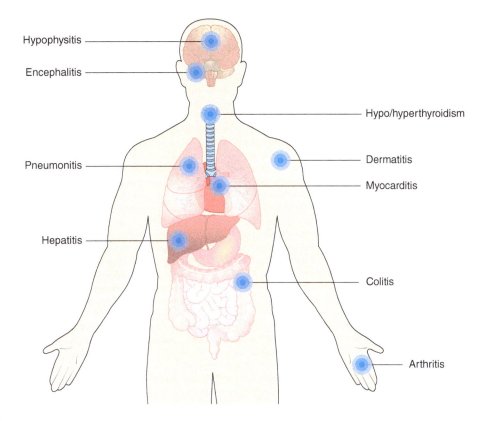

FIGURE 18.5 Immune checkpoint molecules such as PD-1 and CTLA-4 maintain immune tolerance to self-antigens, and the use of immune checkpoint-blocking antibodies can result in immunity against normal host tissues.

CTLA-4, cytotoxic T lymphocyte-associated protein 4; PD-1, programmed cell death protein 1.

Unlike preventive cancer vaccines, which prevent infection with viruses that cause cancer such as the human papillomavirus (HPV), therapeutic cancer vaccines seek to treat cancers (Figure 18.6). The development of therapeutic cancer vaccines has been challenging, and most therapeutic cancer vaccines have failed to demonstrate meaningful clinical responses when used as monotherapy in patients with HPV cancers. Only one therapeutic cancer vaccine is approved in the United States, an autologous dendritic cell-based vaccine called sipuleucel-T (Provenge). It was approved on the basis of a small survival benefit for patients with castration-resistant prostate cancer, but it rarely causes visible tumor regression or symptomatic benefit. Newer therapeutic cancer vaccines are primarily investigated in combination with other systemic immunotherapies, such as immune checkpoint inhibitors. Vaccines can increase the number of tumor infiltrating lymphocytes, and may be able to prime a tumor for immune checkpoint therapy.

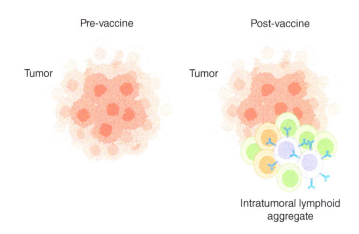

Pre-vaccine   Post-vaccine

Tumor   Tumor

Intratumoral lymphoid
aggregate

FIGURE 18.6 Therapeutic vaccines.

Following their remarkable success against SARS-CoV-2 (severe acute respiratory syndrome coronavirus 2), messenger RNA (mRNA) vaccines have become a promising therapeutic tool against cancer (Figure 18.7). Although therapeutic mRNA cancer vaccines are not yet approved for any cancer, they have demonstrated the potential to generate robust antigen-specific CD8$^+$ and Th1-type CD4$^+$ T cell responses, and many ongoing clinical trials are studying their effectiveness alone or in combination with checkpoint inhibitors. As mRNA vaccines can be rapidly generated, this enables the generation of personalized mRNA vaccines targeting the neoantigens expressed by an individual patient's tumor. First, whole-exome sequencing is carried out on tumor cells and matched normal tissue to identify the tumor-specific mutations. Next, software algorithms are used to prioritize potential neoantigens, usually based on neoantigen binding affinity to major histocompatibility complex (MHC). Next, an mRNA vaccine is designed and produced to target the highest priority neoantigens in the tumor. This vaccine can be given with immune checkpoint inhibitors and other immune-based therapies to overcome immunosuppressive mechanisms in the tumor. While prior therapeutic cancer vaccines have generally targeted tumor-associated antigens (normal proteins that are overexpressed on tumor cells), simultaneous targeting of multiple cancer neoantigens may result in more robust antitumor immune responses.

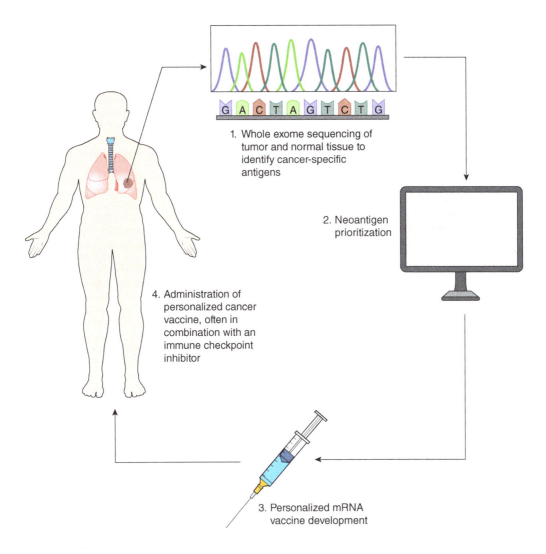

1. Whole exome sequencing of tumor and normal tissue to identify cancer-specific antigens

2. Neoantigen prioritization

4. Administration of personalized cancer vaccine, often in combination with an immune checkpoint inhibitor

3. Personalized mRNA vaccine development

FIGURE 18.7 **Messenger RNA (mRNA) vaccines for cancer therapy.**

Bispecific antibodies, chimeric antigen receptor (CAR) T cell therapy, and T cell receptor (TCR) T cells are cancer immunotherapies that redirect T cells against tumor antigens, resulting in tumor killing (**Figure 18.8**). Bispecific antibodies have the capacity to simultaneously bind to two different antigens and are used to connect the CD3 antigen in the T cell receptor complex to surface antigens on cancer cells. Blinatumomab (Blincyto) is an example of a bispecific antibody. It binds to CD3 (on T cells) and CD19 (expressed on acute lymphoblastic leukemia tumor cells), thereby resulting in T cell killing of leukemia cells. TCR T cell therapies and CAR T cell therapies are two forms of engineered T cell therapy in which the body's own T cells are reprogrammed and expanded ex vivo, and then readministered back into the body to attack cancer cells. However, engineered TCRs and CAR T cells recognize different kinds of tumor antigens. CAR T cells use antibody fragments to recognize specific antigens on the cell surface, and therefore recognize the same kinds of antigens as conventional antibodies and bispecific antibodies. Tisagenlecleucel

(Kymriah) is an example of a CAR T cell therapy in which T cells are modified to recognize CD19 expressed on the surface of acute lymphoblastic leukemia tumor cells; this is the same antigen that is targeted by the bispecific antibody blinatumomab. By contrast, engineered TCRs can be designed to recognize intracellular proteins that are presented by tumor MHC molecules, including neoantigens (see Figure 18.2). Bispecific antibodies and CAR T cells have improved outcomes for patients with a small number of cancers, but it has been challenging to identify cell surface antigens to target for all cancers, and these therapies have been unable to overcome the immunosuppressive TiME of some solid tumors. TCR T cells are not yet approved for any cancer, but are in clinical trials for several tumor types in patients with specific human leukocyte antigen (HLA) types. With bispecific antibody therapy and CAR T cell therapy, T cells directed against tumor antigens can rapidly proliferate and release inflammatory cytokines resulting in a systemic inflammatory syndrome called cytokine release syndrome. Symptoms of cytokine release syndrome can include fever, headache, encephalopathy, and in severe cases, acute respiratory distress syndrome (ARDS) and hypotensive shock. The interleukin (IL) 6R antagonist tocilizumab has been used to treat severe cases of cytokine release syndrome.

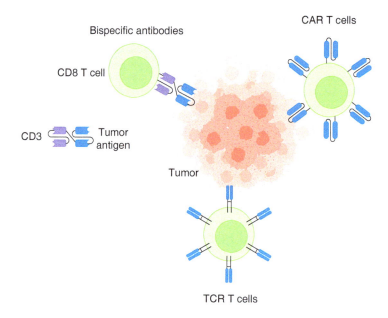

FIGURE 18.8 Novel approaches to cancer immanotherapy: T cell redirection.

CAR, chimeric antigen receptor; TCR, T cell receptor.

CHAPTER SUMMARY

Immuno-oncology is a form of cancer therapy that helps the body's own immune system fight cancer. Immune checkpoint inhibitors, which "take the breaks" off of the immune system, have demonstrated unprecedented activity against certain cancers, but some cancers have been resistant to this form of cancer therapy. Ongoing research efforts seek to better identify which patients are likely to respond to these therapies, and to anticipate and manage immune-related adverse events that can result from their use. CAR T cells, bispecific T cell engaging antibodies, and therapeutic cancer vaccines have demonstrated clinical activity in a small number of cancers but may figure more prominently in the future of cancer care. A major goal of immuno-oncology research is to extend the benefit of immunotherapy to cancer types that have thus far proved to be resistant to these treatments.

CLINICAL PEARLS

- Tumors that exhibit microsatellite instability (MSI) and/or mismatch repair deficiencies are characterized by large numbers of gene mutations. A high TMB may confer increased tumor antigenicity which, in turn, may lead to enhanced antitumor efficacy of immune checkpoint inhibitors.
- The presence of underlying autoimmune disorders is a presumptive contraindication to the use of immune checkpoint inhibitors and such patients are currently excluded from checkpoint inhibitor clinical trials.
- The immune-related adverse events (irAEs) resemble and are treated similarly to GVHD in allogeneic hematopoietic stem cell transplantation (HSCT). Prophylaxis against irAEs is not currently recommended. Immunosuppression to treat irAEs does not reduce the antitumor efficacy of treatment of immune checkpoint inhibitors. The frequency, but not the type or quality, of irAEs may increase with dose and may vary among different cancers. Neither the occurrence of irAEs (irrespective of the grade) nor the use of systemic corticosteroids to treat irAEs affected overall survival or time to failure in patients treated with ipilimumab (and possibly other checkpoint inhibitors).
- Management of patients with grade 2 (moderate), grade 3 or 4 (severe or life-threatening) irAE diarrhea:
  - Hold immunotherapy.
  - Start methylprednisolone (or prednisone) 1 mg/kg/day.
  - If no response in 2 to 3 days, then increase the dose to 2 mg/kg/day and consider infliximab (5 mg/kg).
  - If symptoms persist after the first dose of infliximab, a second dose of infliximab (5 mg/kg) can be given 2 weeks after the first dose.
  - If a patient is infliximab-refractory, consider vedolizumab.
- Blinatumomab, the bispecific monoclonal antibody that is directed against the T-cell antigen CD3 and the B-cell antigen CD19 is approved for relapsed or refractory B cell acute lymphocytic leukemia (ALL) therapy and for treatment of minimal residual disease (MRD) present following antileukemia chemotherapy for B-cell ALL.
- Both blinatumomab and CD-19-directed CAR T cells can be associated with neurotoxicity as well as cytokine release syndromes. Close monitoring is required and rapid intervention with IL-6 inhibitors (e.g., IL-6 receptor–directed monoclonal antibody tocilizumab) is indicated.

MULTIPLE-CHOICE QUESTIONS

1. Which of the following tumor biomarkers can be used to identify patients who can benefit from the PD-1 inhibitor pembrolizumab, regardless of tumor site or histology?

    A. Mismatch repair deficiency (MMRd)
    B. Low tumor mutational burden (low TMB)
    C. High PD-L1 expression (>1% tumor staining by immunohistochemistry)
    D. Presence of a KRAS mutation

2. Which one of the following is a stimulatory receptor on T cells?

    A. CTLA4
    B. PD-1
    C. PD-L1
    D. OX40

3. All of the following are examples of genomic alterations within tumors that create tumor-specific antigens (neoantigens), EXCEPT

    A. Viral transforming genes E6 and E7 of human papillomavirus (HPV)
    B. FGFR2 rearrangement
    C. Amplification of HER2
    D. KRAS G12V mutation

4. CD19-directed CAR T cell therapy is commonly associated with which of the following adverse events?

    A. Colitis
    B. Dermatitis
    C. Hypophysitis
    D. Cytokine release syndrome

5. A 56-year-old male with a history of chronic hepatitis B and cirrhosis develops hepatocellular carcinoma confined to the liver. He undergoes a successful liver transplant, but 2 years after receiving the liver transplant he develops a cancer recurrence with new metastasis to the lungs and bone. He has had no episodes of liver transplant rejection and continues on tacrolimus-based immunosuppression. He also has diabetes and hyperlipidemia. Which of the following aspects of his medical history likely precludes the use of immune checkpoint inhibitor therapy?

    A. Diabetes
    B. Hepatitis B
    C. Liver transplant
    D. Hyperlipidemia

6. Tumors recruit immunosuppressive cells to the tumor microenvironment. Which of the following is an example of an immunosuppressive cell type that expands in cancer?

    A. Myeloid-derived suppressor cell (MDSC)
    B. Naïve CD8 T cell
    C. Activated dendritic cell
    D. Th1 CD4 T cell

7. Which of the following lung cancers is more likely to respond to a PD-1 inhibitor?

    A. Lung cancer in a patient who never smoked
    B. Lung cancer in a patient with an extensive cigarette smoking history
    C. Lung cancer with PD-L1 expression of 0% (negative PD-L1 expression)

8. KRAS is the most frequently mutated cancer gene, but direct inhibition of oncogenic Ras mutants with small molecules has been challenging. Immune targeting of KRAS, an intracellular protein, may be feasible with which of the following targeted immunotherapy approaches?

    A. CD3-mutant KRAS bispecific antibody
    B. Chimeric antigen receptor (CAR) T cell targeting mutant KRAS
    C. T cell receptor (TCR) T cells targeting mutant KRAS

9. Which of the following is approved to treat cytokine release syndrome in patients receiving chimeric antigen receptor (CAR) T cell therapy?

    A. Tocilizumab (IL-6R antagonist)
    B. Anakinra (IL-1 receptor antagonist)
    C. Omalizumab (IgE inhibitor)
    D. Belimumab (BAFF inhibitor)

ANSWERS TO MULTIPLE-CHOICE QUESTIONS

1. **A.** See Figure 18.3. In 2017, the FDA granted accelerated approval to pembrolizumab for mismatch repair deficient (MMRd) solid tumors, the first time that a cancer drug received a tissue/site-agnostic drug approval. Pembrolizumab later received a tissue/site-agnostic approval from the FDA for tumors with a high TMB. High tumor PD-L1 expression is also associated with improved benefit from pembrolizumab within certain tumor types, but is not a tumor-agnostic biomarker.

2. **D.** See Figure 18.4. CTLA4, PD-1, and PD-L1 inhibit T cell activation, and can be targeted with inhibitory antibodies to enhance antitumor immunity. OX40 is a stimulatory receptor, and can potentially be targeted by an agonist antibody to enhance T cell activation.

3. **C.** See Figure 18.2. Viral infections (A), gene rearrangements (B), and mutations (D) create abnormal proteins in tumor cells that are not found in any normal human cell (neoantigens). Such neoantigens are thought to be optimal antigens for targeted immunotherapy because an immune response against a neoantigen is not subjected to central tolerance, and the selective expression of neoantigens on tumor cells may also limit autoimmunity. By contrast, amplification of HER2 within tumors results in higher expression of HER2 in tumors, but this normal protein is also found at lower levels in normal human tissues.

4. **D.** See Figure 18.8. CAR T cells can release inflammatory cytokines resulting in a systemic inflammatory syndrome called cytokine release syndrome. Symptoms of cytokine release syndrome can include fever, headache, encephalopathy, and in severe cases, acute respiratory distress syndrome (ARDS) and hypotensive shock.

5. **C.** Immune checkpoint molecules such as PD-1 and CTLA-4 maintain immune tolerance, and use can be associated with organ transplant rejection.

6. **A.** See Figure 18.1. MDSCs are myeloid cells that often expand in cancers, and can suppress antitumor immune responses.

7. **B.** See Figure 18.3. Hypermutated tumors have higher numbers of neoantigens and may appear to be more "foreign" to the immune system, resulting in greater efficacy with a PD-1 inhibitor. Smoking is a mutagen, and lung cancers occurring in patients who smoke cigarettes tend to have a higher tumor mutational burden (TMB) and are associated with greater efficacy from a PD-1 inhibitor.

8. **C.** See Figure 18.8. Bispecific antibodies and CAR T cells recognize antigens on the cell surface such as CD19, whereas HLA-restricted T cell receptor (TCR) therapies can be designed to recognize intracellular proteins that are presented on the tumor surface in the context of MHC.

9. **A.** See Figure 18.8. The IL-6R antagonist tocilizumab is used to treat severe cases of cytokine release syndrome.

SELECTED REFERENCES

Chalmers ZR, Connelly CF, Fabrizio D, et al. Analysis of 100,000 human cancer genomes reveals the landscape of tumor mutational burden. Genome Med. 2017 Dec;9(1):34. https://doi.org/10.1186/s13073-017-0424-2

Crespo J, Sun H, Welling TH, et al. T cell anergy, exhaustion, senescence, and stemness in the tumor microenvironment. Curr Opin Immunol. 2013 Apr;25(2):214–21. https://doi.org/10.1016/j.coi.2012.12.003

Faje A. Immunotherapy and hypophysitis: Clinical presentation, treatment, and biologic insights. Pituitary. 2016;19(1):82–92. https://doi.org/10.1007/s11102-015-0671-4

Hamid O, Robert C, Daud A, et al. Safety and tumor responses with lambrolizumab (anti–PD-1) in melanoma. N Engl J Med. 2013;369(2):134–44. https://doi.org/10.1056/NEJMoa1305133

Hellmann MD, Ciuleanu TE, Pluzanski A, et al. Nivolumab plus ipilimumab in lung cancer with a high tumor mutational burden. N Engl J Med. 2018 Apr;378(22):2093–104. https://doi.org/10.1056/NEJMoa1801946

Kantarjian H, Stein A, Gökbuget N, et al. Blinatumomab versus chemotherapy for advanced acute lymphoblastic leukemia. N Engl J Med. 2017 Mar 2;376(9):836–47. https://doi.org/10.1056/NEJMoa1609783

Kantoff PW, Higano CS, Shore ND, et al. Sipuleucel-T immunotherapy for castration-resistant prostate cancer. N Engl J Med. 2010 Jul;363(5):411–22. https://doi.org/10.1056/NEJMoa1001294

Kim KW, Ramaiya NH, Krajewski KM, et al. Ipilimumab associated hepatitis: Imaging and clinicopathologic findings. Investig New Drugs. 2013;31(4):1071–7. https://doi.org/10.1007/s10637-013-9939-6

Larkin J, Chiarion-Sileni V, Gonzalez R, et al. Combined nivolumab and ipilimumab or monotherapy in untreated melanoma. N Engl J Med. 2015 May;373(1):23–34. https://doi.org/10.1056/NEJMoa1504030

Le DT, Uram JN, Wang H, et al. PD-1 blockade in tumors with mismatch-repair deficiency. N Engl J Med. 2015 May;372(26):2509–20. https://doi.org/10.1056/NEJMoa1500596

Marabelle A, Fakih M, Lopez J, et al. Association of tumour mutational burden with outcomes in patients with advanced solid tumours treated with pembrolizumab: Prospective biomarker analysis of the multicohort, open-label, phase 2 KEYNOTE-158 study. Lancet Oncol. 2020 Oct 1;21(10):1353–65. https://doi.org/10.1016/S1470-2045(20)30445-9

Maude SL, Frey N, Shaw PA, et al. Chimeric antigen receptor T cells for sustained remissions in leukemia. N Engl J Med. 2014 Oct 16;371(16):1507–17. https://doi.org/10.1056/NEJMoa1407222

Melero I, Gaudernack G, Gerritsen W, et al. Therapeutic vaccines for cancer: An overview of clinical trials. Nat Rev Clin Oncol. 2014 Sep;11(9):509–24. https://doi.org/10.1038/nrclinonc.2014.111

Miao L, Zhang Y, Huang L. mRNA vaccine for cancer immunotherapy. Mol Cancer. 2021;20(1):1–23. https://doi.org/10.1186/s12943-021-01335-5

Michot JM, Bigenwald C, Champiat S, et al. Immune-related adverse events with immune checkpoint blockade: A comprehensive review. Eur J Cancer. 2016;54:139–48. https://doi.org/10.1016/j.ejca.2015.11.016

Mittal D, Gubin MM, Schreiber RD, Smyth MJ. New insights into cancer immunoediting and its three component phases—Elimination, equilibrium and escape. Curr Opin Immunol. 2014 Apr;27:16–25. https://doi.org/10.1016/j.coi.2014.01.004

Nghiem PT, Bhatia S, Lipson EJ, et al. PD-1 blockade with pembrolizumab in advanced merkel-cell carcinoma. N Engl J Med. 2016 Jun 30;374(26):2542–52. https://doi.org/10.1056/nejmoa1603702

Popovic A, Jaffee EM, Zaidi N. Emerging strategies for combination checkpoint modulators in cancer immunotherapy. J Clin Invest. 2018;128(8):3209–18. https://doi.org/10.1172/JCI120775

Robert C, Long GV, Brady B, et al. Nivolumab in previously untreated melanoma without BRAF mutation. N Engl J Med. 2015;372(4):320–30. https://doi.org/10.1056/NEJMoa1412082

Robert C, Schachter J, Long GV, et al. Pembrolizumab versus ipilimumab in advanced melanoma. N Engl J Med. 2015;372(26):2521–32. https://doi.org/10.1056/NEJMoa1503093

Rosenberg SA, Yang JC, Restifo NP. Cancer immunotherapy: Moving beyond current vaccines. Nat Med. 2004 Sep;10(9):909–15. https://doi.org/10.1038/nm1100

Ryder M, Callahan M, Postow MA, et al. Endocrine-related adverse events following ipilimumab in patients with advanced melanoma: A comprehensive retrospective review from a single institution. Endocr Relat Cancer. 2014;21(2):371–81. https://doi.org/10.1530/ERC-13-0499

Topalian SL, Sznol M, McDermott DF, et al. Survival, durable tumor remission, and long-term safety in patients with advanced melanoma receiving nivolumab. J Clin Oncol. 2014;32(10):1020–30. https://doi.org/10.1200/JCO.2013.53.0105

Voskens CJ, Goldinger SM, Loquai C, et al. The price of tumor control: An analysis of rare side effects of anti-CTLA-4 therapy in metastatic melanoma from the ipilimumab network. PLoS One. 2013;8(1):e53745. https://doi.org/10.1371/journal.pone.0053745

Wang DY, Salem JE, Cohen JV, et al. Fatal toxic effects associated with immune checkpoint inhibitors: A systematic review and meta-analysis. JAMA Oncol. 2018 Sep 13;4(12):1721–8. https://doi.org/10.1001/jamaoncol.2018.3923

Weber JS, Kähler KC, Hauschild A. Management of immune-related adverse events and kinetics of response with ipilimumab. J Clin Oncol. 2012;30(21):2691–7. https://doi.org/10.1200/JCO .2012.41.6750

Wolchok JD, Neyns B, Linette G, et al. Ipilimumab monotherapy in patients with pretreated advanced melanoma: A randomised, double-blind, multicentre, phase 2, dose-ranging study. Lancet Oncol. 2010;11(2):155–64. https://doi.org/10.1016/S1470-2045(09)70334-1

Yarchoan M, Johnson BA, Lutz ER, et al. Targeting neoantigens to augment antitumour immunity. Nat Rev Cancer. 2017;17(4):209–22. https://doi.org/10.1038/nrc.2016.154

Index